I0813738

The Harris College of NURSING & Health Sciences

Embracing the Past, Welcoming the Future

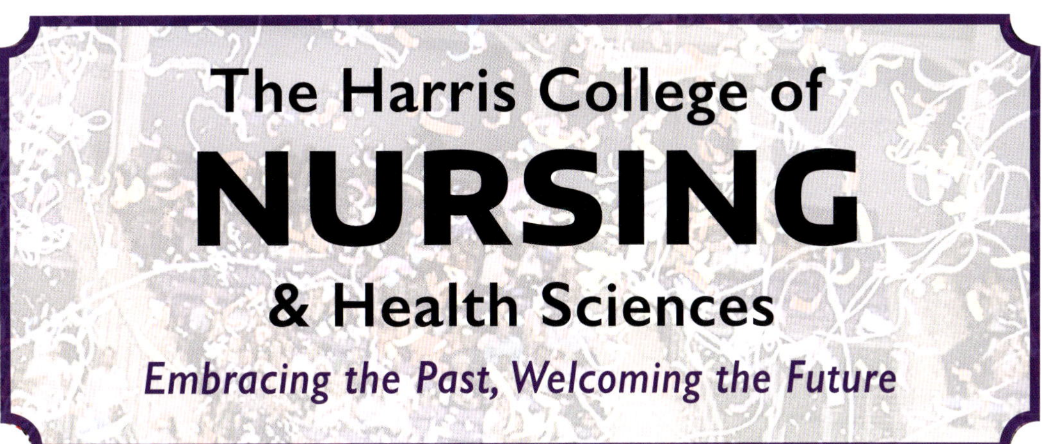

The Harris College of NURSING & Health Sciences

Embracing the Past, Welcoming the Future

Mary Lou Bond

Rhonda Keen-Payne

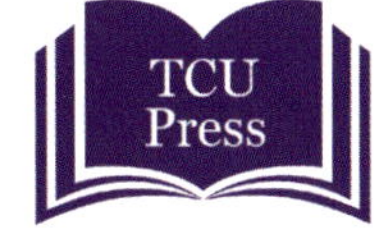

Fort Worth, Texas

Library of Congress Cataloging-in-Publication Data

Names: Bond, Mary Lou, 1937- author. | Keen-Payne, Rhonda, author.
Title: The Harris College of Nursing and Health Sciences : embracing the past, welcoming the future / Mary Lou Bond, Rhonda Keen-Payne.
Description: Fort Worth, Texas : TCU Press, [2019] | Includes bibliographical references and index. | Summary: "Harris College of Nursing and Health Sciences: Embracing the Past, Welcoming the Future details the history of Harris College from 1946 to 2019. The initial history, presented in 1973 by the founding dean Lucy Harris in The Harris College of Nursing: Five Decades of Struggle for a Cause, described the evolution of nursing education from a traditional apprenticeship into an academic program that prepares professional nurses. The current book describes how subsequent generations of faculty, students, and alumnae have responded to the challenges posed by Dean Harris in 1973 to provide a clear definition of nursing roles and functions and to research the effects that variables in nursing care have on the health of people"-- Provided by publisher.
Identifiers: LCCN 2019032071 | ISBN 9780875657264 (cloth)
Subjects: LCSH: Harris College of Nursing and Health Sciences (Texas Christian University)--History. | Harris College of Nursing (Texas Christian University)--History. | Nursing schools--Texas--Fort Worth--History. | Health occupations schools--Texas--Fort Worth--History.
Classification: LCC RT80.T4 B66 2019 | DDC 610.73071/07645315--dc23
LC record available at https://lccn.loc.gov/2019032071

Design by Elizabeth Cruce Alvarez, Southlake, Texas.

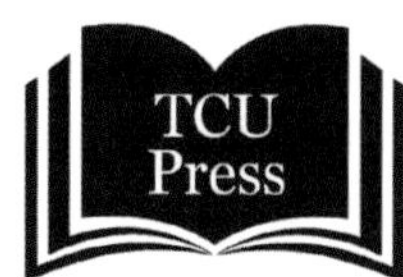

TCU Box 298300
Fort Worth, Texas 76129
817.257.7822
www.prs.tcu.edu
To order books: 1.800.826.8911

Dedication

This book is dedicated to the lasting legacy of Lucy Harris Linn, founding dean of Harris College of Nursing. Dean Harris offered knowledge, compassion, leadership, and persistence; she demonstrated the belief of Florence Nightingale, the founder of modern nursing, who said, "Unless we are making progress in our nursing every year, every month, every week, take my word for it we are going back. . . . The more experience we gain, the more progress we can make." In May 1967, the *Harris Hospital News* recognized Dean Harris as "The Lady with the Lamp in Texas."

Harris, who was awarded an honorary doctorate of law by Texas Christian University in 1968, had distinguished herself throughout her nursing career. In 1965 she was appointed by Governor John Connally to the Texas Board of Nurse Examiners for a six-year term. She received the Ella Goldthwaite Award for Outstanding Leadership and Achievement in Nursing Education from the University of Texas Medical Branch School of Nursing in 1967. She served as president of the Texas League for Nursing and as a board of review member of the National League for Nursing.

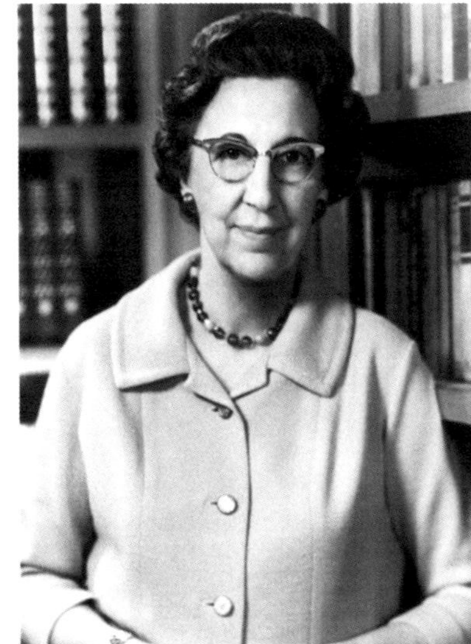

Dr. Harris's contributions were not limited to the nursing profession. She served on the board of directors for the Young Women's Christian Association and as president of Altrusa Fort Worth, a service organization for executive women.

None of the accomplishments of Harris College would have been possible without the dedication and continuous contributions of the early faculty members. These pioneers accepted the challenge posed by Dean Harris when she noted that "tradition was a handicap" and thus moved the college forward to contribute to the ever-changing health care system.

Contents

Foreword

It all began over a piece of Black Forest cake! Seriously!

I first learned of Mary Lou Bond when I became a nursing faculty member at TCU in 1994, but I didn't have the pleasure of getting to know her personally until many years later. I had heard about her sage wisdom, seasoned administrative abilities, and fun spirit. What I didn't realize when I first met her was the extent to which I would come to treasure her commitment to my own professional development. I was named the Acting Dean of Harris College of Nursing & Health Sciences at the end of 2013 following the very unfortunate, serious illness of our prior dean, Paulette Burns. That illness led to Dr. Burns's death, and following a national search for a permanent dean, I was named the dean of Harris College in the spring of 2015. Throughout my time as an acting dean, and continuing throughout my role as the permanent dean and now as vice provost, I often turned to Mary Lou Bond as a mentor, confidante, and trusted colleague. What I didn't initially realize was how quickly she would also become my treasured friend. In fact, our friendship is such that we now call one another "sister"!

During one of my lunch dates with Mary Lou, I was asking her if she had known some of the former deans, and after a moment of reflection, she stated, "I have known every dean of Harris College including the founding dean who admitted me in 1960!" I immediately replied with, "Do I have a deal for you!" For several months I had been mulling over a desire to update the prior history of Harris College that was first documented by Dean Harris. The previous book chronicled the history of Harris College from its establishment at TCU in 1946 until 1973, the centennial of TCU. As TCU began to discuss preparation for its 150th anniversary in 2023, I had a nagging desire to update the Harris College history; however, I felt unable to commit time to the project. The idea of Mary Lou Bond undertaking this project was beyond thrilling to me, as I knew she would be the ideal person—one who had not only observed the history of Harris College, but had participated in many significant moments in the college's history. As we enjoyed our Black Forest cake, we agreed to pursue the idea of this book further.

As we discussed the book, we quickly decided it would be helpful to include another individual who has been significant to both Dr. Bond and me in this project. Rhonda Keen-Payne, a former student of Dr. Bond, is also a former dean of Harris College, and her area of scholarship includes the history of nursing. What better expertise could we possibly add to this project! In addition to her role as a prior dean of Harris College and her relevant scholarly background, Dr. Keen-Payne has also been a significant mentor to me. I've often stated that I would not have survived my early days as a nursing faculty member if it had not been for Dr. Keen-Payne's guidance, patience, and willingness to answer hard questions about how things were done in an academic setting.

Although the early history of Harris College is rooted in the profession of nursing, the college has since expanded to include a vibrant mix of multiple health disciplines. While the history that threads its way through much of this book relates to nursing at TCU, you will also find chapters detailing the history of each of the other departments represented in Harris College. Each of these departments has a unique story to tell, and their particular journeys add greatly to the scope and breadth of Harris College.

In addition to the story of Harris College, you will find interesting descriptions of how individual students and faculty members have used their formative experiences within the college to launch their own successful professional journeys. These narratives allow the broader impact of Harris College to be felt in a palpable way.

I am confident that readers of this book will find themselves reflecting on their own educational experiences and ways their education has enriched their own lives. Although this is the story of a college, it is much more. It tells of the impact a single institution can have.

As educators, we have the opportunity to make a meaningful difference through the students we teach, the colleagues we mentor, and the communities we impact through our graduates. It is indeed a privilege to be an educator, and this book helps solidify the place of Harris College in making a difference in the lives of its students, faculty, and staff members as well as the communities served by the graduates.

I am most grateful for the dedication and commitment Mary Lou Bond and Rhonda Keen-Payne have shown to this project. They have each had challenges to overcome during the preparation of this manuscript, yet they remained focused on the goal of documenting the history of a significant contributor to Texas Christian University, the North Texas region, and the broader professions represented in Harris College.

Susan Mace Weeks, DNP, RN, CNS, FNAP, FAAN
Acting Dean of Harris College, 2013–2015
Dean of Harris College, 2015–2018
Vice Provost, 2018–present
Executive Director, Health Innovation Institute at TCU

Foreword

When professors Susan Weeks and Mary Lou Bond approached me in 2017 about updating the original book of Harris College of Nursing's history written by our first dean, Lucy Harris Linn, I was immediately sold on the idea.

In 2013, I facilitated the seventieth gala of the nursing program and spent much time exploring Linn's text, contacting alums, and gathering historical pictures for the event. As a 1983 Harris College of Nursing (HCN) graduate, I found myself reconnecting not only with peers but also with the rich history and importance that our nursing program has had. The display of our various uniforms, our "designer" cap, and our Texas Christian University (TCU) nursing pins as they evolved in style provided tangible evidence of the evolution of the degree program through the decades. The opportunity to hear the stories from alums that evening was magnificent and made me even more proud to be a TCU nursing alum.

So here we are in 2020, and I can see that several of those same people who were sharing stories in 2013 are the alums highlighted in this text. TCU nursing has met, and in many ways exceeded, the challenges that our first dean believed lay ahead for the professional nurse. TCU nursing has been able to do this because of the extraordinary resources it has received from the university, from alums who have given back, and from the partnerships it has established locally, regionally, nationally, and globally. TCU nursing students engage daily in classroom, lab, and clinical settings with nursing faculty who model daily, lifelong learning for students. The strong integration of the teacher-scholar model that values both faculty practice and innovative scholarship has led to an alumni base that is making a difference.

Sitting in the Annie Richardson Bass Building almost forty years ago, I never imagined I would be writing a foreword to a history book for my alma mater co-authored by one of my former professors and the dean who offered me a faculty position. How many of you recall the "graduation celebration" that the bachelor of science in nursing (BSN) students participated in at commencement each year? Silly string, confetti, paper streamers, and all! A mess that is reserved for our graduating students and enjoyed by all in so many pictures over the years! I worked hard and put in long hours to earn my TCU degree, and I was always in awe of the faculty who taught me. To this day, I am well aware that being a TCU alum means something special.

Today as associate dean for nursing, I still feel that way. I learn each day from my faculty colleagues; now more than ever, they are an interdisciplinary team. I still work hard each day, but it is to ensure that Harris College is the best it can be and the college Dean Harris imagined it could be.

Finally, being part of Harris College of Nursing & Health Sciences is a special privilege because of our alumni, partners, and the communities they serve. Together, we are excelling at the challenges Dean Harris said were ahead. I am excited for you to read how we have contributed not just to the nursing profession and scholarship but also to the health professions throughout our history of growth at TCU.

Suzy Lockwood, PhD, MSN, RN, OCN, FAAN
Associate Dean, TCU Nursing, 2015–2019
Associate Dean, TCU Nursing and School of Nurse Anesthesia, 2019–present
Division Director, Undergraduate Nursing, 2014–2015
Director, Center for Oncology Education and Research, 2007–present
Interim Dean of Harris College, 2018–June 1, 2019

A Few More Words

Since the publication of *The Harris College of Nursing: Five Decades of Struggle for a Cause* in 1973 by Lucy Harris, the health care industry has seen an explosion of technology; increasing demand for highly trained health care professionals; governmental, public, and private industry requirements for improved quality of health care and safe delivery of services; cost effectiveness of care; and the need for health care facilities and providers to obtain a competitive edge and demonstrate excellence while facing significant financial constraints placed on them by payers. Additionally, the aging population and increases in chronic health conditions in the United States have challenged the industry's ability to manage service provision and cost of care. These driving forces have contributed to the demand for strong partnerships between health care institutions, service providers, and academic and technical training programs to achieve the individual and mutual goals of all entities.

The impact of the frontline nurse has been recognized as one of the most important factors in patient outcomes. This was recognized in the Institute of Medicine (IOM) report in 2010 *(The Future of Nursing: Leading Change, Advancing Health),* which included recommendations for the nursing profession to effectively overcome barriers in meeting the complexity of the current health care environment. These recommendations include the need for (1) nurses to practice at the highest level of their education and training and (2) nurses to achieve higher levels of nursing education and training through an improved education system that promotes seamless academic progression. (Institute of Medicine. [2010]. *The Future of Nursing: Leading Change, Advancing Health.* Retrieved from https://www.nap.edu/read/12956/chapter/1.)

Historically, as the need for registered nurses has increased, Texas Health Harris Methodist Hospital Fort Worth (THFW) relied heavily on its strong relationship with TCU Harris College of Nursing to meet the needs of our patients and our community. Additionally, as nursing roles have expanded and specialization has increased, the partnership between THFW and TCU has been critical in developing future academic and professional development programs. Innovative and partnered programs that have grown the nursing profession and offered nurses the opportunity to practice at the top of their licenses and to advance practice include: certified registered nurse anesthetist (CRNA), clinical nurse specialist (CNS), clinical nurse practice (CNL), and doctor of nurse practice (DNP). These programs have led to the proliferation of nurses with advanced degrees in all areas of nursing at THFW. The academic excellence and faculty resources at TCU have had a strong impact on the growth and quality of research at THFW through the years. Research and evidence-based practice (EBP), once seen as academic endeavors only, have now been sewn into the fabric of TCU nursing's professional practice. The TCU Evidence-Based Practice Consortium, cocreated to instruct frontline nursing staff in EBP, has increased in size and scope in the ten years since the inception of the program. This foundational work often leads nurses to conduct research and to answer fundamental questions about the patient experience, patient outcomes, and the work of nursing. Research partnerships (a foundational component of nursing excellence) have grown through the years through the Joanna Briggs Institute (JBI) and the use of TCU faculty as nurse scientists helping to research issues and concerns at THFW.

THFW has always had a reputation for excellent patient care, and a large part of that reputation is related to the TCU connection. THFW became the first hospital in Fort Worth to receive the prestigious Magnet designation for nursing excellence, and there is no doubt that TCU helped THFW achieve Magnet designation and maintain it over the past twenty years. Collaboration on advisory boards and setting mutual goals with THFW have been key to setting a standard for nursing excellence and positive patient outcomes.

There is no doubt that the historical connection between TCU and THFW, which began one hundred years ago, has had a tremendous impact on nursing and patient care in our community, and it has been a great pleasure to be a part of this relationship and see the growth and all the positive changes in our profession over much of the last fifty years. Continued collaboration will be the key as we chart the next fifty!

Phyllis Norman, RN, MBA, NEA-BC
Vice President, Patient Care Services (retired)
Texas Health Harris Methodist Fort Worth Hospital

Mary Robinson, PhD, RN, NEA-BC
Vice President for Professional Practice, Research and Magnet
Texas Health Resources

Preface

The *Harris College of Nursing & Health Sciences: Embracing the Past, Welcoming the Future* provides a historical account of the mission, goals, and outcomes of the Harris College of Nursing, in existence from 1946 until 2000, the renamed College of Health and Human Sciences from 2000 until 2005, and the evolution of the current Harris College of Nursing & Health Sciences (HCNHS), founded in 2005. Today, HCNHS is composed of TCU Nursing, the Davies School of Communication Sciences and Disorders, the Department of Kinesiology, the School of Nurse Anesthesia, and the Department of Social Work. Together, their efforts are motivated by the desire to enhance global health.

In 1973, *The Harris College of Nursing: Five Decades of Struggle for a Cause* was published by the founding dean, Lucy Harris, with the goal of providing an understanding of the development of nursing education from a traditional apprenticeship system into an academic program that prepared nurses for professional careers. Challenged to update the book through the current decade, we have attempted to provide a chronicle of events within the context of a changing health care system that has helped precipitate changes in nursing education.

We have also described how the nursing faculty members have attempted to meet the two challenges posed by Dean Harris in 1973: (1) "to clearly define nursing roles and functions and (2) to conduct research that would serve to determine what effects variables in nursing care can have on the health of people" (Lucy Harris, 1973, 85).

This book is offered with the hope that readers may recognize the significant contributions made by former and current deans, faculty and staff members, and students and graduates. It is presented as validation of the significant ways in which the professions of nursing, anesthesia, communication sciences and disorders, kinesiology, and social work collaborate to meet the health care needs of an increasing global society and to reaffirm former dean Susan Weeks's comment: "After graduating from TCU, Horned Frogs turn possibility into reality."

Acknowledgments

The authors acknowledge the consistent and unwavering assistance provided by the Harris College of Nursing & Health Sciences and the Texas Christian University family during the development of this book, *The Harris College of Nursing & Health Sciences: Embracing the Past, Welcoming the Future.* Without the support of numerous individuals and groups, the completion of this project would not have been possible.

Thank you to Susan Weeks, former dean and vice provost for academic affairs, for offering the opportunity to serve the college through the updating of the original history of Harris College of Nursing, entitled *The Harris College of Nursing: Five Decades of Struggle for a Cause,* and for providing the needed resources to accomplish the task. Appreciation is further extended to Dr. Suzy Lockwood, former interim dean (April 2018–May 31, 2019) of Harris College of Nursing & Health Sciences and current associate dean for nursing and nurse anesthesia, for her continuation of support and resources.

To all the faculty members and emeritus faculty who have provided information, artifacts, and encouragement, thank you! Appreciation is extended to Laura Patton for helping us connect with a number of graduates. Without the ongoing assistance of all staff members, we could not have completed the book. Charles Dewar provided ongoing technical assistance throughout this writing process. Scott Murdock assisted with the organization of photos. A special thank you is in order to Susan Moore, who undertook the challenge of formatting the final revisions, and to Mary Morton, who took on the tedious task of providing day-to-day access to documents and printed needed materials.

We acknowledge the contribution of a TCU nursing honors student, Katelyn Jones, who researched events over the decades in which the story of TCU's nursing program unfolded. Her findings provided the context and trends within nursing and the health care system at national and international levels that occurred from the 1970s to 2018. Thank you to Dr. Lisa Bashore, chair of Katelyn's honors thesis committee, who provided guidance for this project.

Thank you to all of the authors from Communication Sciences and Disorders,

Kinesiology, Nurse Anesthesia, and Social Work. Their contributions have showcased the nature of the collaborative work that is done between departments.

Support from individuals of the larger TCU community has been invaluable. Appreciation is extended to Dr. Philip S. Hartman, dean and professor of biology in the College of Science & Engineering and to Dr. Andrea Smith, adjunct faculty, TCU Nursing, for their review of the initial prospectus of the book and for their recommendations for development. Alysha Sapp, TCU Nursing's and Nurse Anesthesia's librarian, has been tireless in assisting us to locate needed references. Additional thanks go to the staff of TCU Press: Dr. Dan Williams, director; Melinda Esco, production manager; Kathy Walton, editor; Molly Spain, assistant editor; and Rebecca Allen, marketing coordinator. They were always available to answer questions and offer suggestions. Thanks also to Ann George and Sara Kelm's editing and publishing students, whose editorial work on the manuscript helped prepare it for publication.

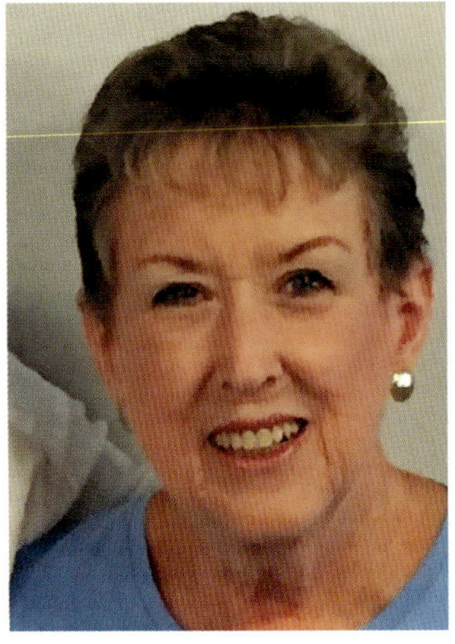

Dr. Kay Avant.

Three external reviewers—Dr. Kay Avant, Dr. Gail Davis, and Dr. Patricia Thompson, all nurse educators and researchers—posed important questions about content within the chapters related to TCU nursing. Their observations and insights strengthened the story of the ongoing work of nursing at TCU.

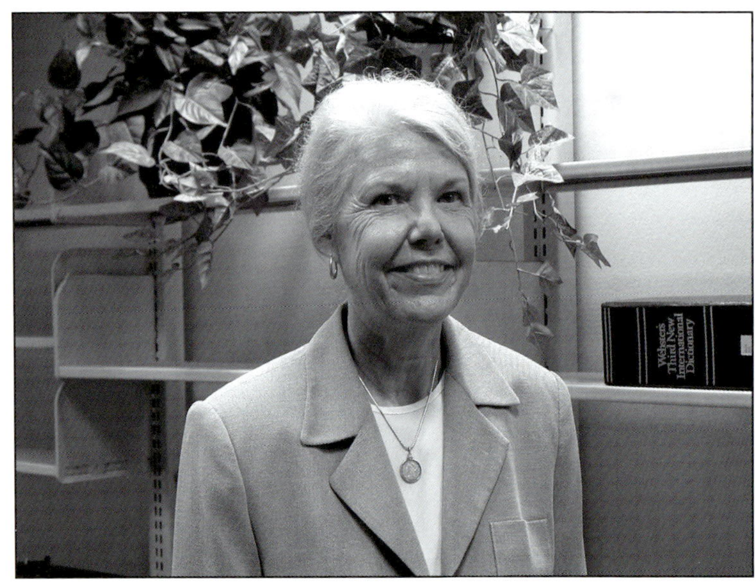

Dr. Gail Davis.

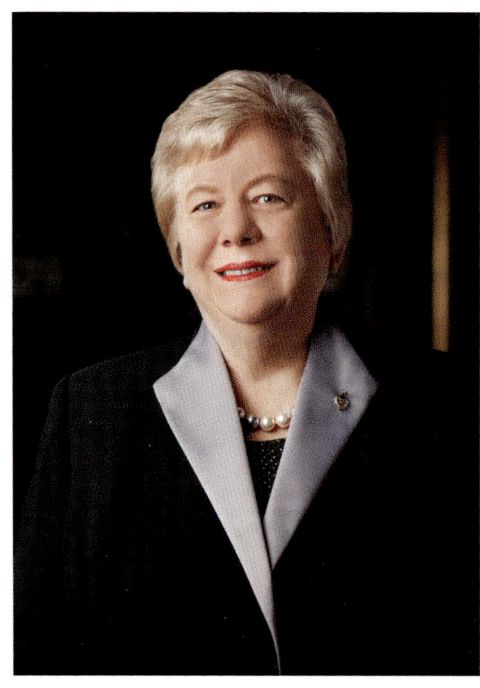

Dr. Patricia Thompson.

Chapter One

Looking Backward

Looking backward into the history of the Harris College of Nursing is an intriguing journey of discovery. In the preface to *The Harris College of Nursing: Five Decades of Struggle for a Cause,* founding dean Lucy Harris stated that the book was offered "in the hope of giving a better understanding of how nursing education has developed from a traditional apprenticeship system into dynamic, innovative, and academically sound programs for professional nursing careers" (Lucy Harris 1973, ix). Throughout the book she describes the multiple challenges faced in moving the nursing educational program from a hospital setting to the university setting.

In the last pages of the book, she commented on the work of the deans and faculty members who developed an outstanding program "despite the burdens of inflexible expectations and demands" (Lucy Harris 1973, 85). She continued by identifying two challenges which "loom for the near future." The first challenge was to clearly define nursing roles and functions. The second was to "conduct research that would serve to determine what effects variables in nursing care can have on the health of people" (Lucy Harris 1973, 85).

The "burdens of inflexible expectations and demands" might seem foreign to nursing students of the current decade—or even to today's younger nursing faculty members who are the recipients of our forerunners' efforts to lay a solid foundation for the systems that are in place today. Obstacles to moving forward, identified by Harris (p. vii), were complex, as described in Table 1.

TABLE 1 Obstacles to Moving Forward

Tradition as a handicap
Finances as a means of control
Nursing shortages and related problems
Antiquated ideas of nursing education
Organizational issues

Source: Harris 1973, 29–45.

Using the phrase "tradition as a handicap," Harris described how early schools operated primarily to provide care for patients within hospitals, with nurses simultaneously providing instruction and supervision for nursing students. She observed that, in many instances, early hospital-based schools were "schools in name only" (Lucy Harris 1973, 1), with students working beside nursing personnel and attending class after long hours of service.

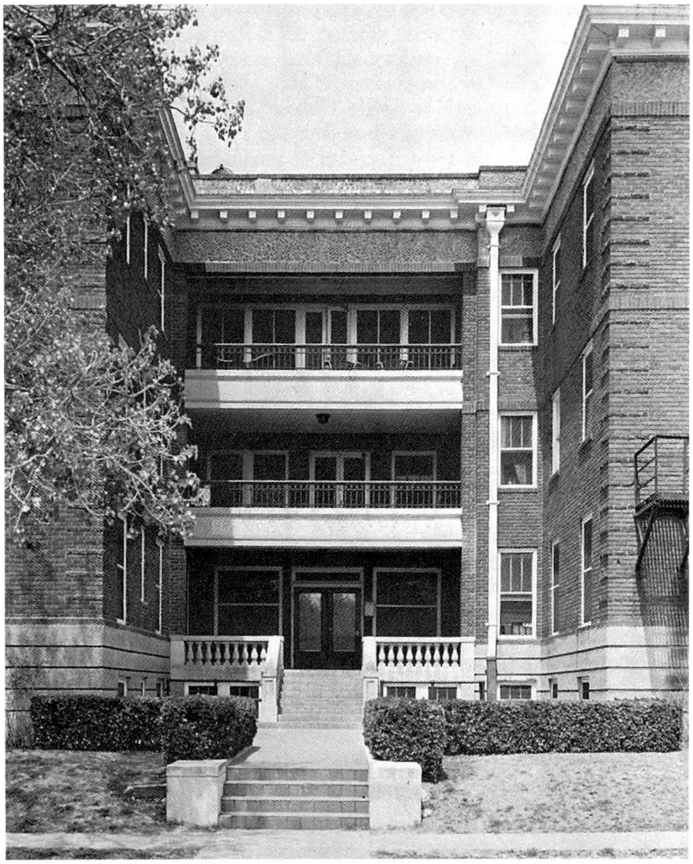

Old Harris Hospital and Clinic Building, 1912.

The chronology of events traced by Dean Harris describes the opening of a twenty-five-bed hospital by Dr. Charles Harris in 1912 with the simultaneous chartering of the Harris School of Nursing, a three-year diploma program. In 1930, in the midst of the Great Depression, the Methodist Hospital and School of Nursing opened and admitted its first students, with the encouragement of (and donations from) Charles Harris. The last students were admitted in 1933, followed by the closure of Methodist Hospital and School of Nursing in 1937 due to bankruptcy (Lucy Harris 1973, 87). After various outside proposals to reopen the hospital, Methodist's board of trustees came to an agreement with Dr. Harris, who closed Harris Hospital and moved its operation, along with the Harris School of Nursing, to Methodist, taking charge of its operations as director. In gratitude for his efforts, Methodist's trustees renamed the hospital Harris Memorial Methodist Hospital.

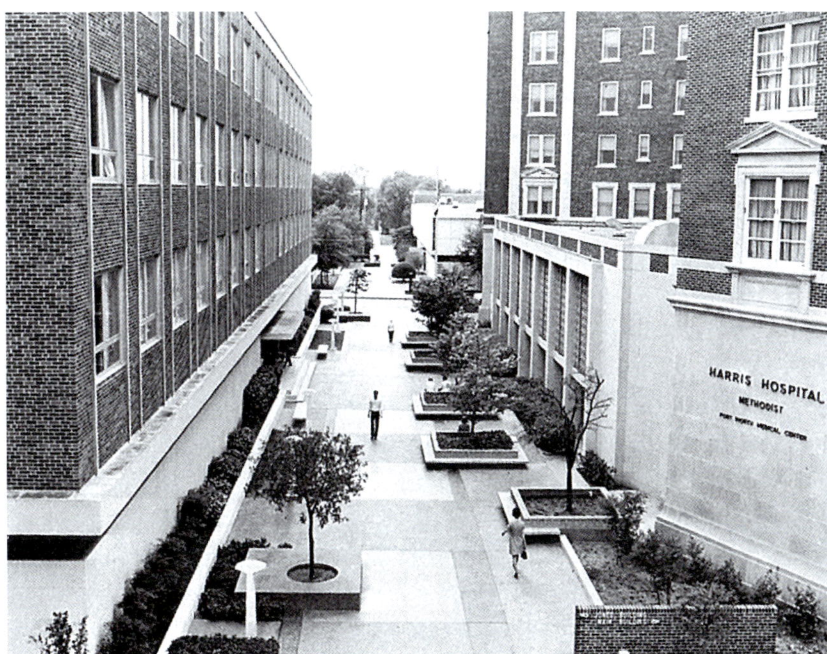

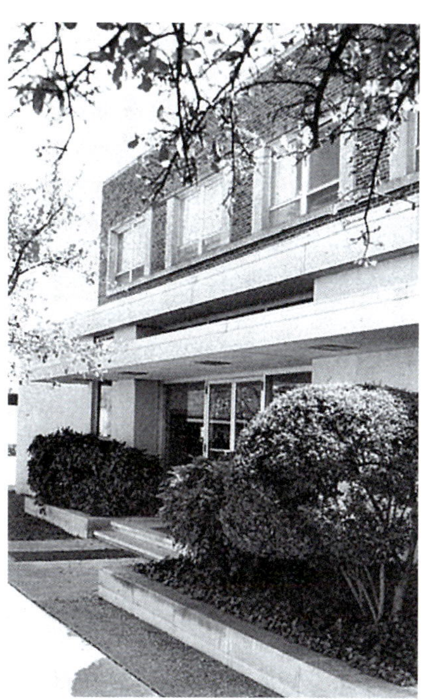

(Left) Walkway between Harris Hospital Buildings.
(Right) Fannie M. Harris Building: Home of Harris College of Nursing 1960–71.

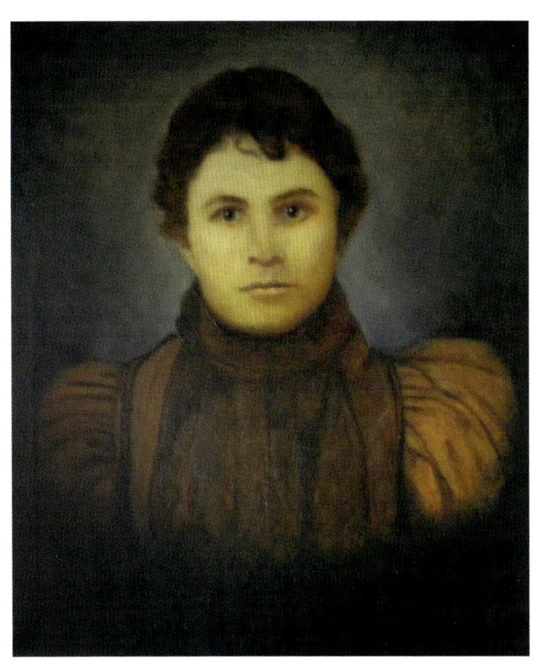

Fannie M. Harris.

In 1942 Charles Harris announced a decision to establish a college of nursing and signed a contract with Texas Christian University (TCU). The following year, Dr. Harris created a trust fund to establish the program, which he deemed necessary due to the "increasing demands being placed on nurses with the rapid increase in scientific knowledge" (*Harris College of Nursing Self-Study Report 1976,* viii).

While the movement to establish a college of nursing within an academic setting was a first step in recognizing the need for professional nursing programs, challenges remained—for example, arrangements for the transfer of funds between the Harris College of Nursing and Harris Hospital, which held responsibility for bookkeeping and "making up any deficit for expenditures previously approved by the two Boards" (Lucy Harris 1973, 30). This financial arrangement was necessary because the contract between Harris College of Nursing and Harris Hospital had not yet been ratified by the Central Texas Methodist Conference and resulted in attempts by the hospital administrator to control the college's policies on faculty salary and vacation time (Lucy Harris 1973, 30). Those policies were subsequently negotiated after TCU's chancellor stated that salary and benefits for nursing faculty would need to be consistent with that of other TCU faculty members.

The struggles for the acceptance of a collegiate program are detailed in excerpts from multiple sources, of which the following are only a few: the dean's report to the Harris College of Nursing Board of Directors in 1948 (Appendix 1), letters exchanged between Dean Lucy Harris and physicians at Harris Hospital who held conflicting opinions (Appendix 2), excerpts from the dean's report to the Harris Hospital medical staff in 1960 (Appendix 3), and the TCU chancellor's letter of appreciation to the medical staff at Harris Hospital in 1960 (Appendix 4) (Harris 1973, 89–110).

One early conflict between Dean Harris and hospital physicians concerned the Harris College of Nursing faculty members having control over students during their clinical practice. Harris noted that the idea of faculty taking responsibility for students in clinical practice as well as in classroom instruction was "too revolutionary for 1946" (Lucy Harris 1973, 34). She continued by saying that during the first fifteen years of operation of the college, "few physicians offered encouragement and many openly opposed [the college]," thus further validating "antiquated ideas about nursing education" (39).

Harris School of Nursing, a three-year diploma program, was granted national accreditation in 1946, the same year that Harris College of Nursing was incorporated (Lucy Harris 1973, 87). During initial stages of development of the four-year program, both a baccalaureate and a diploma program were in existence (*Harris College of Nursing Self-Study Report 1970*). In 1952, Harris College of Nursing was granted national accreditation as the college administration moved to the science building on the TCU campus. The diploma program admitted its last students in 1955 (*Harris College of Nursing Self-Study Report 1970*). Lucy Harris noted that in 1952, the Harris College of Nursing was one of fifty schools offering a baccalaureate program in nursing and one of ninety holding national accreditation (Harris 1973, 82).

The progression of events at the Harris College of Nursing during the early years paralleled many of the events unfolding at the national level. The American Society of Superintendents of Training Schools for Nurses was founded in 1893 to establish and maintain a universal standard for the training of nurses. The organization published standards of curricula, initiated accreditation for programs of nursing education, and later, in 1952, became recognized by the US Department of Education under its current name, the National League for Nursing. During these same years, Harris College of Nursing moved from an apprenticeship model to a professional model, which was reflected in curricular changes and continuous attainment of accreditation.

Movement to the professional model was also accompanied by movement from the hospital setting to an educational setting. In the early years of the Harris College

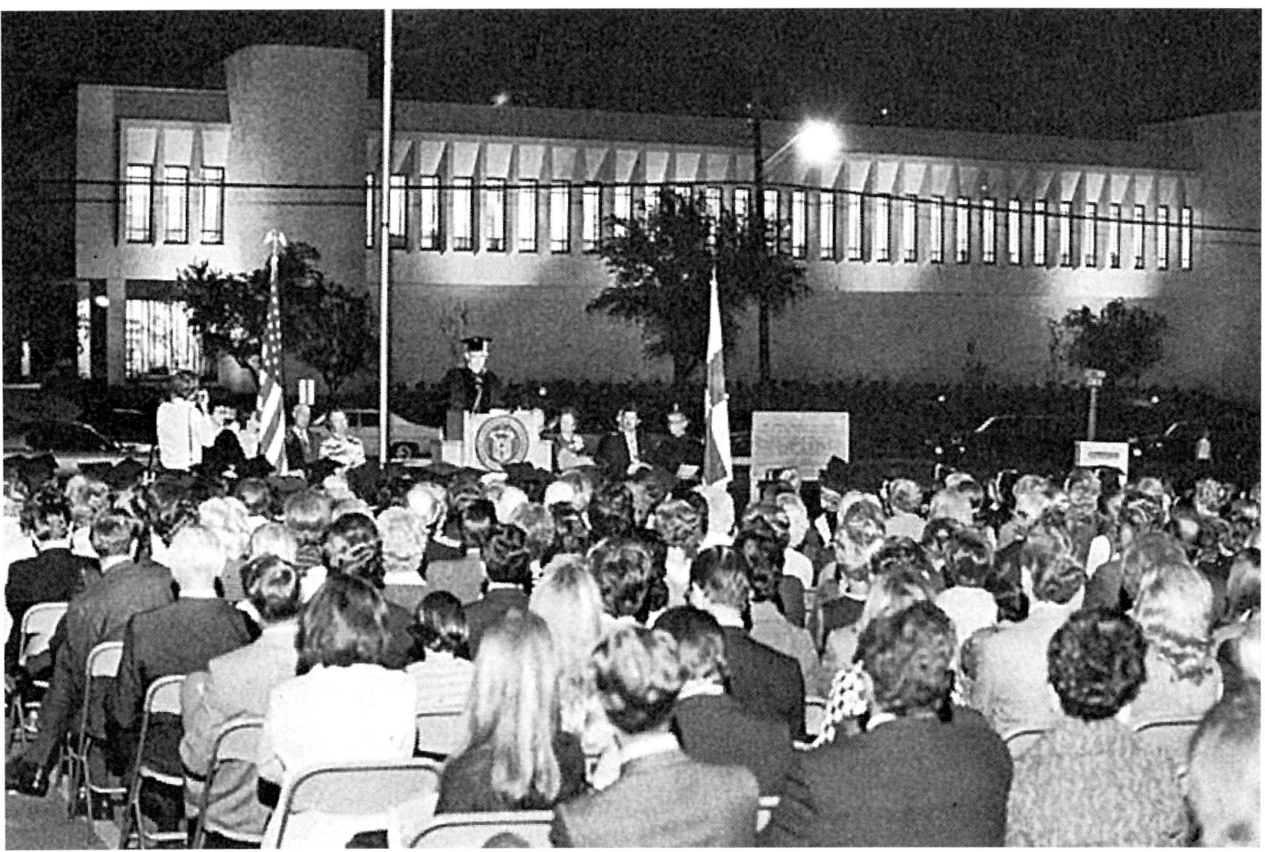

Annie Richardson Bass Building. New home of Harris College of Nursing: Dedication Ceremony, 1971.

of Nursing, students attended classes on the TCU campus, but faculty members remained off campus. In 1971 the Annie Richardson Bass Building became the new home of Harris College of Nursing faculty members, who had been housed in a former dormitory near Harris Hospital. New classrooms and laboratories offered students state-of-the-art equipment and access to all resources on the university campus. The 34,600-square-foot building was characterized by "graceful and strong-lined architecture" (Lucy Harris 1973, 73), with provisions for closed-circuit television and computer-assisted instruction, along with independent study carrels. Harris also noted that the building "gave heart to faculty and students . . . and will surely result in improvement in teaching and learning" (74).

Mary Hill, acting chief of the Nursing Education Branch, Division of Nursing, Department of Health, Education, and Welfare, said at the dedication, "A building is tangible evidence of many unseen things . . . a place where skills are learned, where attitudes are molded, where knowledge is cultivated, where sensitivities are attuned and where the habit of inquiry is encouraged" (*This Is TCU* 1972, 9).

CHALLENGE ONE

A Clear Definition of Nursing Roles and Functions

The new building became the physical setting in which faculty members would continue to respond to the challenge of providing "a clear definition of nursing roles and functions" (Lucy Harris 1973, 85). An organized structure and collaboration with clinical agencies helped provide students with a variety of experiences that facilitated their learning and helped them achieve goals.

The Harris College of Nursing continued to function under the direction of both the Harris College of Nursing Board of Directors (an independent organization) and the TCU Board of Trustees (*Harris College of Nursing Self-Study Report 1976*, 8). From 1967 to 1979, the college was administered by Dean Virginia Jarratt, a nurse educator with a doctoral degree. The college was organized into four clinical departments: medical-surgical nursing, maternal- and child-health nursing, psychiatric- and mental-health nursing, and public-health nursing.

Curricular changes in 1946, 1955, 1964, and 1971 show continuing clarification of nursing roles and functions (Lucy Harris 1973, 89–131). As roles changed, registered nurses who were graduates of diploma programs were admitted to the college in small numbers, as they had been since "the beginning" (Lucy Harris 1973, 65). Harris noted that upon her retirement in 1967, the faculty, led by Dean Jarratt, conducted a "detailed analysis of the strengths

Curriculum 1971

Course	Semester Hours
Freshman Year:	
English 1113 and 1123	6
Chemistry 1153 and 1163	6
Nursing 1114 (Intro. to Psychological and Physiological Aspects of Human Behavior)	4
Social Science 1053 or History	3
Religion 1203	3
Fine Arts (Music, Art, or Theatre Arts)	3
Government 1113	3
Physical Education	2
Sophomore Year:	
English 2253 or 2263	6
Biology 2204-2214 (Anat. & Physiol.)	8
Biology (Microbiology)	3
Home Economics Nutrition 2103	3
History 2603 or 2703	3
Nursing 2104 (Nursing I)	4
Nursing 2203 (Nursing IIA Theory)	3
Nursing 2202 (Nursing IIA Practicum)	2
Nursing 2201 (Nursing IIA Seminar)	1
Summer Session:	
Sociology 2213	3
Psychology 2213	3
Junior Year:	
Nursing (Nursing IIB Theory)	6
Nursing 3316 (Nursing IIB Practicum)	6
Nursing 3314 (Nursing IIB Seminar)	4
Nursing 3404 (Nursing IIIA Theory)	4
Nursing 3406 (Nursing IIIA Practicum)	6
Nursing 3402 (Nursing IIIA Seminar)	2
Elective	3
Senior Year:	
Nursing 3504 (Nursing IIIB Theory)	4
Nursing 3506 (Nursing IIIB Practicum)	6
Nursing 3502 (Nursing IIIB Seminar)	2
Nursing 4603 (Nursing IV Seminar)	3
Nursing 4613 (Nursing IV Practicum)	3
Nursing 3330 (Elective)	3-6
Religion 3103	3
Electives	6

131

Nursing Curriculum Plan, 1971.

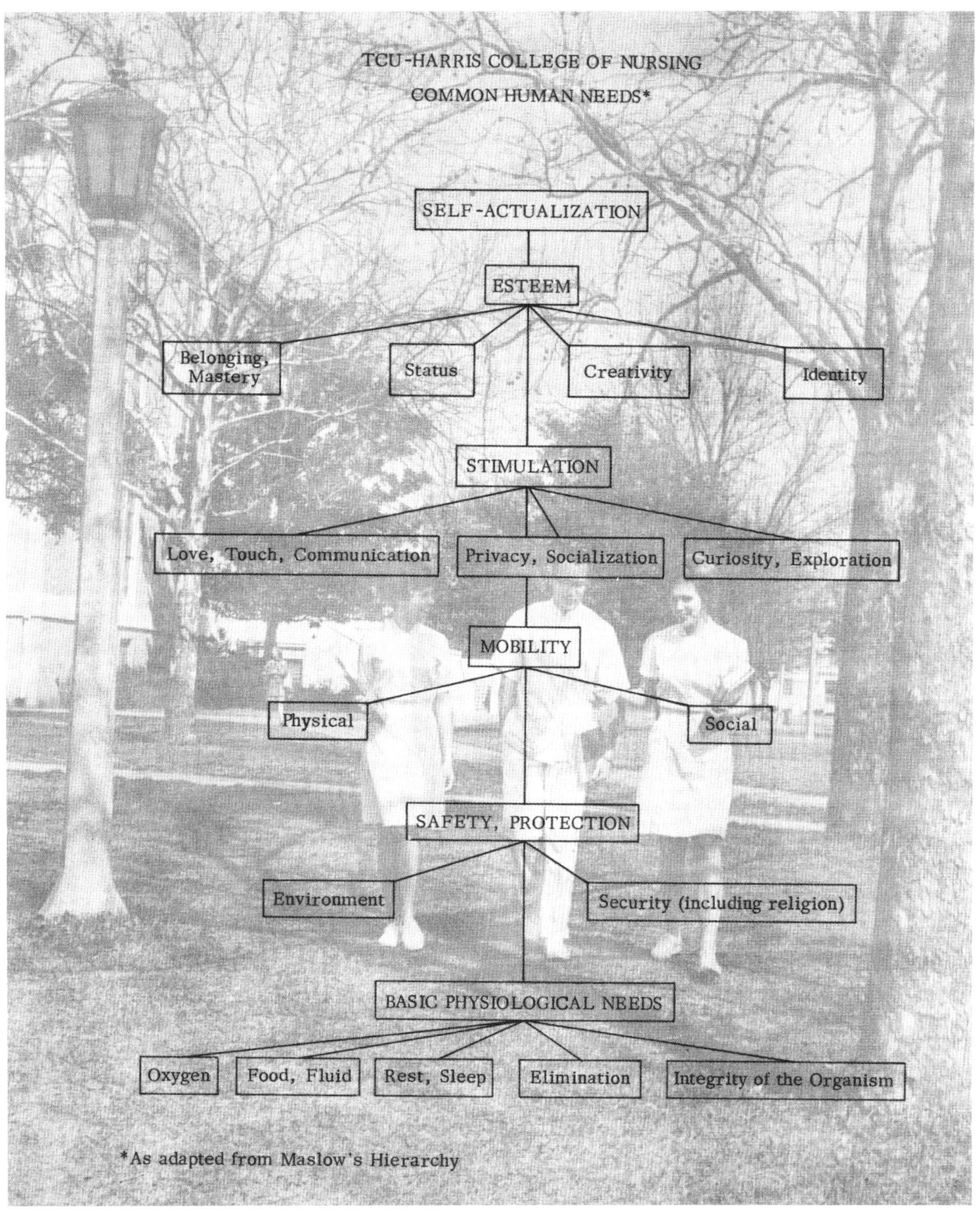

Maslow's Hierarchy of Needs.

and weaknesses of the course of study" (Lucy Harris 1973, 84). As a result, a new integrated curriculum based on common human needs (Lucy Harris 1973, 131) was implemented in 1971. As noted in the 1972 *Harris College of Nursing Self-Study Report,* the primary purpose of the program in the early seventies was to "prepare a graduate who has a broad base of knowledge and skills which can be utilized for identifying health needs, in prescribing measures for health promotion and maintenance, and for assisting patients and families to reach optimum health" (Harris College of Nursing Archives).

Dean Jarratt commented that the new curriculum represented a look to the future of nursing practice. She said that by focusing on the entire person, with his or her unique individual experiences, the student's learning "is a directed discovery experience" (*This Is TCU* 1972, 6). Underlying the new curriculum was the assumption that "all nursing actions can be derived from common human needs" (*This Is TCU* 1972, 6). Classroom and clinical teaching emphasized critical thinking, logical reasoning, and decision-making.

Core classes with a focus on common human needs as experienced by patients provided the opportunity for students to compare all clinical areas. Team teaching, computer-assisted instruction, and the expanded learning resource center emerged as strengths in the '70s. Curricular changes, the use of new teaching strategies, and the creativity of the faculty members demonstrated how the Harris College of Nursing indeed moved forward from an apprenticeship program, where nursing students served long hours as hospital staff members to solve the problem of a shortage of registered nurses (Lucy Harris 1973, 89), to a "dynamic, innovative and academically sound program" (ix).

At the beginning of the fall semester in 1970, there were eighteen faculty members with master's degrees, one with a doctorate, and two who were enrolled in part-time graduate study. It was expected that by 1972 all faculty members would have at minimum a master's degree in an area of specialization, although the possibility of employing faculty assistants with baccalaureate degrees was not ruled out. The 1970 *Harris College of Nursing Self-Study Report* recommended that there should be one or more faculty members with the appropriate doctoral degree for each clinical specialty area by 1975 (Harris College of Nursing Archives). New roles in nursing had moved beyond the scope of the apprenticeship model of the past and required advanced, specialized education.

While a variety of clinical facilities were available for student experiences, additional community health facilities, such as other major hospitals, nursing homes, outpatient departments, and community centers, were investigated for future use. The *Harris College of Nursing Self-Study Report* from 1970 noted that more professional role models were needed in some facilities to strengthen the learning opportunities for the students (Harris College of Nursing Archives).

Faculty members in the early '70s also recognized the need to increase the diversity of the student body to include all socioeconomic groups as well as a variety of cultural backgrounds and places of origin. The heterogeneous mix of students in 1971 included students from thirty-three states. Of these, 27 students were male and 290 female; 10 students were of African American descent and 307 were Caucasian; 58 were married and 259 were single. Harris noted that the "student body had lost much of the provincialism which characterized earlier schools of nursing" (Harris 1973, 65).

CHALLENGE TWO

Research to Determine What Effects Variables in Nursing Care Can Have on the Health of People

Dean Harris believed that "the primary responsibility of the faculty in a baccalaureate program in nursing was the preparation of competent nurses" (Lucy Harris 1973, 77). She acknowledged that future faculty "must assume responsibility for research to achieve more effective nursing services" (77). Ruth Eloise Sperry, a faculty member from 1942 to 1976, was engaged in research early, recording on her 1975 curriculum vitae her "participation in a cooperative research project with the University of Texas" between 1961 and 1966 (Harris College of Nursing Archives).

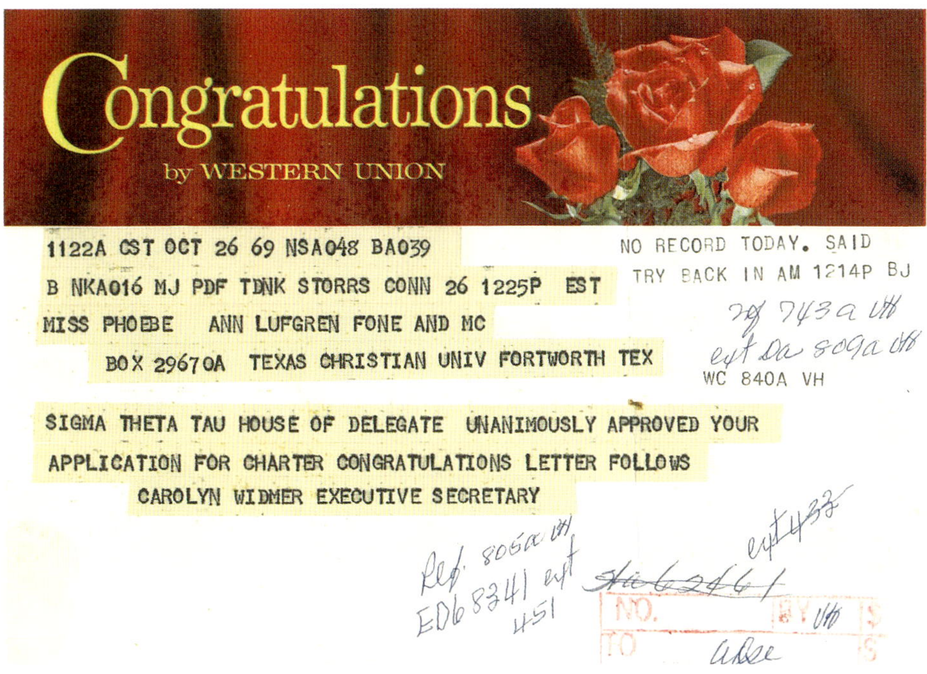
Congratulations
by WESTERN UNION

1122A CST OCT 26 69 NSA048 BA039
B NKA016 MJ PDF TDNK STORRS CONN 26 1225P EST
MISS PHOEBE ANN LUFGREN FONE AND MC
BOX 29670A TEXAS CHRISTIAN UNIV FORTWORTH TEX

NO RECORD TODAY. SAID TRY BACK IN AM 1214P BJ
WC 840A VH

SIGMA THETA TAU HOUSE OF DELEGATE UNANIMOUSLY APPROVED YOUR APPLICATION FOR CHARTER CONGRATULATIONS LETTER FOLLOWS
CAROLYN WIDMER EXECUTIVE SECRETARY

Western Union Telegram with approval of application for charter of Beta Alpha, STTI.

An important step toward meeting the challenge of conducting research was the formation of a TCU chapter of Sigma Theta Tau International Honor Society of Nursing (STTI). With its mission of "advancing world health and recognition of excellence in nursing through scholarship, leadership and service" (Sigma Theta Tau International), the induction of faculty members and students would signify the college's commitment to making research a priority. On October 26, 1969, Phoebe Ann Lufgren, a faculty sponsor for the proposed chapter, received a Western Union telegram notifying her that the STTI House of Delegates had unanimously approved the application for chartering.

According to the *Harris College of Nursing Self-Study Report* for 1976, fifty-five students and fifteen faculty members were initiated as charter members of the Beta Alpha chapter of STTI on April 12, 1970 (Harris College of Nursing Archives).

The coat of arms for Sigma Theta Tau International symbolizes the ideals of the honor society. The eye represents wisdom and discernment, and the stars are in recognition of the six founders. The founding words—storga, tharos, tima (love, courage, honor)—appear on the scroll. The lamp represents the lamp of knowledge,

SIGMA THETA TAU, INC. BETA ALPHA CHAPTER

INSTALLATION CEREMONY

Presentation of Charter..................Dr. Lois Meier
Second Vice President, National Council

Response........................Dr. Virginia Jarratt
Dean, Harris College of Nursing

Response..............................LaVern Marsh
Chairman, Steering Committee

Congratulatory Statement......Dr. James Newcomer
Vice Chancellor for Academic Affairs

Congratulatory Statement...Dr. Ted E. Klein, Jr.
Director, Honors Program

Induction Ritual ....Dr. Lois Meier

Recognition of Transfer Members

Initiation of New Members

Response ....Phoebe Ann Lufgren
Faculty Advisor, Steering Committee

Installation of Officers................Dr. Lois Meier

President..................................Sue Kidd
Vice President.........................Cherry Jones
Secretary ....Susan Wilkinson
Treasurer ....Dorothy Westfall
Senior Counselor.........................Anne Lane
Junior Counselor......................Allene Jones

Response....................................Sue Kidd
President, Beta Alpha Chapter

Charge to the Chapter....................Dr. Lois Meier

TRANSFER MEMBERS

Dr. Virginia Jarratt
Alpha Delta Chapter, University of Texas
Mona Fields....Alpha Kappa Chapter, University of Colorado
Mildred Hogstel...Alpha Delta Chapter, University of Texas

NEW INDUCTEES

Phyllis Joy Anderson
Joyce M. Baldwin
Kathleen Alison Barthel
Nancy Lynne Beatty
Millie Hill Beavers
Toni Jane Bennett
Dolores O. Berkovsky
Barbara Ann Bickley
Jo Ellen Bogert
Mary Lou Bond
Dixie Lee Brown
Joanne Bodnar Burch
Mary Melissa Cadenhead
Merry Jahn Chandler
Karen Elizabeth Cupp
Kay Dawn Deaton
Mary Ann Flood
Aurian Frances Forrester
Hazel Marie Garrett
Mary Susan Gilligan
Wanda Ruth Gipson
O. Monette Graves
Robert T. Hadley
Gail Jean Hargrave
Patricia Anne Harrison
Reta Estelle Higgins
Lucile Houston
Jan Michelle Hunter
Margaret Anne Irby
Rebecca James
Sharon Estelle Jimenez
Allene Jones
Cherry Rue Jones
Mary Catherine Junge
Sue Monk Kidd
M. Anne Lane
Madgelyn Ann LaVallee
Diane Frances Lowe
Phoebe Ann Lufgren
Adra Mae McConnell
Patricia Ann McLean
Frances LaVern Marsh
Peggy Marie Mayfield
Nancy Elizabeth Miller
Jeanette Elaine Mill
Mary Frances Mullins
Dorothy Ellen Parker
Nicki Lee Potts
Anita Lynn Presley
Paula Lorraine Pressley
Judy Ann Quereau
Frances Ann Ratheal
Frances Kathryn Richardson
Margaret Elaine Salisbury
Betty Jean Shockey
Ruth Eloise Sperry
Pettey Caldwell Steele
Fay M. Stephenson
Nancy Lee Stewart
Danna Clyde Strength
Linda Joyce Thorn
Shirley Nichols Trowbridge
Judith Ann Ward
Sharon Elizabeth Watson
Susan Elizabeth West
Dorothy Lucile Westfall
Cordelia Nelson Wetsel
Cynthia Lee Wiegand
Sandra Sue Wilkerson
Susan Helen Wilkinson

Installation Ceremony, Beta Alpha, 1970.

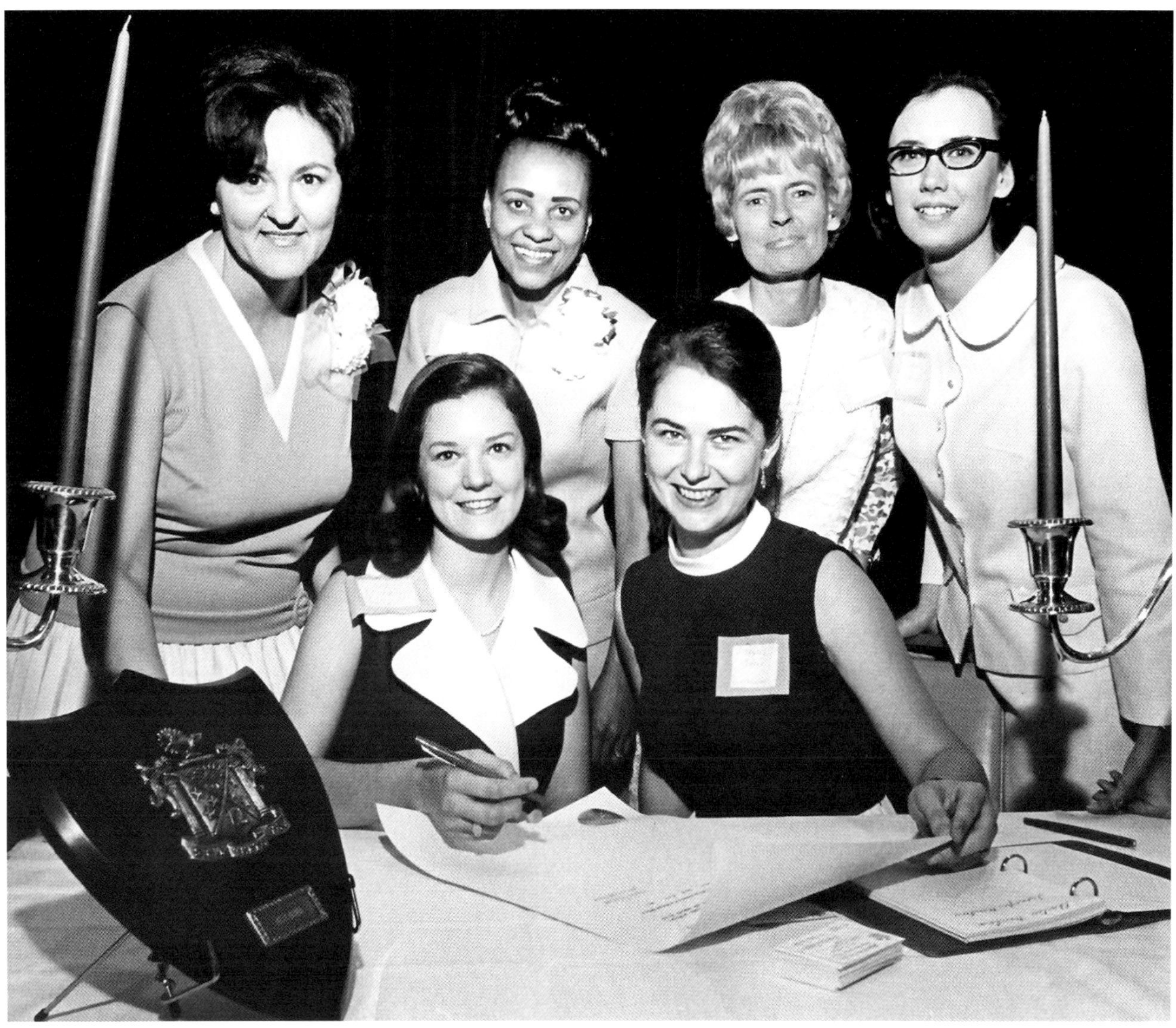

Beta Alpha Officers, 1970; L-R (seated) Sue Kidd and Cherry Jones; L-R (standing) Anne Lane, Allene Jones, Dorothy Westfall, and Susan Wilkerson.

and the pillars denote service, professional endeavor, and strength of leadership. The 1976 *Harris College of Nursing Self-Study Report* shows that early activities of Beta Alpha included sponsoring a member's attendance at the Third Regional STTI Conference (1970), cosponsoring a symposium with Beta Beta Chapter of Texas Woman's University entitled "Nurse Involvement in Health Care in the 80s" (1973), and establishing a scholarship fund in 1975 (Harris College of Nursing Archives).

From 1946 until 1967, then, the preparation of nurses moved from an apprenticeship model to a dynamic, innovative, and sound program of professional nursing at the Harris College of Nursing. This forward movement was facilitated under the extraordinary leadership of Lucy Harris, a visionary for her time, and the continuing dynamic leadership of Virginia Jarratt.

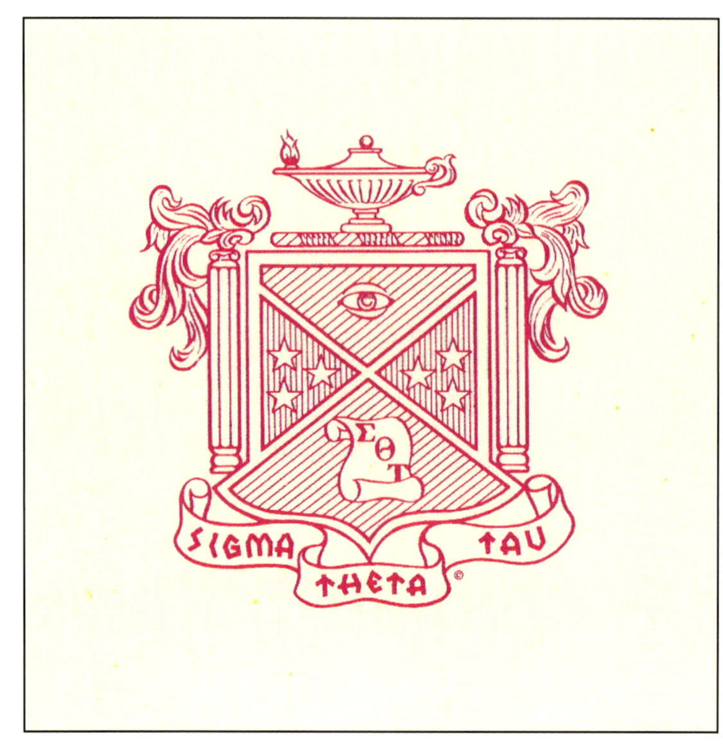

(Right) The Sigma Theta Tau coat of arms.

(Below) Congratulatory note from national STTI Officers.

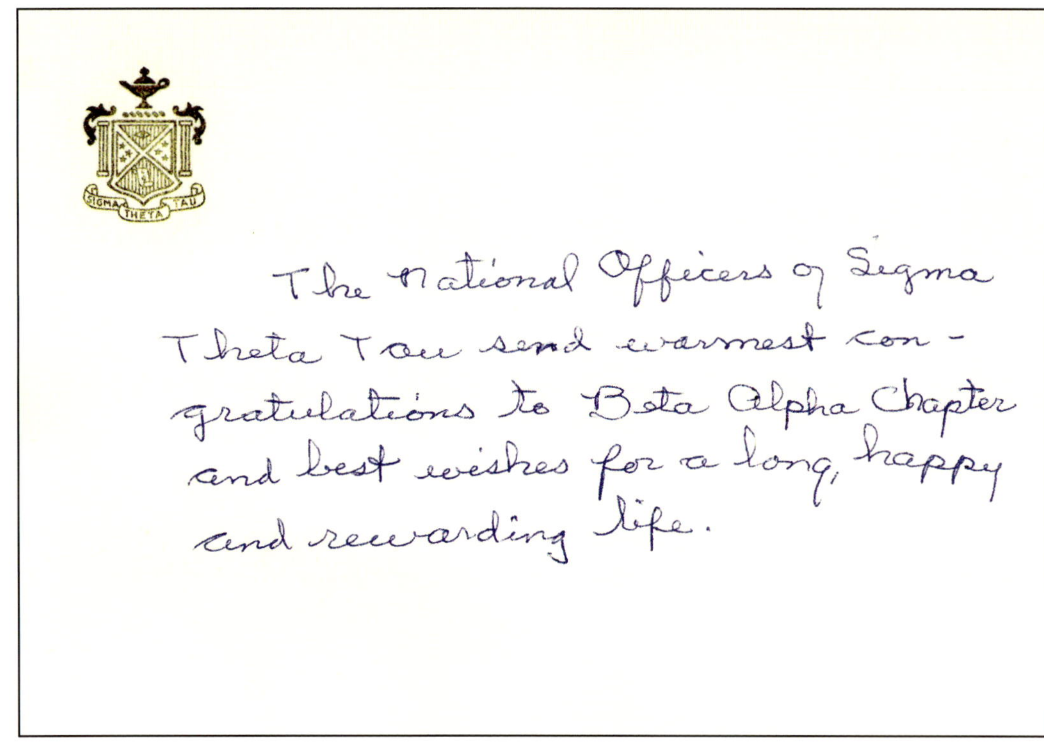

The National Officers of Sigma Theta Tau send warmest con-gratulations to Beta Alpha Chapter and best wishes for a long, happy and rewarding life.

CHAPTER TWO

Moving Forward

1973–1979

As she looked back in her 1974 *Harris College of Nursing Report to the Board of Directors,* Dean Virginia Jarratt reviewed the college's progress, changes, and continuing concerns and determined that it required "careful decisions about future direction" at many critical points. Constant change, burgeoning enrollment, adjustments in clinical facilities, and faculty workload contributed to making the early 1970s, and especially 1974, difficult (Harris College of Nursing Archives).

CHALLENGE ONE
A Clear Definition of Nursing Roles and Functions

Context and Trends

In 1971 a committee developed by the secretary of the US Department of Health, Education, and Welfare released a statement to assure the medical community that there were no barriers to role expansion for registered nurses (Bullough 1976). This, along with the gradual adoption of the American Nurses Association's 1955 example definition of nursing as "any act of observation, care, and counsel of the ill," bolstered the states in their efforts to expand nursing practice (Bullough 1976, 1, 478). Between 1971 and 1975 these efforts included over half of the states changing board guidelines, expanding definitions of registered nurses, encouraging more delegation by physicians, or standardizing nursing procedures in nurse practice acts. Included in these changes were the adoption of physical assessments and nursing diagnoses into nursing and nursing education, further promoting the autonomy of registered nurses (Lynaugh and Bates 1984).

The role expansion for nursing was accompanied by major changes in health care in the United States. In 1973 President Nixon signed the Health Maintenance

Organization Act to encourage the growth of Health Maintenance Organizations and to curb health care costs, which had doubled in the 1970s after the adoption of Medicaid and Medicare (Moseley 2008). To top off the decade, medical developments such as organ transplants, in vitro fertilization, and genetic experimentation required a deeper look into the ethical side of health care (Silvia 1974). These health care advances included the development of the first living will statute in California in 1974, beginning the patient movement, in which patients advocated both for their rights and to be a part of their own care (Sabatino 2010). This became known as the legal transactional approach, which was later replaced by the communications approach (224). While the patient movement allowed patients to develop a living will, the communications approach included discussions with family members and physicians about the future of individuals with serious illnesses and the way in which they wished their preferences to guide medical decisions. These discussions may have included all aspects of the patient's life: family matters, spiritual questions, concerns about finance, and any other issues experienced by seriously ill patients and their families (Institute of Medicine 1997, 198–99).

Harris College of Nursing

The new curriculum based on common human needs, which was first offered in 1971, had been fully implemented. "One Integrated Curriculum—An Empirical Evaluation" was conducted in 1975 by a Harris College of Nursing faculty member, M. Ann Richards, who later published the results in *Nursing Research.* Initial findings demonstrated a higher degree of leadership and empathy "without sacrifice of knowledge" among students under the new curriculum, but less critical-thinking ability than previous students who had undertaken the older "block" curriculum (Richards 1977, 90).

Nursing students also had the opportunity to participate in the honors program, launched at TCU in 1962 to identify, motivate, and challenge the superior student. Pre-honors courses were taken during students' first and second years in honors sections of general education courses such as English, religion, political science, history, and fine arts. During the junior and senior years, students enrolled in upper-division honors courses being offered in their major fields of study. The 1976 *Harris College of Nursing Self-Study Report* indicates that this included a two-credit seminar in the junior year and an individual two-semester project in the senior year. The Junior Honors Seminar was designed to allow students to discuss issues and topics of concern to nursing, such as abortion, child abuse, alcoholism, and the ethical and legal aspects of organ transplants, along with the expanding role of the nurse. The senior honors project was available to students who completed the Junior Honors Seminar and maintained a grade point average of 3.4 or above. Projects, selected by the student and approved by the faculty, involved such topics as the nurse as a family therapist, postpartum blues, attitudes of nurses toward disabled people, and a phenomenological explication of the experience of empathy. Requirements included a comprehensive study of a problem, a formal paper, and an oral presentation based on the results. In 1976 one student who was enrolled in the junior honors course and another enrolled for a senior honors project served as voting members of the college Honors Committee (*Harris College of Nursing Self-Study Report 1976,* 162).

Students learned the process of nursing primarily by developing and writing nursing care plans. They went to the hospital or place of their clinical assignment the evening before their shift to find the patient(s) to whom they had been assigned. Then they wrote a care plan that would guide their care of the patient(s) the next day. When appropriate, nursing diagnoses were used as the problem statement.

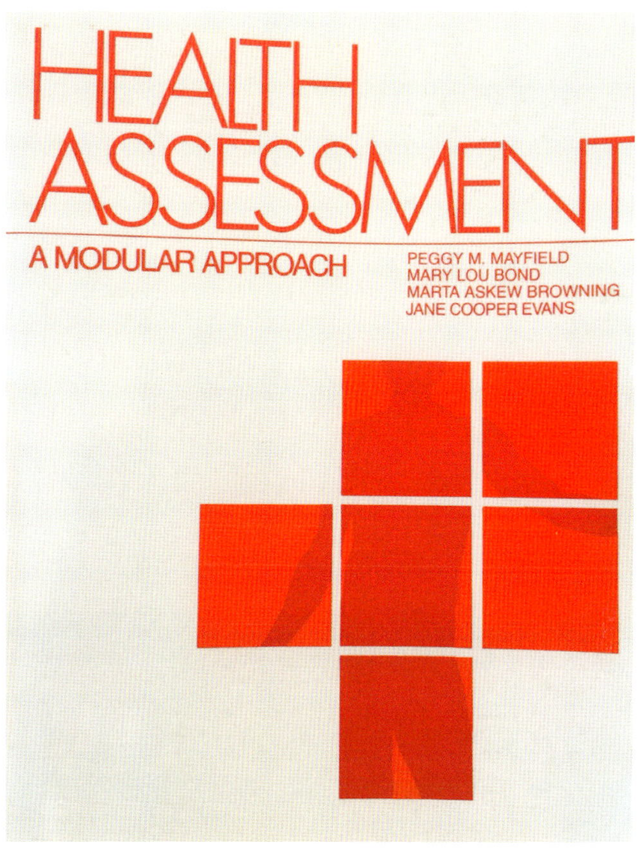

Health Assessment Textbook, 1980.

Faculty members continued to explore new teaching methods and prepared instructional modules to reinforce learning. For example, the *Harris College of Nursing Self-Study Report* for 1976 noted that team teaching had been increasing since the inception of the integrated curriculum. Team endeavors, including full engagement among faculty members serving as resources for the lead teacher, who implemented and evaluated the course, were thought to "enrich the classes, promote curriculum goals and tap and expand faculty expertise" (Harris College of Nursing Archives).

Additionally, in response to the rapidly expanding role of the nurse and the need for incorporating additional assessment skills into the curriculum, Peggy Mayfield, a faculty member, enrolled in a health assessment course at the University of California, Los Angeles (UCLA) to gain additional knowledge and skills not previously taught in nursing programs. Upon her return, she and three other faculty members (Mary Lou Bond, Marta Askew Browning, and Jane Cooper Evans) developed modules for independent study throughout the curriculum. Students were to complete these modules, which focused on clinical specialties, prior to conducting health assessments. The modules were later offered in an elective first taught by Mayfield in 1978 and offered to students, faculty members, and alumnae (Peggy Mayfield, pers. comm., August 9, 2017). In 1980, a book derived from their work entitled *Health Assessment: A Modular Approach* by Mayfield, Bond, Browning, and Evans was published by McGraw-Hill.

A second curricular development, an elective entitled A Comparative Analysis of Two Cultures: Considerations for Nursing, was offered as the first study abroad course in May 1978. Under the direction of Mary Lou Bond and Frances Richardson, students spent three weeks in Aguascalientes and Cuernavaca, Mexico, to help them learn about cultural considerations for nursing care. Activities included cultural lectures on health beliefs and practices, tours of local hospitals, a visit to a *curandero* (lay healer), and selected health-assessment activities with other medical and nursing students in Mexican hospitals.

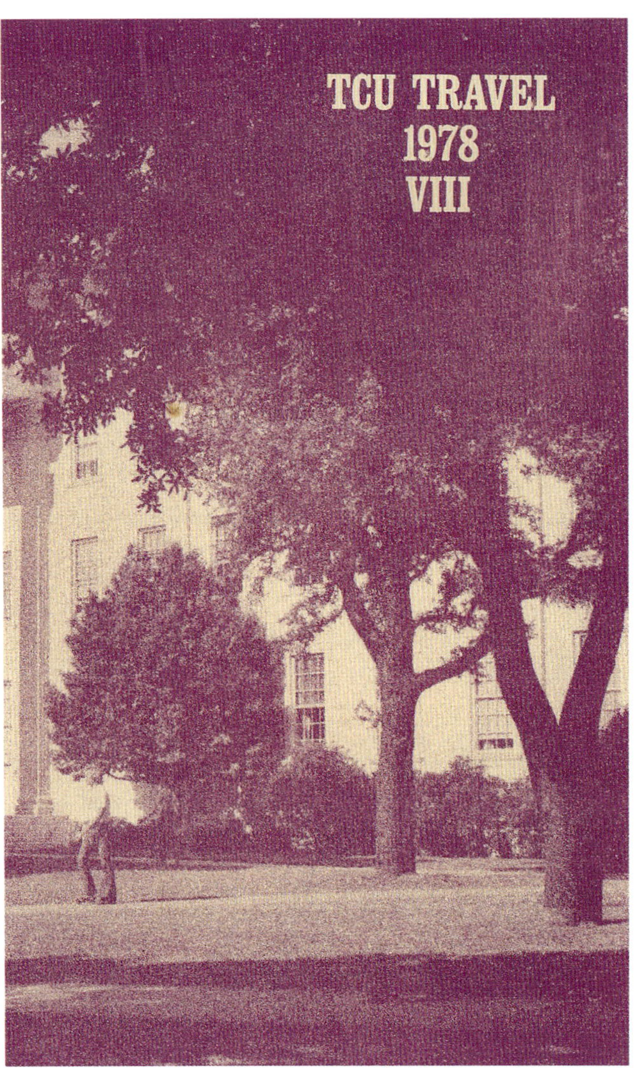

Study Abroad brochure.

This was followed by a local component working with Mexican Americans in the Dallas–Fort Worth metroplex, including individuals in the large Hispanic population on Fort Worth's north side and patients at John Peter Smith Hospital and at Los Barrios Unidos Community Clinic in Dallas.

Students commented that language barriers, cultural traditions, and health beliefs had major implications for the delivery of nursing care. One student who became ill in Mexico and tried to communicate in limited Spanish with Mexican doctors stated, "It was a sort of reverse culture shock and opened my eyes" (Miller July 18, 1978).

Nearly forty years later, a former student remembered selecting the course because of an "ongoing fascination with anthropology, sociology, archaeology, and museum sciences." Another motivating factor for this student was learning what might be useful in treating the increasing number of Hispanic patients in the US. Visits to the National Museum of Anthropology in Mexico City and the Metropolitan Cathedral impressed this student because of the "hordes of impoverished people who came

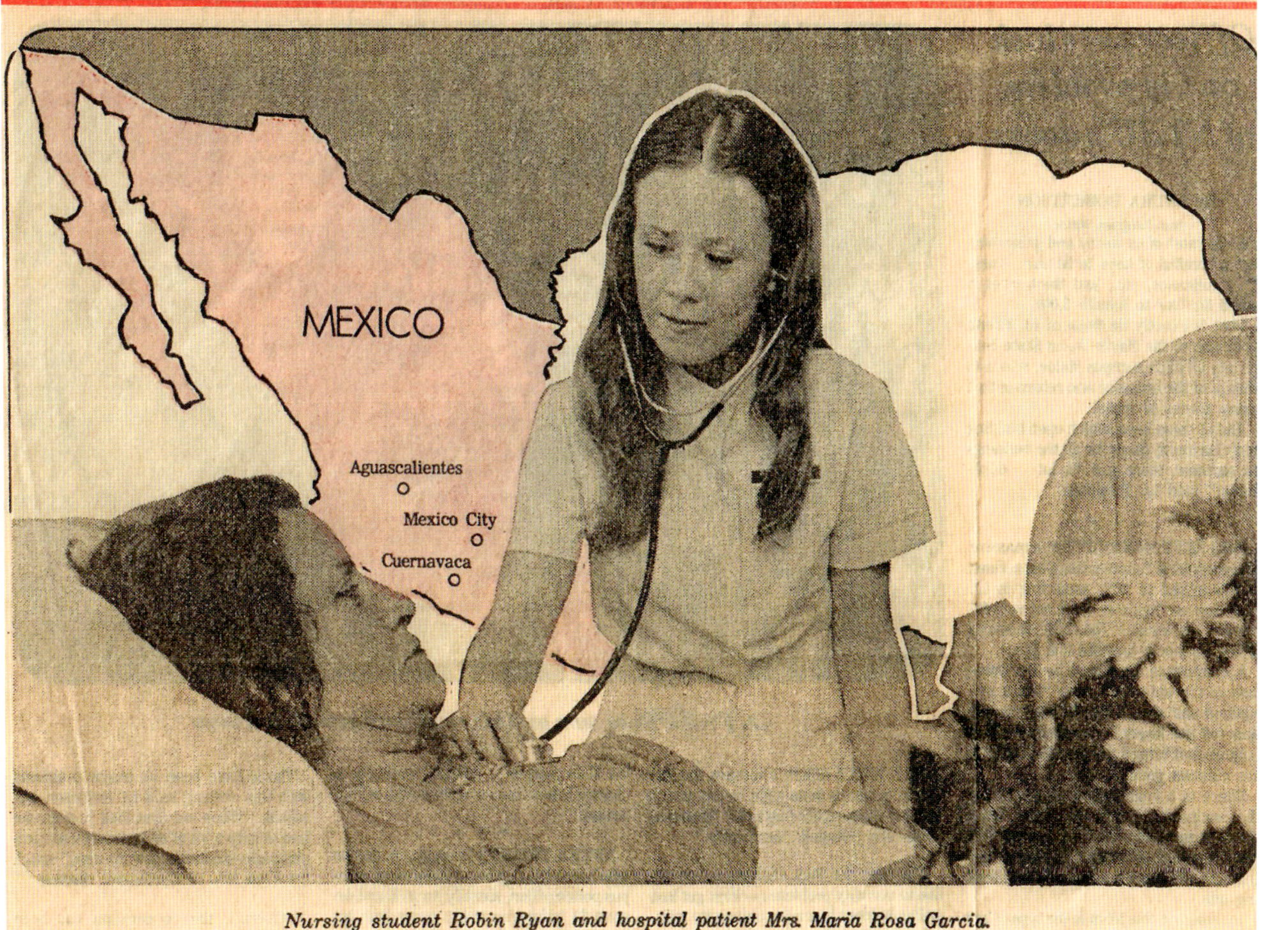
morning Star-Telegram TUESDAY, JULY 18, 1978

Nursing student Robin Ryan and hospital patient Mrs. Maria Rosa Garcia.

TCU Nursing student Robin Ryan in Study Abroad in Aguascalientes, Mexico, 1978.

to worship in such an opulent cathedral." Other memorable experiences included: (1) getting to see a midwife's clinic in a home setting, (2) receiving a blessing from a *curandero,* and (3) traveling to a remote Mexican village with a medical team and seeing firsthand traditional Mexican medicine practices in a rural area. "No book, class, or documentary film could ever provide me with this type of learning experience." Over the years, this student has found an added benefit to be an enhanced cultural sensitivity to nurses from other countries with whom the student has worked (Anonymous former student, pers. comm., August 8, 2017).

As nursing roles continued to change and expand, the roles of faculty members

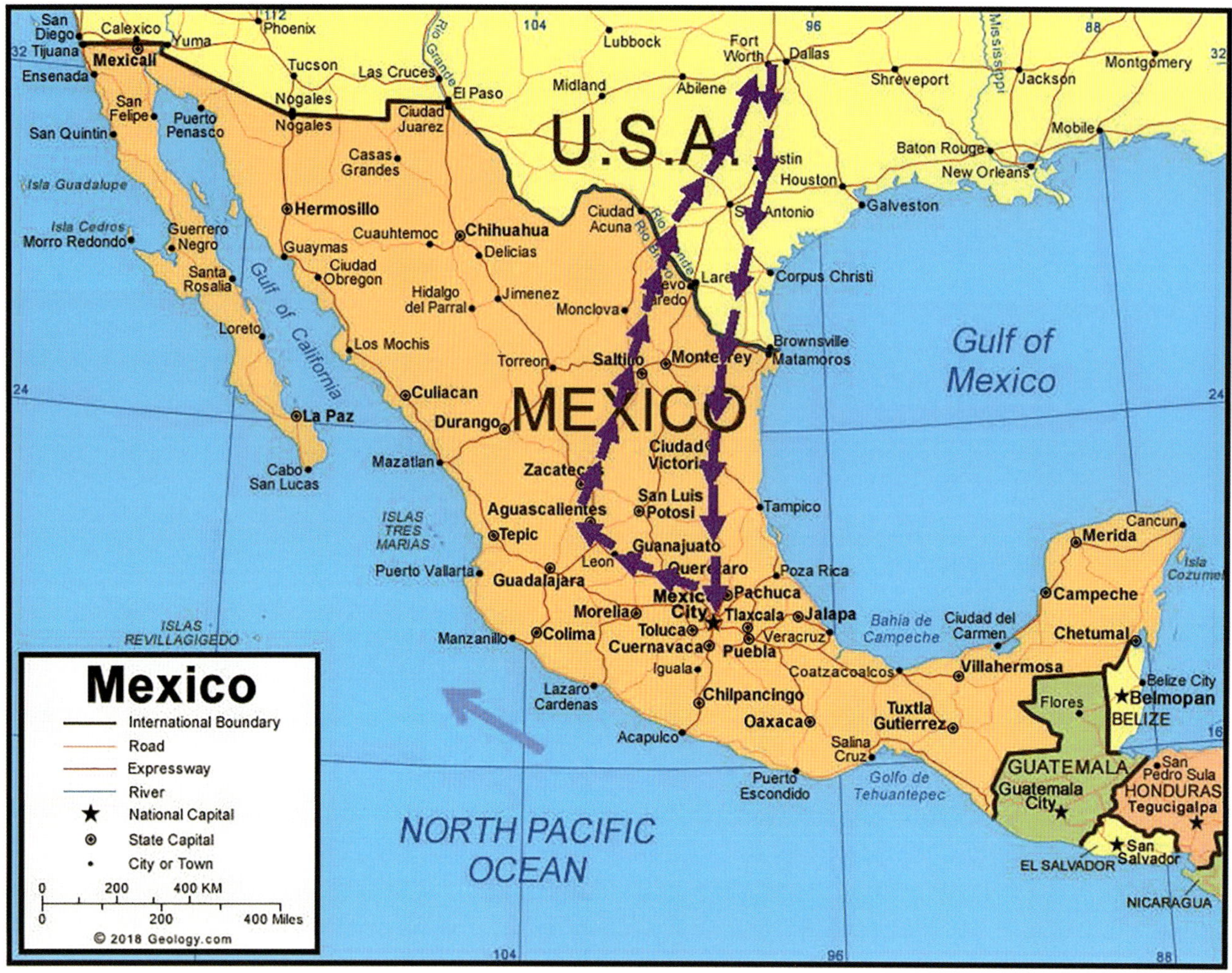

Map of students' journey in Mexico.

also increased. In 1974 Dean Jarratt noted in the *Harris College of Nursing Report to the Board of Directors* that the university evaluation plan did not include instruments for evaluating clinical teaching and omitted the "essential consideration" of professional involvement which is required of nursing faculty. In turn, this "penalizes" nursing faculty members, who are held to different standards from those of other faculty members (Harris College of Nursing Archives). Heavy workloads and differing criteria continued to limit robust engagement in research and scholarship. Jarratt's reports to the board from 1978–80 show that this problem continued throughout the '70s (Harris College of Nursing Archives). Despite heavy teaching loads and heavy involvement in community and professional activities, members of the faculty remained dedicated. For example, Katy Nichols's 1989 curriculum vitae shows that she served as the first vice president of district three of Texas Nurses Association (TNA) from 1970 to 1972 and was president of TNA from 1974 to 1975. Dr. Gail Davis's professional leadership, detailed on her 1997 curriculum vitae, included serving as president of district three of TNA from 1978 to 1979 and as president-elect and a board member from 1977 to 1978. She also served as secretary for the Texas League for Nursing from 1978 to 1980. In addition, Davis published an article for the Texas League for Nursing newsletter in 1976 titled "The Improvement of Nursing and Health Care through a Changed Nurse Practice Act" (Harris College of Nursing Archives). Patricia Eichelberger Thompson, a clinical instructor, published an article describing her experience of becoming an adoptive mother while holding a full-time teaching position (Thompson 1978).

Despite such burdens, faculty members began to accept the challenge of conducting research. Willadean Ball's 1997 curriculum vitae indicates that she conducted a study in 1975 to explore the attitudes of pediatric nurses toward abusive parents (Harris College of Nursing Archives). Mildred Hogstel conducted a study "Use of Reality Orientation with Aging Confused Patients," which was published in *Nursing Research* (1979b). She published a second study that focused on attitudes of hospital nursing service personnel toward caring for elderly parents in the *Journal of Nursing Administration* (1979a).

In 1976 the *Harris College of Nursing Self-Study Report* explains that the college was reorganized on departmental lines with level coordinators "who fulfill roles similar to those of department chairs in other colleges" (Harris College of Nursing Archives). Along with the level coordinators, an assistant to the dean (who had been in place since 1973), a clinical facilities coordinator, and an electives coordinator served as members of the Nursing Administrative Council. According to Dean Jarratt's 1978 and 1979 reports to the board of directors, goals and objectives for those years focused on the ongoing evaluation of the curriculum and the initiation of factors influencing performance on the State Board Examination. A second major goal was to appoint a committee to study the feasibility of a graduate program (Harris College of Nursing Archives).

Student Characteristics and Organizations

The *Harris College of Nursing Self-Study Report* for 1976 included a profile of students based on a questionnaire given that year to 359 students in all core nursing classes. It showed that most students were Protestant, Caucasian, single females between the ages of eighteen and twenty-two. The typical student came from a family with two or three siblings, a father engaged in a business or profession, and a mother who was a homemaker. However, thirty-one of the students listed their mother's occupation as nursing. Most students were from Texas, and some had transferred from another college or university. Minorities in the student body in 1976 included males (10 percent), African Americans (10 percent), Native Americans, Hispanics, and Asian Americans (together 6.6 percent). Dean Jarratt's 1974 report to the board of directors noted that the percentage of students participating in armed forces programs was high (Harris College of Nursing Archives). A systematic plan for recruiting disadvantaged students was completed in 1978 by Hogstel, and a cluster of factors predicting dropouts was identified.

Preparation for the role of the professional nurse was also enhanced through student organizations. According to the 1976 *Harris College of Nursing Self-Study Report,* the Nursing Student Association (NSA) at TCU Harris College of Nursing was part of the Texas Nursing Students' Association and the National Student Nurses' Association (NSNA) and sent a representative to the TCU House of Representatives. Between 1973 and 1976, the number of NSA members increased from 63 to 132. During this period, four elected state officers were Harris College of Nursing students. Student nurses also participated in annual blood pressure screenings, fund-raising activities, the TCU campus blood drive, and Christmas parties for an orphanage (Harris College of Nursing Archives).

Alumni

The Harris College of Nursing Association (composed of alumni) was reorganized between 1970 and 1975. Activities of the Alumni Association included an annual banquet that promoted membership and provided and maintained scholarship funds. A major accomplishment during this period was the establishment of the Ruth Eloise Sperry Award for Teaching Excellence, which recognized a faculty member who demonstrated excellence in classroom or clinical teaching. Recipients of the award are identified in Appendix 5.

Changing Nursing Roles and Challenges

While nursing roles in the United States continued to change, the employment of many nurses from Ireland and England, who had been recruited to respond to the nursing shortage at Harris Hospital and other clinical facilities, brought new challenges to the college. Because of different curricula in Ireland and England, where psychiatric and obstetric nursing were not part of the programs, nurses from these countries were ineligible to write state board nursing exams. As a result, the college was placed on warning by the Board of Nurse Examiners (BNE) for allowing students to work under the supervision of unlicensed nurses employed by the hospital who served as preceptors for students. In collaboration with Harris Hospital, two faculty members from Harris College of Nursing, Anne Lind and Mary Lou Bond, designed and received approval from the BNE to provide courses in psychiatric and obstetric nursing for foreign nurses, who subsequently passed licensure exams, adding to the health care workforce.

Fort Worth, the official publication of the Fort Worth Chamber of Commerce, ran a feature in 1978 titled "Nursing Has Caught Up with the Times." The article noted the profession had "broadened in scope and specialization," and cited nurse anesthetist and a nurse practitioner programs. It also cited Dean Jarratt, who observed that the expanded role "includes broadened activities for specialists, the assessment of biological and psychosocial factors in health and disease, the opportunity to monitor patients, teach, and provide professional awareness" (Fort Worth Chamber of Commerce 1978, 29).

Gary Force, the first male nurse in obstetrics at Harris Hospital and a graduate of the Harris College of Nursing, was also featured. "People thought I was a fruitcake!" he said. "It wasn't easy going to nursing school in the beginning." He also said that although male nurses (in obstetrics) get a "certain amount of flak," he found great satisfaction in helping patients cope with their problems. After serving as patient education director for maternity patients and teaching childbirth education classes, he reflected on his job and noted "a high degree of autonomy" (Fort Worth Chamber of Commerce 1978, 30).

Dean Jarratt described these scenarios as examples of how nurses' roles were in a period of transition, which she believed would continue into the 1980s. "The nurse of today needs educational experiences providing development of leadership, collaborative skills, priority setting, and such things as decision making ability as well as accountability" (Fort Worth Chamber of Commerce 1978, 29).

Jarratt provided an example of leadership through her service on the National League for Nursing Board of Review for Baccalaureate and Higher Degree Programs between 1967 and 1972. In 1976 her contributions were recognized by her alma mater, which designated her a Distinguished Alumni of the University of Texas system. The following year, 1977, she was inducted into the American Academy of Nursing (see Appendices 6 and 7). In the following years she served as president of the National League for Nursing and the Commission on Graduates of Foreign Nursing Schools.

Nursing education was still evolving. Fast forward to the 1980s.

ALUMNI EXAMPLES OF CHANGING ROLES

Defining the Role of the Nurse as a Clinical Nurse Specialist:

An Interview with Rebecca Crane-Okada, BSN 1976

Crane-Okada's original plan was to become an interior designer, but her volunteer work as a candy striper at a local hospital while she was in high school and her "love of biology, math, and science in general" persuaded her to study nursing instead. Although she did not know how she wanted to specialize upon graduation, when she interviewed for staff positions in orthopedic, urology surgery, and oncology, she related most to a young head nurse on the oncology unit "who had lots of energy and talked of the team approach" (Crane-Okada, pers. comm., 2018). She also credits Mildred Hogstel, Carol Reynolds, and Nancy Ackley as teachers and role models who influenced her future work.

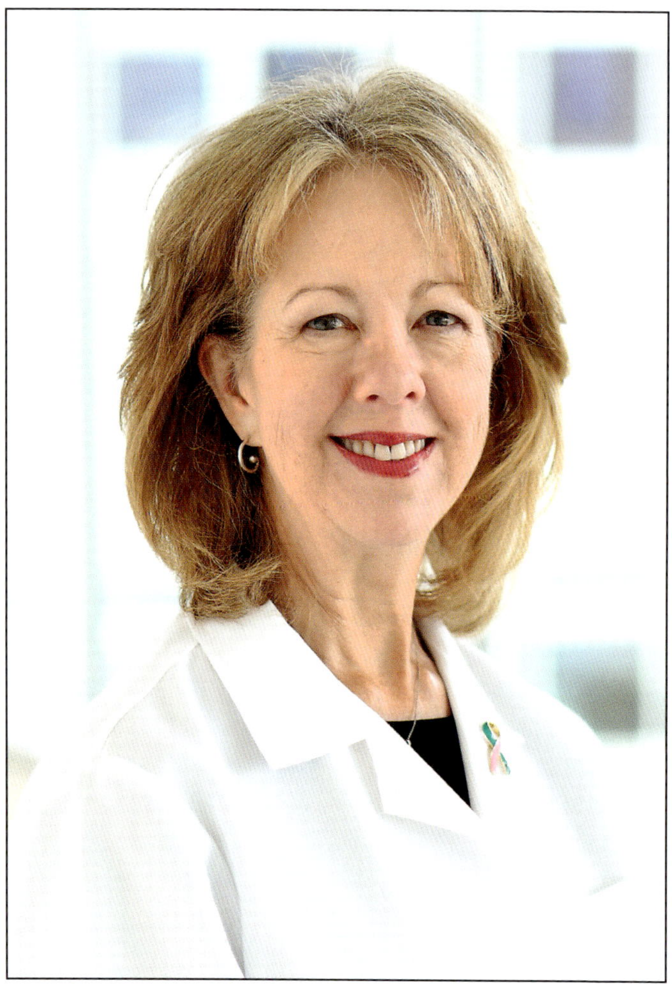

Rebecca Crane-Okada.

Following completion of her master's degree at UCLA, Crane-Okada began working as an oncology clinical specialist at Harbor-UCLA Medical Center. There she focused on balancing a caseload of underserved patients with pain management, vascular access, and terminal care needs. She established programs to support patients' psychological and physical rehabilitation after diagnosis. After learning about the research of Dr. Harold Freeman, president of the American Cancer Society, who had discovered important issues related to her patient population, she obtained her PhD in nursing from UCLA in 1999. Her dissertation focused on the specific issues of women facing an undiagnosed breast problem.

Today, Crane-Okada is the director of Patient Navigation and Willow Sage Wellness Programs at Saint John's Health Center in Santa Monica, CA. In this role, she is responsible for navigation and wellness services—nutrition, yoga, and mindfulness, among others—offered to breast and gynecologic cancer patients. Concurrently, she has participated in research focused on the impact of the Mindful Movement Program (a combination of mindfulness and movement or dance) on fear of recurrence, mindfulness in everyday life, and immune function. In the initial study, it was determined that participation in the Mindful Movement Program reduced fear of recurrence and improved mindfulness.

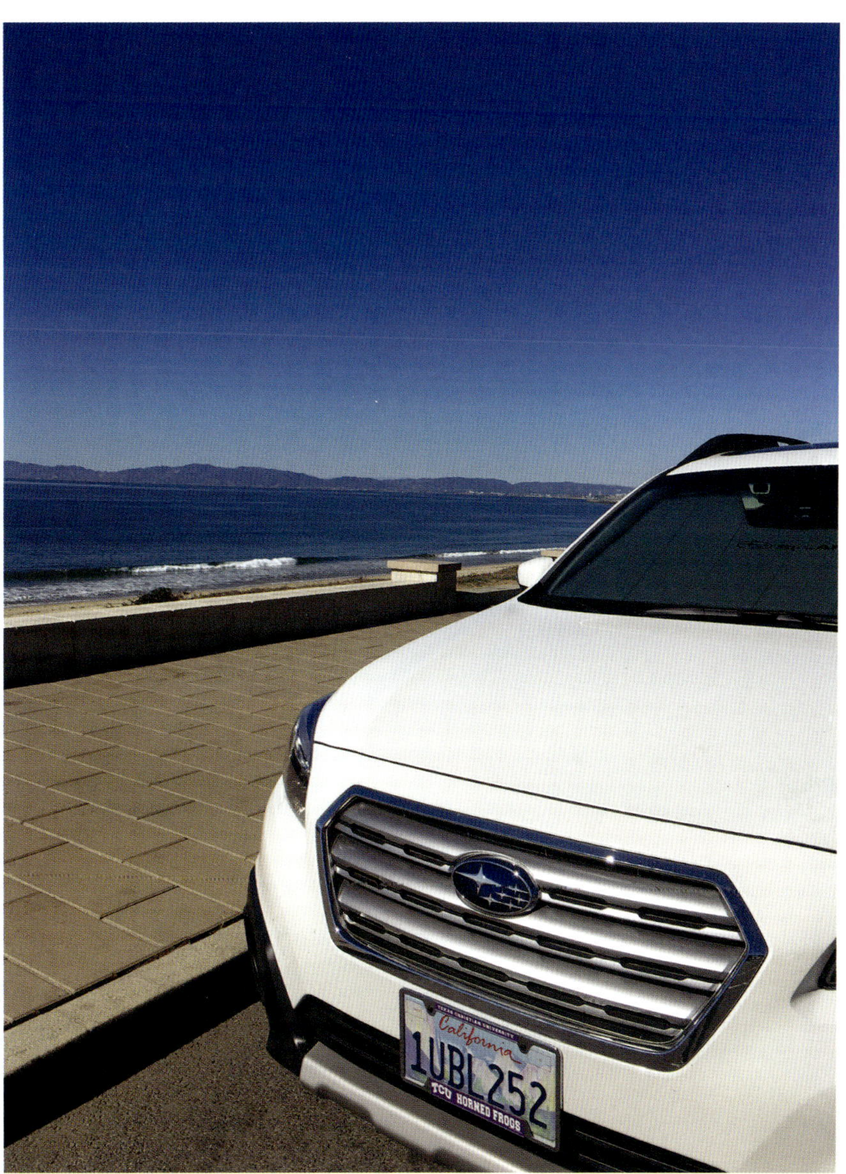

Rebecca's car in Redondo Beach, California, with TCU displayed on license plates.

Major challenges to her ongoing work include dividing her time between clinical practice, education, and research, and obtaining funding for nursing research. She believes her skill set enables her to see a bigger picture and to develop and implement programs and services that can impact a larger group of patients. She also states that "nursing still struggles with role definition" but that "nurses are the glue holding patients together." In closing, she observed, "I still get to be an interior designer of sorts, as my passion for the psychosocial and spiritual care of patients with cancer helps them attend to their interior" (Crane-Okada, pers. comm., 2018).

Defining the Role of the Nurse with the Centers for Disease Control and Prevention:

An Interview with Joyce A. Goff, BSN 1973

Joyce Goff, who obtained her bachelor of science in nursing (BSN) in 1973, was born to a working-class family and raised in Lubbock, Texas, in the days of the civil rights movement. She recalls that her high school teachers labeled her "least likely to succeed." As she thought about what motivated her to become a nurse, she stated that no matter how "old and ugly" she became she would always be able to get a job and take care of her parents (Goff, pers. comm., 2018).

Goff has not only succeeded but has surpassed all expectations. In high school, Goff was accepted into the US Department of Education's Upward Bound Program at Texas Tech University. After graduating from high school, she attended Hardin Simmons University in Abilene, Texas, in their diploma nursing program. She later enrolled in the nursing program at TCU, where she received her BSN.

Following graduation, Goff worked at Harris and John Peter Smith Hospitals in Fort Worth but soon decided that it was time to broaden her experiences, so she moved to Atlanta. While working at Grady Memorial Hospital in Atlanta, she attended Georgia State University, where she obtained her master's degree in education to become a health educator. She believes that "if [young women were] educated,

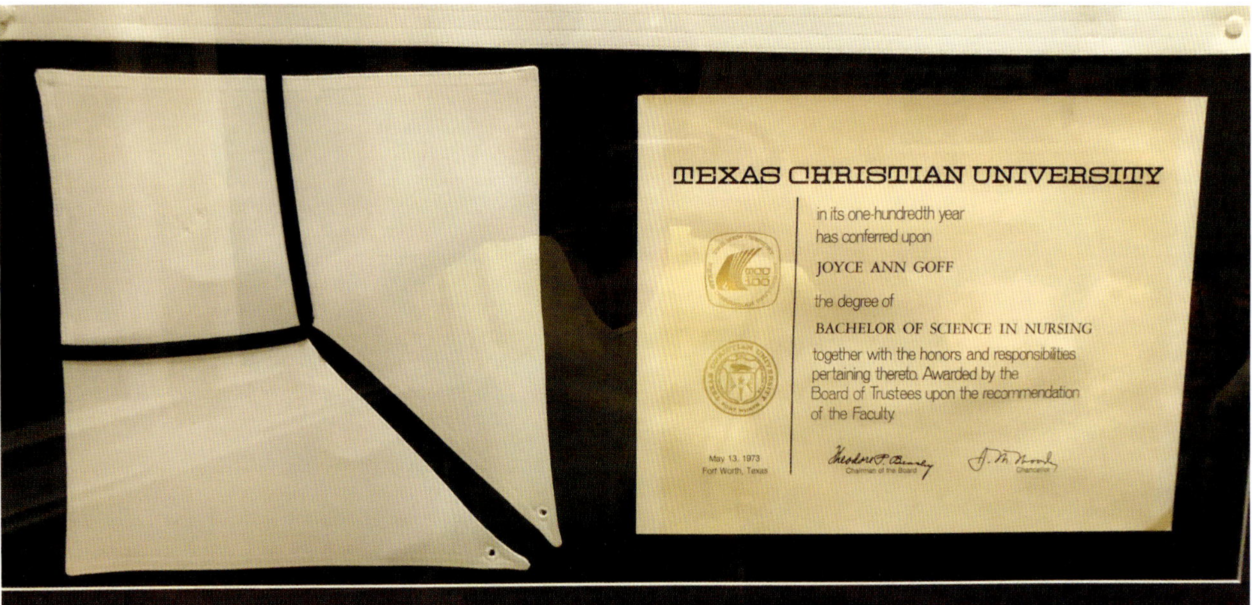

Nursing cap and diploma.

unhealthy behaviors would change" (Goff, pers. comm., 2018), and she wanted to educate the many single teenage mothers she cared for. While she was at Grady, someone suggested that the Department of Health and Human Services would be a good opportunity for her to develop her skills as a health educator. This was the beginning of her twenty-six-year career with the United States Public Health Service (USPHS). During her career, Goff rose through the ranks and became Captain Joyce Goff, serving at the CDC as Nurse Director, Health Education Specialist, and Nurse Epidemiologist. In these roles she responded to and investigated vaccine-preventable disease outbreaks and addressed public concerns about vaccine safety and efficacy. She also developed and managed continuing nurse education (CNE) programs for nurses at the CDC.

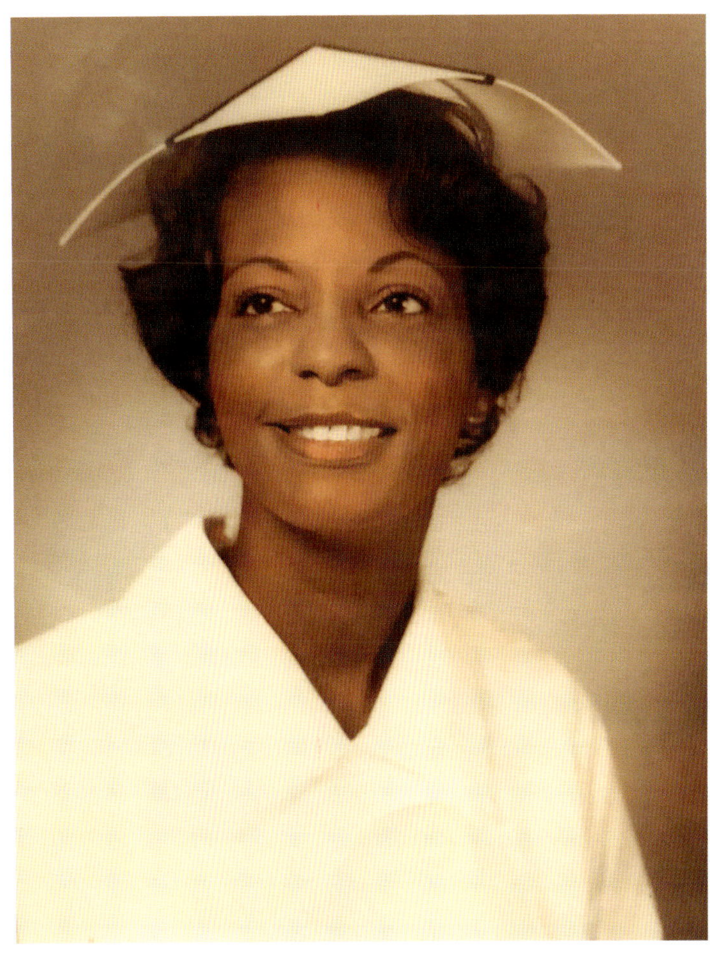

Joyce Goff graduation picture.

As her career developed, Goff became aware of legal ramifications and public concern over vaccines. So that she could help address some of these concerns, Goff obtained a master's degree in health law in 2003 and more recently, in 2017, a PhD in conflict analysis and resolution from Nova Southeastern University. She believes that these credentials further empowered her to communicate with lawyers and judges on public health issues and to view conflict and dispute from various perspectives (Goff, pers. comm., 2018).

Goff has served as a consultant to numerous organizations at the national and international levels. She was a nurse consultant and educator to the anthrax vaccine projects collaboration between the CDC and the Department of Defense at Walter Reed Army Medical Center, as well as to the World Health Organization Country Office for India for polio eradication efforts. She collaborated with the American Nurses Association to organize a committee of professional nurses to review and make recommendations on a curriculum designed to educate medical and nursing students about vaccine-preventable diseases in adults; she also served as a

COMMISSIONED CORPS AWARDS

COMMENDATION MEDAL

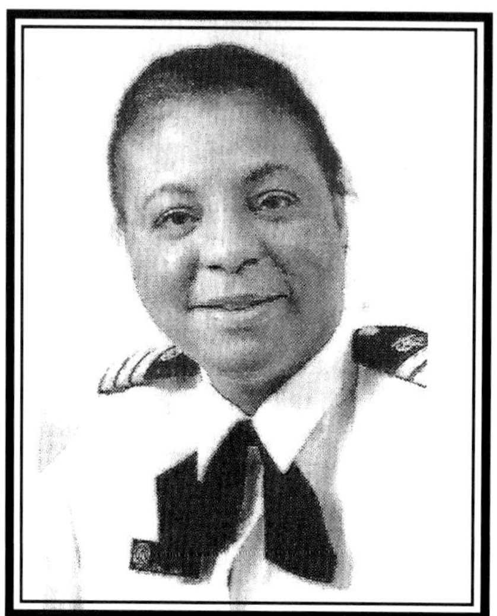

JOYCE A. GOFF
NURSE EPIDEMIOLOGIST
EPIDEMIOLOGY AND SURVEILLANCE DIVISION

FOR OUTSTANDING LEADERSHIP IN LAUNCHING CDC'S CONTINUING NURSING EDUCATION PROVIDER UNIT, EARNING CDC'S FIRST ACCREDITATION AS A NATIONALLY RECOGNIZED PROVIDER OF CONTINUING NURSING EDUCATION.

Commissioned Corps Awards Commendation Medal, 1973.

consultant to the American College of Occupational and Environmental Medicine and the American Association of Occupational Health Nurses to promote adult vaccines in the workplace.

Goff credits Allene Jones, one of the first African American TCU nursing student and later the first African American TCU nursing faculty member, as being her mentor during her student days at Harris College of Nursing. She found the faculty at TCU to be supportive and the experiences at Harris Hospital and John Peter Smith

Hospital to be instrumental in establishing the foundation for her career. Several years after her graduation, Goff was inducted into Beta Alpha Chapter of Sigma Theta Tau International (STTI).

When asked about the major challenges, rewards, and impacts of her role, she states that the biggest challenge was to "break through some professional barriers and be recognized and be respected" in a primarily male, physician-dominated environment such as the CDC. Rewards of her career were "to gain the respect of her peers and professional colleagues, the friendships, the opportunities to travel outside of the United States and to work with international organizations." The greatest reward was "to work for the premier federal agency in the world and the American people." Goff sees the impact of her career as having "made a difference in other people's lives" (Goff, pers, comm,, 2018).

In 2005, *Nursing Spectrum* paid tribute to nurses coast-to-coast who had made significant contributions. Goff was recognized as a health education specialist in the National Immunization Program.

"It was a lifelong dream to work for the Centers for Disease Control. . . . It is the utopia of a career. We help the world identify disease and do various things to control and prevent diseases. Who wouldn't want to be a part of that?" (*Nursing Spectrum* 2005).

Defining the Role of the Nurse in Many Settings:

An Interview with James R. (Ron) Hilliard, BSN 1972

Ron Hilliard, a biology and chemistry minor at MacMurray College, did not hesitate when he was asked what motivated him to become a nurse. He "needed a job!" His mother was a high school biology teacher, and his father was a college professor of biology. His mother said, "Ron, you like working with people. Go get a job at the hospital." He did and began working as a nursing assistant at a local hospital in Abilene. This was his introduction to health care. One day when the director of nursing was walking down the hall, she approached him and asked if he had ever considered going into nursing. After receiving several bulletins from schools, including TCU, Hilliard got a call from the army recruiter in Fort Worth, who told him about the Army Student Nurse Program and set up an appointment with him and the dean at TCU. By that afternoon, he had been accepted into both the army program and the Harris College of Nursing. While at Harris College, he worked as an orderly at Harris Hospital in Fort Worth and as a student nurse at All Saints Hospital, also in Fort Worth. He credits these experiences with allowing him to apply the skills he was learning, to see how a hospital operated, and to understand the role of the nurse. Looking back, he realized that nursing was his calling, and at the Harris College of Nursing he

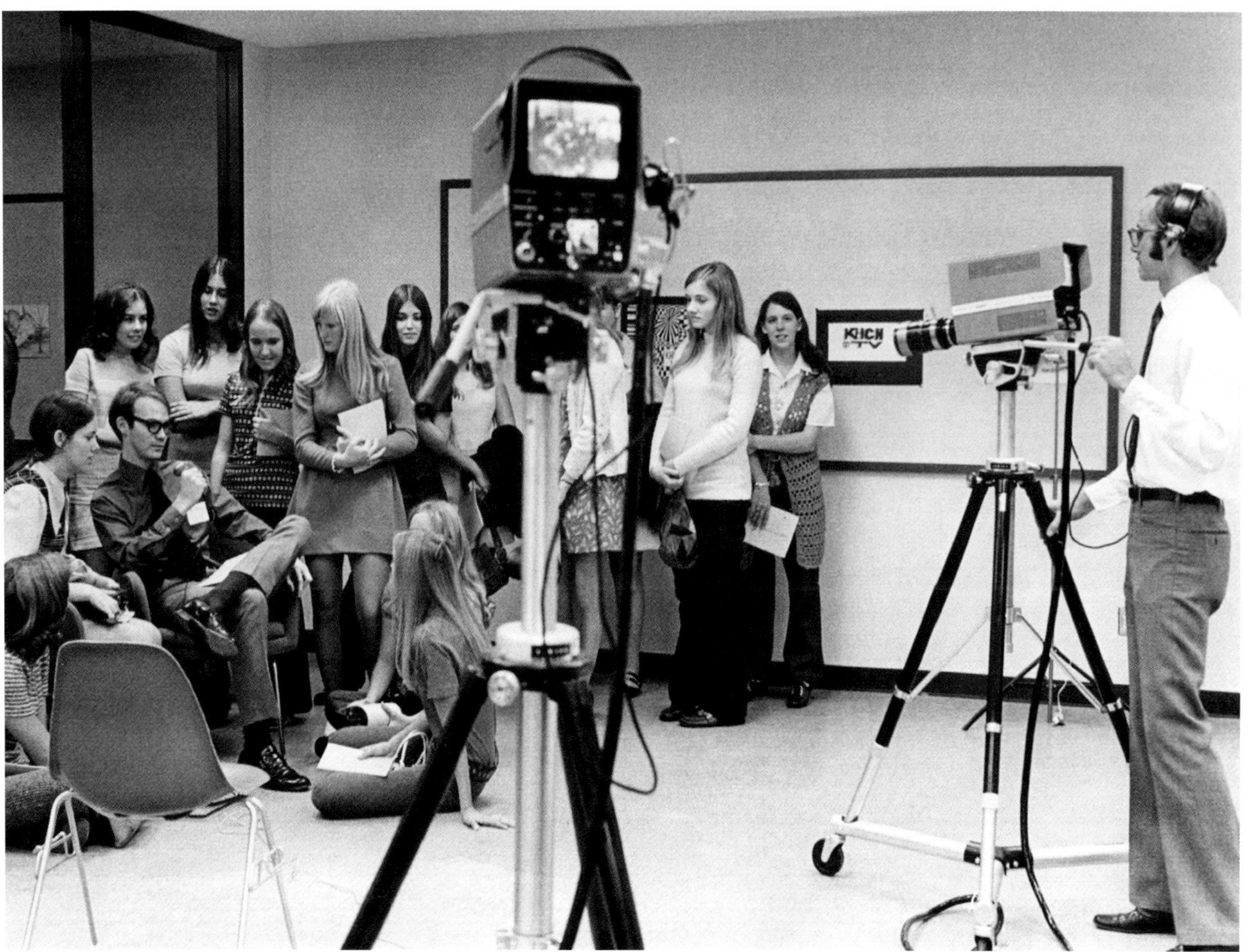

Ron Hilliard in Skills Lab, 1972.

learned not only the science but also the art of nursing. The members of the faculty were role models of how to be a professional nurse and guided him throughout his career (Hilliard, pers. comm., 2018).

Following graduation and receiving his license as a registered nurse in 1972, Hilliard served in the US Army Nurse Corps as a medical-surgical nurse and was transferred from California to Honolulu, where he worked in elective surgery orthopedics, which he found "boring." Again, he was given an opportunity: the chief nurse asked him to help feed babies in the neonatal intensive care unit (NICU) for ninety days until more NICU nurses arrived and promised him a position in the surgical intensive care unit. He spent two and a half years in the NICU working with high-risk infants and loved it. Later in his career, he had the opportunity to work in the world-famous burn unit for a short time, and he set up the first pediatric ICU at Brooke Army Medical Center. After twenty years of service, during which he held several positions as a clinical head nurse, Hilliard retired from the army (Hilliard, pers. comm., 2018).

After the army, he worked in prehospital emergency care, training EMTs and paramedics at the University of Texas Health Science Center-San Antonio, and he set up the First Responder Network in Bexar County. While doing this, he worked in the ER at University Hospital in San Antonio, a Level I Trauma Center. After meeting and marrying Debby, he then moved to Pflugerville, Texas, and was the director of the ICU at Round Rock Hospital. Here he became one of the first "nurse informaticists" when he was tasked to oversee the installation of a computer system and EDITECH software in the hospital. Following that project, he became the trauma coordinator in the ER at Round Rock. After several years, he moved to the Texas Department of State Health Services and oversaw the state trauma program. After 9/11, he was tasked to set up and manage Texas's Hospital Preparedness Program, working with 582 hospitals and an annual budget of $33 million. He was later recruited by the National Emergency Response and Recovery Training Center at Texas A&M University to bring health and medical into the planning, training, and implementation of programs against terrorism and weapons of mass destruction. Hilliard then retired from the state.

Although again retired, Hilliard did not become inactive. While he was teaching shelter management in the Red Cross Student Nurse Program pilot project at Concordia University Texas in Austin, Dr. Joy Penticuff, the director of the newly established nursing program, invited him to become part of the faculty. Seeing this as another opportunity and something he had dreamed of doing, he accepted the position. While teaching in the nursing lab, he discovered simulation and integrated it throughout the curriculum and became the simulation coordinator. He began by developing scenarios for use in the laboratory. With the realization that "mannequins don't do everything" (Hilliard, pers. comm., 2018), he wrote a scenario about alcohol withdrawal and made himself the binge-drinking patient who began hallucinating after being admitted for dehydration, nausea, and vomiting for three days. Seeing the memorable impact this role-playing had on students, he went on to develop other real-life scenarios and integrating MASK-ED into the program. The goal was to develop critical thinking and decision-making skills related to the roles of nursing and to integrate that into their practice.

The challenges of his role as a faculty member were to educate new nurses in the roles of nursing and to demonstrate how being a member of the profession was key to their responsibility as nurses. He taught them that "the only constant in nursing is change" and that becoming engaged is essential to moving the profession forward.

Hilliard found observing change in students over time was one of the major rewards of his most recent position and believed that his impact on the profession increased his passion for nursing. He hoped that his passion would affect his students and help mold them into future nurses. In April 2018, Hilliard retired from Concordia (Hilliard, pers. comm., 2018).

While in Austin, Hilliard became a member of the Texas State Guard and worked in the headquarters to support mass care during Texas disasters. His responses included Operation Lone Star, the lead for the response to Hurricane Alex, and working the State Operations Center of the Texas Division of Emergency Management. As always, his focus was on health and medical services and the role nurses play in providing care in disasters. After writing response plans, training guardsmen in mass care, and assisting Texas in major disaster responses, Ron retired as a Lieutenant Colonel in May 2018.

As if there wasn't enough on his plate, Hilliard was a volunteer firefighter for thirty-five years. He was an organizer and chief of the Northeast Volunteer Fire Department in Bexar County and president of the Bexar County Firefighters Association while in San Antonio. After moving to Pflugerville, he spent ten years as an officer at the Pflugerville Fire Department as both firefighter and first responder.

Like most nurses, Hilliard continues to be engaged in the profession despite being retired. Currently, he is a coleader in the Texas Team Coalition for Central Texas and is active in the Texas Nurses Association Governmental Affairs Committee and part of their Capitol Corps. He is also a past president of Texas Nurses Association district five and is the regional nursing lead for the American Red Cross Central and South Texas Region out of Austin. Hilliard has never forgotten the role Harris College of Nursing and the faculty played in developing him as a professional nurse and enabling him to fulfill the many roles he has had as a professional nurse over the past forty-six years.

CHALLENGE TWO

Research to Determine What Effects Variables in Nursing Care Have on the Health of People

Context and Trends

Before 1970, universities in which nurses studied received funds from the Division of Nursing to support graduate-level and postdoctoral interdisciplinary research. A focus on better-prepared nurses and improvement of patient care resulted in funding for research through the Nurse Training Act (Judd 2014, 245).

During the 1970s the American Nurses Association Commission on Nursing Research recommended recognition of nursing research in the mainstream of biomedical and behavioral sciences (National Institute of Nursing Research 2016). Martha Rogers (1970), an early nurse theorist, identified nursing as a science which was "translated into nursing practice" (Judd 2014, 246). Other nurses developed nursing theories which were intended to define nursing, what nurses do, and how they influence patient care outcomes (Judd 2014).

Long before the decade of the 1970s, STTI funded the first nursing research grant. These small grants have been awarded through 2018. In the 1970s, STTI furthered its commitment to research by adding new conferences and research sessions at major nursing conferences (Sigma Theta Tau International 2016).

Harris College of Nursing

The second challenge noted by Dean Harris, to conduct research "to determine what variables in nursing care can have on the health of people" (Harris 1976, 85), was further realized as several faculty members (Gail Davis, Mildred Hogstel, Myrlene Kiker, Ann Kirkham, and Willadean Williams) engaged in research projects *(Harris College of Nursing Self-Study Report 1976).* In the following years, both research and publication began to increase significantly. During the academic year of 1977–78, sixteen faculty members had manuscripts published or accepted for publication *(Harris College of Nursing Annual Report 1977–78).* One faculty member, Mildred Hogstel, took Dean Harris's challenge to heart and published nine manuscripts between 1976 and 1979.

Faculty members from the Harris College of Nursing were active in establishing the Inter-University Research Council and participating in it with Baylor University and the University of Texas at Arlington School of Nursing. The purposes of the council were (1) to encourage research and the use of findings in practice, (2) to provide consultation on research, (3) to provide a forum for presentation and analysis of clinical nursing research, and (4) to publish the clinical nursing research presented at the forums *(Harris College of Nursing Self-Study Report 1976,* 67).

The second half of the decade of the '70s was also marked by the founding of the Lucy Harris Linn Institute. The purpose of the institute was to honor the first dean of the Harris College of Nursing, who had become a nationally recognized leader involved with the development of nursing and nursing education for nearly fifty years. Established by the Texas Nurses Association district three, the first institute was held in 1976 and was cosponsored by the Beta Alpha Chapter of STTI. Dr. Madeleine Leininger, dean and professor at the University of Utah as well as a well-known nurse anthropologist, was the speaker. Leininger's topic, "Cultural Shock and Change in Nursing," reflected rapid changes both within society and in the culture of nursing. The institute continued with nationally known speakers who shared their perceptions about the history of nursing and nursing education and their predictions for the future (Appendix 8). In 1975 the Harris College of Nursing was honored to have Mary Tolle Wright, one of the student founders of STTI, as the guest speaker for the STTI induction ceremony. Her topic, "Visions of Sigma Theta Tau—Yesterday and Today," focused on the history of the organization and its opportunities and responsibilities in the future.

To summarize, moving forward through the '70s called for change in roles of both faculty and students. Faculty members embraced team teaching in an integrated curriculum as a method to bring perspectives from various clinical areas to students. The expansion of nursing roles, which included new content related to health assessment, necessitated continuing education for faculty and additional content for students.

During this decade there was also an emerging focus on global health. While nurses from Ireland and England worked side by side with faculty and students in local clinical facilities, students from Harris College of Nursing participated in the first nursing study abroad course to Mexico.

Moving from the apprenticeship model of teaching and service for nursing faculty, new expectations emerged within the academic setting. Harris College of Nursing faculty responded to the challenge to begin research and dissemination of findings with the purpose of improving nursing care and patient outcomes.

Chapter Three

The Eighties

A Decade of Transition

The spring of 1980 was a period of transition that began with the resignation of Dean Virginia Jarratt. This was followed by the appointment of Interim Dean Dr. Joan Goe, who served in this role until August 1, when Dr. Patricia Scearse assumed the role as the third dean of the Harris College of Nursing. In Dean Scearse's initial report to the Board of Directors in November of 1980, she commented, "I was struck as I reviewed the minutes of previous board meetings by the numerous times it has been reported to you that the Harris College of Nursing faculty is conscientious, dedicated, heavily involved in community and professional services, and largely understaffed and overloaded" (Scearse 1980, 3).

Early observations made by Dean Scearse included not only the commitment of the faculty, but the challenges that the college would face in the years ahead: recruiting and maintaining a core group of faculty members, keeping the curriculum pertinent to ongoing changes in the health care system, providing financial support for students, and increasing faculty professional growth and scholarship. These observations echoed the challenges posed by the founding dean, Lucy Harris, as she considered the future.

CHALLENGE ONE
A Clear Definition of Nursing Roles and Functions

Context and Trends

Early in the decade of the '80s, the American Nurses Association (ANA) published *Nursing: A Social Policy Statement,* in which nurses were charged to answer the question, "What is nursing?" (ANA 1980, 1). They were further charged to "define and establish the scope and trends of nursing practice and the characteristics of nursing specialization" (American Nurses Association, 1980, 1). The National League for Nursing (NLN) subsequently released a credentialing document, *Nursing Roles—Scope and Practice* (1984), which became a standard for the preparation of nursing professionals. Patricia Benner's research on the role of the nurse, *From Novice to Expert,* also published in 1984, identified specific functions that nurses assume as they move from "novice to expert."

While Benner, the ANA, and the NLN were defining nursing roles, changes in the health care system itself were altering nursing practices. Patient's illnesses were increased in acuity, but hospitals were shortening lengths of stay, forcing nurses to develop new strategies to continue to ensure a high quality of care (Detmer 1986). These changes were followed by the development of Diagnosis Related Groups (DRGs) by Medicare in 1983, which contributed to an acute decline in the number of practicing licensed vocational nurses, in turn putting more pressure on associate- and bachelor-trained registered nurses to provide increasingly efficient patient care (*American Journal of Nursing* 1985). Also, the increasing fragmentation of care required nurses to take on the role of viewing the patient holistically rather than for just a single diagnosis (Field and Winslow 1985). Throughout the decade, nurses would continue to be challenged by both new nursing standards and changes in the health care system that paved the way for an improved and expanded scope of practice for all future nurses.

Harris College of Nursing

Harris College of Nursing and the characteristics of faculty, students, and alumni continued to evolve during the 1980s as the curriculum underwent continuous evaluation to produce graduates equipped for evolving roles in a changing health care system. In 1984 the faculty noted that the foci of professional nursing included "the promotion of wellness, prevention of illness, care of the ill and injured, restoration of health, rehabilitation. and supportive care for reduction of suffering when restoration of health is impossible" (*Harris College of Nursing Self-Study Report 1984,* 56a).

After several years of "careful study," the Harris College Board of Directors requested that the Texas Christian University Board of Trustees be the "sole survivor" of the Harris College Board of Directors (*Harris College of Nursing Self-Study Report 1984,* 9). This change was approved and became effective on June 1, 1985. The Harris College of Nursing was an integral part of TCU and "subject to the identical personnel policies and curriculum policies as all other academic units" (9). In 1984 Dean Scearse noted that the "internal structure" of the Harris College was more formalized than that of many other academic units on campus (9), which suggested the increasing complexity of nursing roles and functions within the academic setting. Significant reorganization of the faculty structure occurred during the '80s with an administrative council functioning in an advisory capacity to the dean, while also acting as a decision-making body for items related to budget, faculty assignments, student progression, and retention (12–13). Faculty members, known collectively as the faculty assembly, held responsibility for development and implementation of the nursing program. Clinical councils, representing all clinical areas, and nine standing committees brought recommendations to the administrative council and the faculty assembly for approval.

Students had the opportunity to serve on selected faculty committees. Student members were selected by the Harris College of Nursing Student Association and had "full voting privileges and responsibilities of membership" (*Harris College of Nursing Self-Study Report 1984,* 37). For example, in 1984, the curriculum committee had three students, the honors committee had four, and the library committee had two student members. Additionally, four students served on the recruitment and retention committee and two on the research committee.

At the time of the reaccreditation visit by the National League for Nursing site evaluators in the fall of 1984, there were a total of twenty-nine faculty members and two administrators (dean and associate dean). Although the faculty was smaller, there had been a decrease in faculty turnover for the preceding three years and an increase in faculty continuity and stability, albeit with "adequate turnover for new suggestions and ideas."

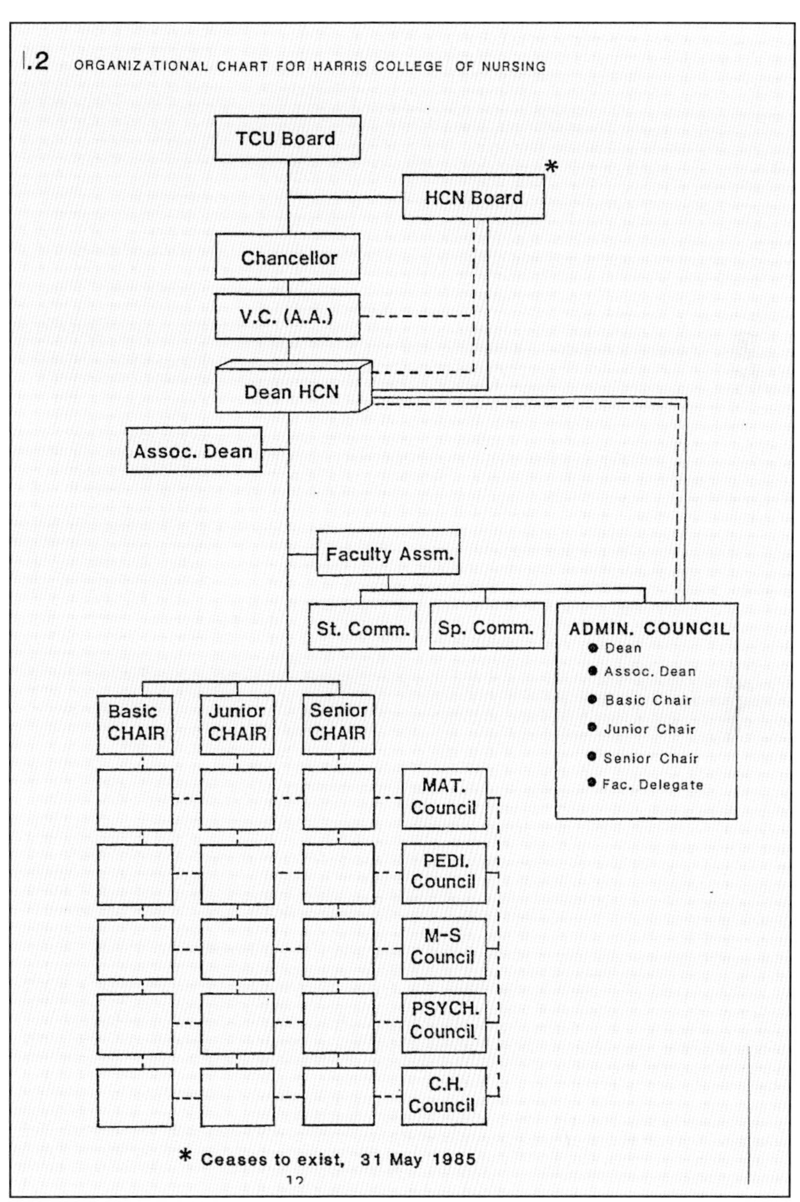

Harris College of Nursing Organizational Chart, 1984.

Seven support staff were in place. Lora Bailey, sister of former dean Lucy Harris, retired after many years of service to the Harris College of Nursing as a staff member who had supported faculty members. During these years, the Harris College of Nursing was housed at the Fannie M. Harris Building next to Harris Hospital before moving to the Annie Richardson Bass Building on the TCU campus.

Diversity among students who enrolled in Harris College of Nursing in the '80s continued to increase. While many were recent high school graduates, a number of older students who sought second degrees in nursing were admitted, along with licensed vocational nurses and registered nurses (RNs) seeking a baccalaureate degree in order to assume increasingly complex nursing roles.

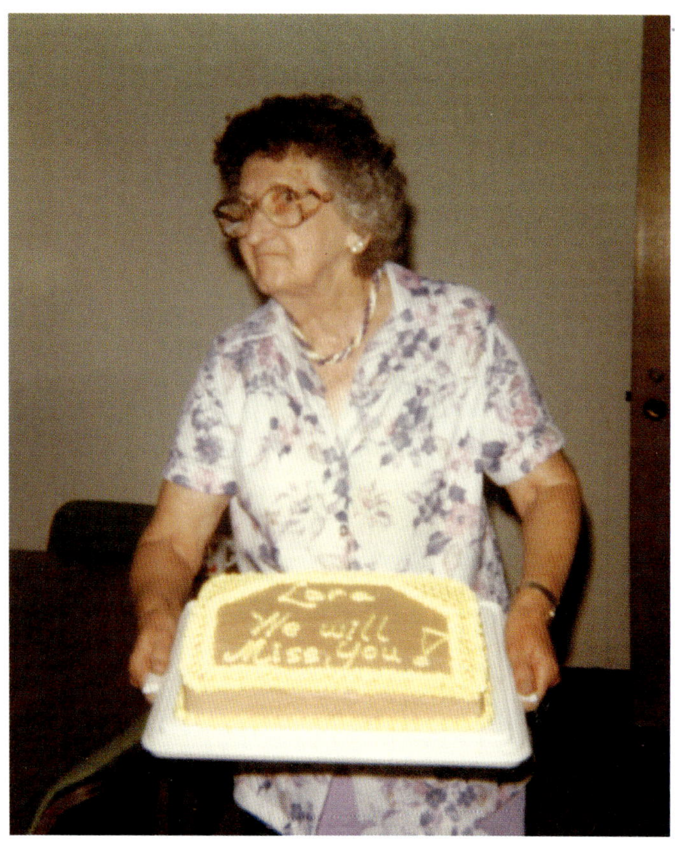

Lora Bailey with retirement cake at her party, 1984.

Changing Nursing Roles and Faculty Responses

As nursing roles continued to evolve, faculty members also sought to maintain expertise in their specialty roles and gain additional skills through a variety of activities: working in private practices, at the University Student Health Center, in joint appointments at local hospitals, and serving in the military reserve. Billie Hightower modeled leadership roles in multiple presentations related to childbearing and healthy lifestyles for young adult women and by serving as a preceptor for graduate students in maternity nursing at the University of Texas (Hightower 1992). Monette Graves published two chapters in a book entitled *Nursing Care of Older Adults;* one chapter described the physiological changes of aging and the other drug use and abuse (Graves 1984). Gail Davis published seven articles, two of which were related to her pain research and five to nursing education. She also published six book chapters and two sets of pediatric nursing questions for nurses' review in preparation for the licensing exam. Nancy Sayner contributed several articles about the conduct of research to the *Journal of Neuroscience Nursing:* (1) "Research in the Clinical Setting: Potential Barriers to Implementation" (1984), (2) "Conceptualizing Researchable Neuroscience Nursing Problems in the Clinical Setting" (1987), and (3) "Observation and Literature Review: The Key and Lock to Research Endeavors" (1989). Dean Scearse's positions demonstrated the variety of roles that a nurse educator or administrator could pursue: accreditation site visitor, board member, assistant editor of the *Journal of Professional Nursing,* and president of the Texas Association of Deans and Directors of Professional Nursing.

The clinical practice experience of faculty in the early part of the decade was diverse, with eleven faculty members holding doctoral degrees from seven different universities. Twenty-eight of the nursing faculty held master's degrees with clinical specialization appropriate to their areas of teaching; one held a master's in nursing education. Another seven faculty members were in the process of obtaining doctoral degrees (*Harris College of Nursing Self-Study Report 1984,* 51).

The preparation of faculty with specializations in specific clinical areas ultimately influenced the curriculum, which had been modified from a predominantly integrated one to a modified block approach (*Harris College of Nursing Self-Study Report 1984,* 3). Faculty believed that there needed to be a more distinct relationship between content and the five major clinical areas: medical-surgical, maternity, pediatric, psychiatric, and community health. "Common human needs" (physiological, safety, love, self-esteem, and self-actualization) continued to be the organizing framework with seven strands (communication, critical thinking, group process, management, professionalism, research, and teaching-learning) being threaded throughout the courses at all levels. The nursing process (assessment, planning, intervention, and evaluation), enabling the nurse to meet the individual's common human needs, continued to be the strategy for role implementation.

With an increasing emphasis on legal and ethical issues in nursing and health care delivery, the nurse's role in resolving these issues became apparent. In addition to the integration of ethical issues into the core curriculum, Dr. Alice Gaul introduced an elective course: Ethical Dilemmas in Health Care. In this course, students had the opportunity to explore ethical problems in nursing settings and consider their roles in ethical decision-making. Gaul subsequently published two articles about the students' experiences. "The Effect of a Course in Nursing Ethics on the Relationship Between Ethical Choice and Ethical Action in Baccalaureate Nursing Students" was featured in the *Journal of Nursing Education* in 1987. A second article, "Ethics Content in Baccalaureate Degree Curricula: Clarifying the Issues" was published in *Nursing Clinics of North America* in 1989. Additional elective courses allowed students to increase their knowledge and skills in selected clinical areas. These electives included courses in emergency nursing, critical-care nursing, pediatric nursing, and intraoperative nursing.

From Horned Frog Oct 31, 1987 Vol. 23 No. 127 p 139

NURSING COLLEGE FIRST TO ADD NEW TECHNOLOGY

Everywhere we turn, computers are there. At the bank, the grocery store, the airport, even now at bedside in hospitals.

To reduce the paperwork burden that limits the time nurses can devote to patient care, hospitals are replacing patient charts with bedside computer terminals. The technology reduces by an hour to an hour-and-a-half the time a nurse spends documenting patient information per eight-hour shift. Besides improving patient care by increasing the time nurses can spend with patients, the new technology provides an accurate, reliable record of patient care, which is particularly important if a court case is filed.

Texas Christian University is believed to be the first university in the country to add this new technology to its nursing school.

Although the transition from paperwork to computer documentation is new and occurring slowly in hospitals throughout the country, it is likely to become universal in urban hospitals within several years. The National League for Nursing already requires its nurses to be computer literate.

To give nursing students an edge on using this developing technology, Harris College of Nursing has installed four terminals and a main computer in its basic skills lab.

"We feel that if our students will be using these computers after they graduate, they need to become familiar with them now," says Dr. Patricia Scearse, dean of Harris College of Nursing. "To our knowledge and the knowledge of the company that installed the system, we are the first nursing school to install these terminals."

Students are introduced to the computers early in their education, typically as sophomores, when they are learning basic nursing skills.

"We want the students to see the computer as a tool, not something mysterious or hard, but something they'll use along with their other tools, like the thermometer," Scearse says.

Purchased from Micro Healthsystems of New Jersey, the system was set up in the nursing lab as it would be installed in a hospital. Placed between two beds, each terminal can record information for two patients. Peggy Mayfield, assistant professor of nursing who uses the terminals in her health assessment course, was not satisfied with the original screen design. To make the computers as useful as possible, Mayfield redesigned the screen to correspond with the workbook she wrote for the lab.

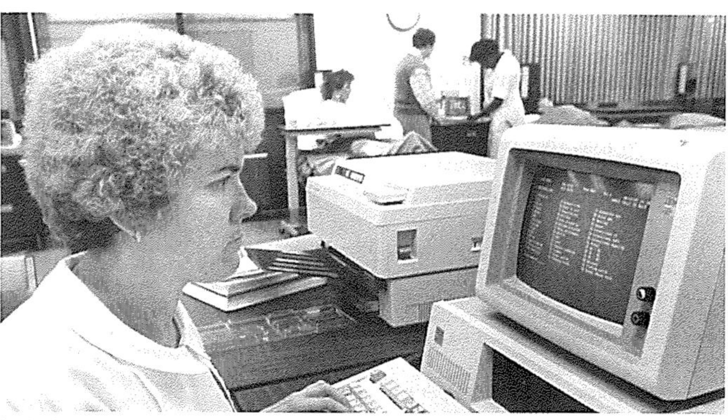

In the foreground Diane Mautone, a hospital employee returning to college to earn her bachelor's degree, reviews patient information on the main computer. Behind her in Harris College of Nursing's basic skills lab, associate professor Peggy Mayfield, center, shows junior Elouise Dawes how to enter information on a bedside terminal. Jaci Probst, a second-degree student who has worked as a surgical technologist, acts the role of the patient.

"As it was originally, the screen didn't meet our needs," she explains. "I asked the company last spring if I could redesign it."

Micro Healthsystems now uses her materials.

In the basic skills lab, nursing students act as patients while other students practice skills – in this case, entering patient information into the specially-designed keyboard. The computers store information such as vital signs, diet, intravenous care, wound care and safety precautions.

Mayfield uses the computers in another way in her health assessment course. Rather than entering data on patients, health assessment students punch up existing data to use in making assessments of particular organs and systems.

"The computers give the course a new dimension, since an important part of health assessment is correct documentation," she says. "One advantage is that the computer already contains the vocabulary they are learning, so they use the words as they learn them. Also we have a laser printer, and being able to print out a neat-looking document encourages students to enjoy using the computer."

Many of Mayfield's students are registered nurses working in hospitals while earning their Bachelor of Science degrees.

"These nurses know that the technology is coming, and they are really excited," Mayfield says. "They share with us ways they can use the computers in the work setting."

Incorporated into the labs since the beginning of the fall semester, the computers are already suggesting additional applications as teaching devices. Dr. Rhonda Keen-Payne, assistant professor of nursing and basic nursing skills instructor, has found that the computer also can be used as a testing device.

"You could, for instance, enter into the patient information an allergy to penicillin, then test to see if the student catches that fact when you assign medication," she said.

As one measure of TCU's quickness in responding to developments in the nursing field, no hospital in Tarrant County has yet implemented a similar system, although at least one is trying a system on an experimental level.

Nursing College Basic Skills Lab, 1987.

Along with changes in the basic curriculum and electives offered, new teaching methodologies were adopted. Texas Christian University was cited as being the "first university in the country to add bedside computer terminals to replace patient care charts" (Texas Christian University 1987, 139). This emerging technology permitted nurses to spend more time with patients and to provide an "accurate, reliable record of patient care" (139).

Nursing students continued to participate in the university's honors program, whose purpose was to identify, motivate, and challenge the superior student. Nine nursing students completed the honors program between 1980 and 1984.

The curriculum was further revised in 1988 to reflect changes in the university's core curriculum and an increased awareness of the diversity of the community. Additional electives were offered to prepare students for expanding roles in women's health, healthy lifestyles, and health care delivery; these were open to all TCU students. The health care delivery course examined health care systems and nursing roles in other countries (*Harris College of Nursing Self-Study Report 1984,* 10).

TABLE 2 Students' Honor Projects, 1980–1984

STUDENT	YEAR	TITLE OF SENIOR HONORS PAPER
Laura Jean Applegate	1980	A Determination and Comparison of the Nurses' and the Public's Definition of the Term *Death with Dignity*
Janet Striplin	1980	Assessing the Knowledge Base of 5–6 Year Old Children Concerning Basic Nutritional Practices
Ainslie Taylor	1980	Job Satisfaction Among Nurse Managers
Cynthia Lawrence	1981	Primiparas' Expectations of Maternal and Infant Care in the Post Partum Hospital Period
Helen Stearns	1981	The Effect of a Nurse's Behavioral Traits on the Formulation of Nursing Diagnosis
Odette Bolano	1981	The Nurse's Knowledge of Nosocomial Infections Secondary to Intravenous Therapy
Barbara Hair	1983	Evaluation of the Efficacy of a Fifteen-Second Scrub with Ten Percent Povidone-Iodine in Reducing Skin Bacteria
Patricia Newcomb	1983	Paternal Experience During Hospitalization of High Risk Neonates
Debra Glidewell	1984	The Perceived and Operationalized Nursing Roles of Associate Degree and Baccalaureate Degree Nursing Graduates

Source: *Harris College of Nursing Self-Study Report 1984.*

The Abell-Hanger Professorship of Gerontological Nursing

The Abell-Hanger Professorship of Gerontological Nursing was established in 1986 by the family foundation of the late Gladys Hanger Abell, a Midland civic leader, and her husband, George T. Abell, an independent oil operator. During the illness that preceded her husband's death in 1979, Mrs. Abell worked side-by-side with the nurses who cared for him, becoming acutely aware of the importance of their expertise and empathy. Her observations motivated her to provide funding for a professorship at TCU's Harris College of Nursing.

Dr. Mildred Hogstel, who was the initial Abell-Hanger Professor of Gerontological Nursing, held the position from 1988 to 1994.

The Abell-Hanger Endowed Professorship

In 1988 the Abell-Hanger Professorship in Gerontological Nursing was created to promote the healthy aging of older adults by educating students, faculty, community professionals, and the public about aging-related issues.

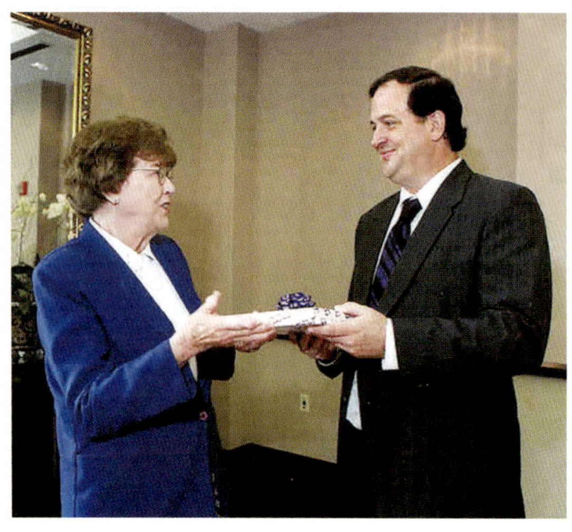

Dr. Mildred Hogstel celebrates the appointment of Dr. Dennis Cheek to the Abell-Hanger Professorship.

The first recipient was Dr. Mildred Hogstel, who held the position until her retirement in 1994. The endowed professorship was later awarded to Dr. Dennis Cheek (2004), who teaches pharmacology and pathophysiology.

Cheek's research has focused on the health of postmenopausal women, specifically, investigating hormones that might influence heart disease development and/or progression. Cheek has also collaborated with faculty members in the Department of Kinesiology on various research activities.

ALUMNI EXAMPLES OF CHANGING ROLES

Defining the Role of the Nurse as Interprofessional:

An Interview with Diane Hawley, BSN 1981

Dr. Diane Hawley, a 1981 graduate from the Harris College of Nursing and a current faculty member, came to TCU with the intention of majoring in music performance. While in high school, she played both the clarinet and oboe and wanted to set the world on fire with her brilliant performances.

She "found her way" into the nursing profession via her mother, who had enrolled her in a co-op program while she was still in high school because Hawley was getting bored and thus finding trouble. During that program, she was assigned to a hospital catheterization lab where she enjoyed the camaraderie of various health care professionals and interacting with

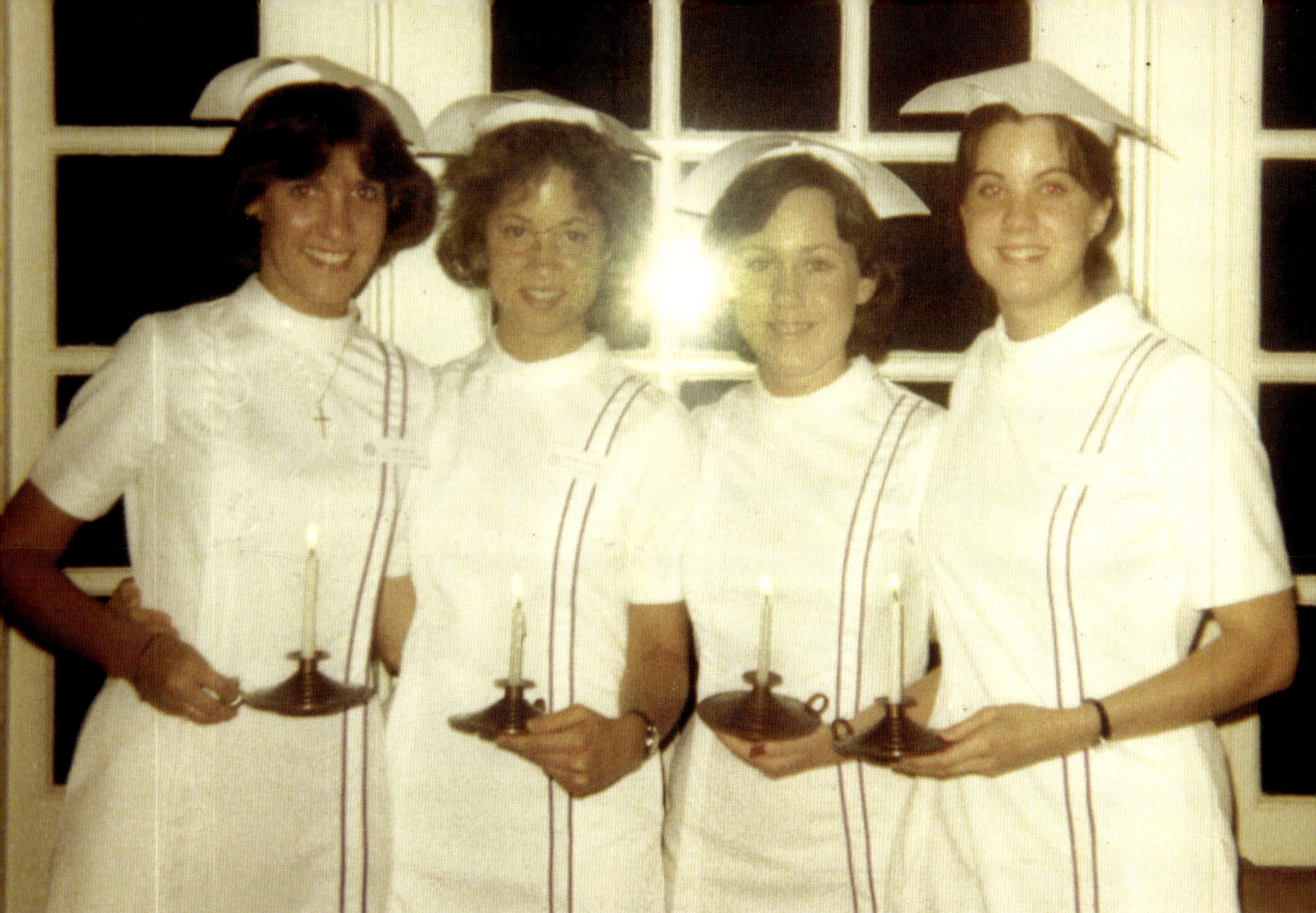

Capping Ceremony. L-R, Diane Hawley, Helen Stearns Huffingham, Kim Ellis Jagoda, and Amy McCurdy McCarty, 1980.

patients as she performed tasks such as running exercise stress treadmill studies for them. Think about that—a seventeen-year-old young woman conducting a potentially very dangerous procedure on individuals who were suspected to have heart disease. She recalls saying that a twelve-lead ECG had "doohickeys."

True to her original intent, Hawley wrote "music performance" for her major on the enrollment forms during orientation at TCU. Her mother grabbed the paper, crossed "music performance" out, and wrote "nursing." Hawley attributes the fact that she is a nurse today to her mother changing her major at orientation. Hawley also went on to say that there was no one better to help guide her path into a career as a nurse than her mother, and she is nothing but grateful for the "nudging." By the time she graduated from the Harris College of Nursing, Hawley knew she wanted to work in critical care because of an elective she took under the guidance of Dr. Alice

Gaul. Following graduation Hawley worked in Dallas at Methodist Hospital for a short time and then at Harris Hospital in Fort Worth, where she says she "grew up" as a cardiac critical-care nurse in the open-heart surgery ICU.

It was during her time as a critical-care nurse that Hawley became aware that nurses "were not educated to be team players" (Hawley, personal communication, 2017). Hawley noted that nurses wrote care plans indicating what they would do for the patient without clearly understanding that much of each plan depended on the assistance of others. This notion haunted her for several years before she decided to do something about it.

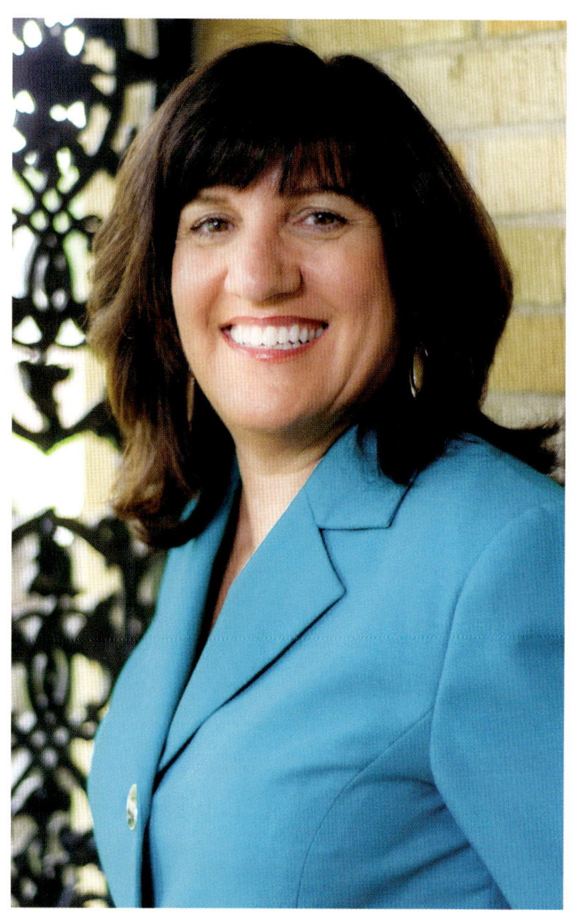

Diane Hawley, faculty member, 2016.

Hawley joined the TCU nursing faculty in 1998, and every semester she has taught code management in a simulated setting to undergraduate nursing students. Hawley regularly impersonated a physician to demonstrate to students the role and responsibilities of a doctor. When she tired of pretending to be a physician, she considering enrolling at the medical school right down the street. In the fall of 2012, Hawley contacted the director of Simulation at the University of North Texas Health Science Center (UNTHSC). The pair explored working together so that the medical, pharmacy, and nursing students could learn from and with each other about how to manage a patient who needed cardiopulmonary resuscitation in a simulated environment. To date, code simulation is an interprofessional learning activity that all health care professional students benefit from.

At this same time, UNTHSC was working on developing an overarching curriculum that focused on incorporating interprofessional education competencies into all programs within the health science center, and Hawley was invited to the discussions. A program initiated by the Division of Gerontology at UNTHSC was another factor in bringing interprofessional education to the forefront of TCU's nursing curriculum. UNTHSC wanted nursing students to participate in the Seniors Assisting in Geriatric Education (SAGE) program. SAGE was implemented to prepare health care professional students to better serve older adults. SAGE partners health care profession students from UNTHSC (physician, physician assistant, physical therapy, pharmacy) and TCU (nursing, social work, and nutrition) with senior citizens who receive home-delivered meals from Meals on Wheels of Tarrant County or who volunteer in the local community. Students make home visits over three semesters as part of an interprofessional team where they apply their classroom education in the care of an older adult. Hawley was instrumental in bringing TCU nursing students to this program, and she coordinates their participation in it. They are members of one of approximately 350 teams composed of 1,300 health care personnel. Over 350 older clients receive care while students gain knowledge about the needs of seniors. Hawley is currently in the midst of a study analyzing whether students have acquired enhanced knowledge, skills, and abilities in working with an interprofessional team and if this work has changed their perceptions of working with older individuals.

In January of 2015, the Geriatric Division at UNTHSC contacted the Harris College of Nursing's dean, Susan Weeks, to solicit a faculty lead in nursing who would be interested in working with the Health Resources and Services Administration (HRSA) on a grant proposal entitled the Geriatric Workforce Enhancement Program (GWEP). Hawley volunteered to participate in the innovations envisioned for this grant, and in July of 2015, UNTHSC, TCU, JPS, and the Area Agency on Aging received notice that they had received the $2.55 million GWEP grant. Hawley has transitioned from critical care to geriatric care based on an increasing need, and under the grant her role is to help improve geriatric primary care with an interdisciplinary workforce.

As a leader, researcher, and author, Hawley's role in interprofessional care today may be quite different from that of nurses when Dean Harris saw the need to clarify their role.

Defining the Role of the Nurse as a Founder of a Specialty:

An Interview with Virginia Lynch, BSN 1982—Founder of Forensic Nursing

Virginia A. Lynch is the preeminent scholar and founder of forensic nursing as a scientific discipline. She received her bachelor of science degree in nursing in 1982 from TCU, where she was introduced to the forensic sciences through a clinical assignment. This project took her into the world of interpersonal crime and the scientific investigation of death. Her first experience in a crime laboratory refocused her professional interest, inspiring her to learn more about the forensic sciences and their application to nursing practice. She learned that many interpersonal crimes are never properly adjudicated, often because evidence was inadvertently discarded or improperly preserved and secured after collection by health care personnel.

Following graduation from TCU, she pursued her master's degree with a focus on forensic nursing, a program she was instrumental in designing at the University of Texas at Arlington (UTA) College of Nursing. During her studies she was credentialed as a sexual assault forensic examiner.

Lynch recognized the need for nurses to be enlightened about the precise preservation and relevance of forensic evidence. She was motivated to establish a rape crisis program in a rural Texas county and to pursue practice changes that led to a new nursing specialty aimed at improving health and legal outcomes for victims of violence.

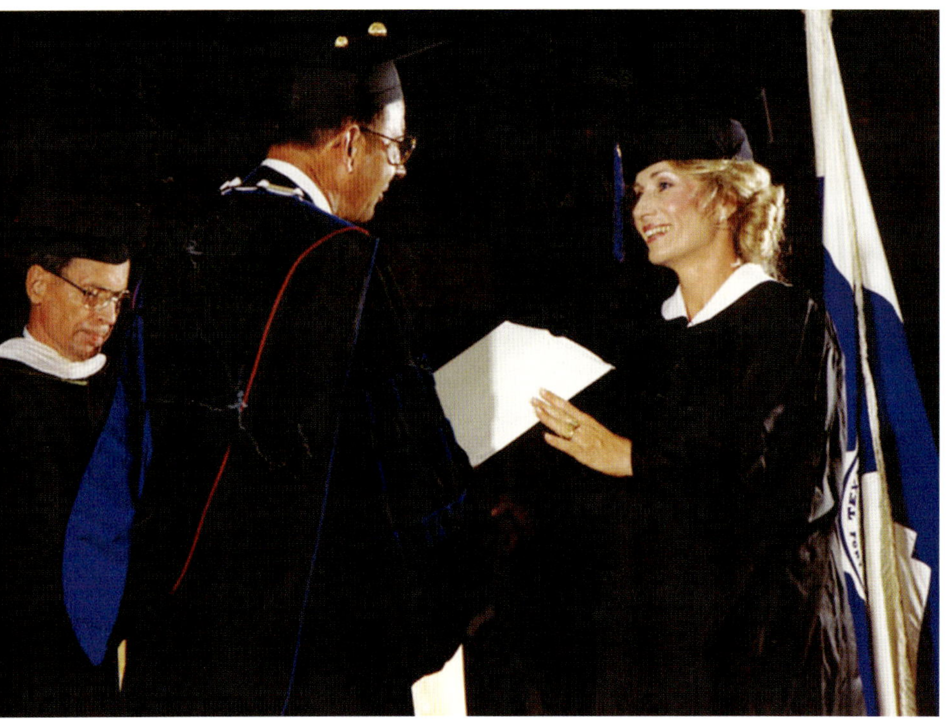

Virginia Lynch at graduation, 1982.

In 1984 Lynch served as a medical death investigator for the Tarrant County Medical Examiner's District in Fort Worth, Texas, and subsequently became a certified coroner in the state of Georgia in 1992, further promoting death investigation as a forensic nursing role. This experience broadened her perspectives about potential contributions of nurses in innovative forensic roles and led her to advocate for the role of the forensic nurse death investigator. In 1993 she accepted a faculty position at the University of Colorado, Colorado Springs, and developed the first course in human rights for forensic nurses. In 2000 she launched a global outreach program in forensic nursing science, involving teaching, consulting, and social advocacy. Lynch was elected to the American Academy of Forensic Sciences (1986), which asked her to define the discipline of forensic nursing. She was honored as a Distinguished Fellow in 2018.

As founding president (1993–1996) of the International Association of Forensic Nurses (IAFN), she was honored by the establishment of the Virginia A. Lynch Pioneer Award, which the IAFN presents annually to a member who has significantly contributed to the advancement of the forensic nursing specialty. Today, the association has 3,700 members representing twenty-four countries. Using Lynch's model and specialty descriptions, the American Nurses Association recognized forensic

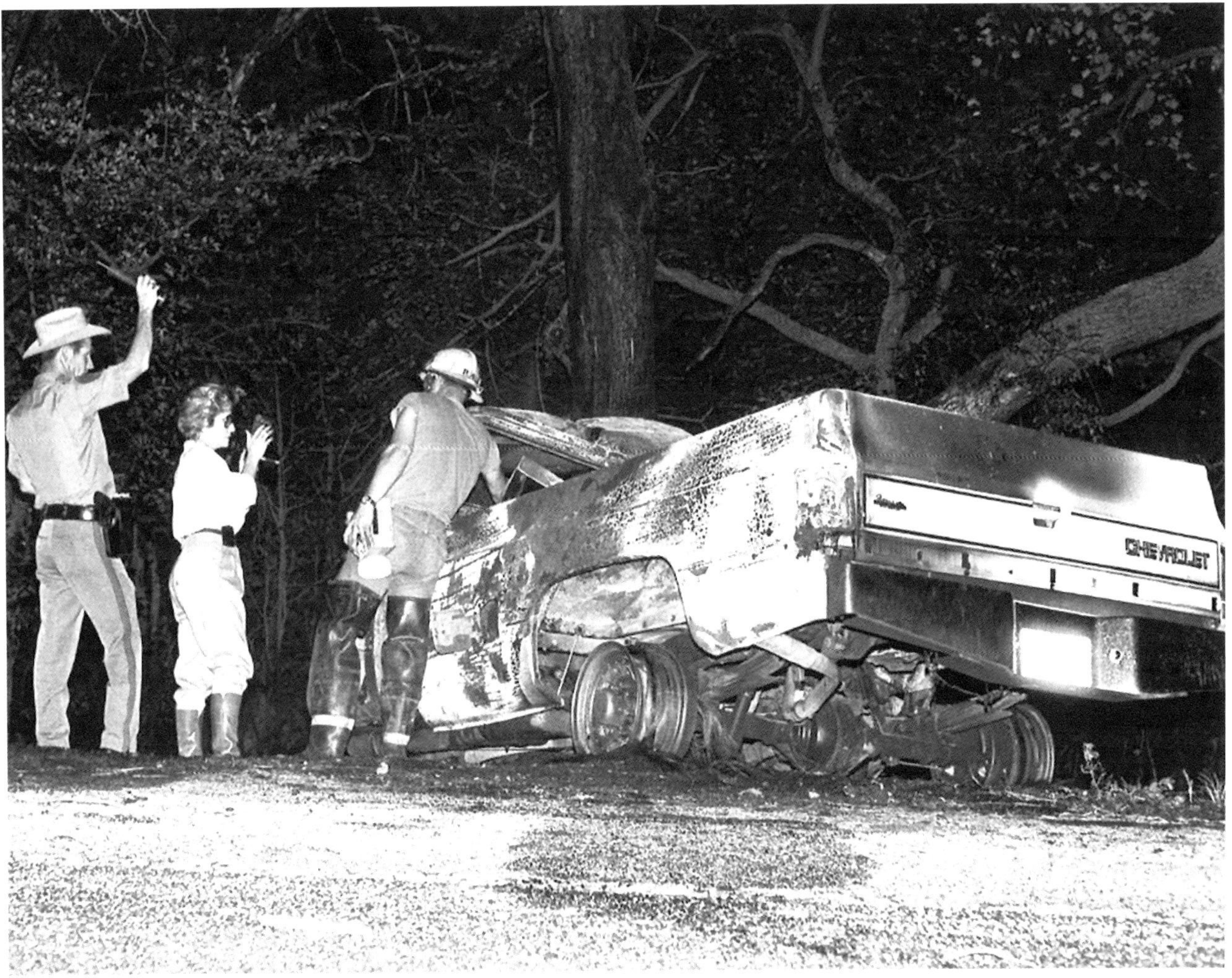

Virginia Lynch at crime scene, 1986.

nursing as a distinct nursing specialty in 1995, paving the way for advanced practice education and credentialing. Her advocacy role with military physicians and nurses was a significant catalyst for new legislation requiring aggressive programming within the Department of Defense to prevent and manage sexual violence.

A member of the American Academy of Nursing, Lynch's expertise is sought globally, taking her to more than thirty countries as a visiting professor and independent consultant. She has participated in numerous global consortiums and conferences, and has received a Fulbright Fellowship in global health at Punjabi University in India. A frequent lecturer and a prolific writer, she wrote the seminal text *Forensic Nursing Science* published by Elsevier in 2006, which was recognized as the "most significant scholarly/professional contribution to nursing and allied health" by the

American Association of Publishers (American Association of Publishers, Inc. 2006) and coauthored the second edition, which was published in 2010.

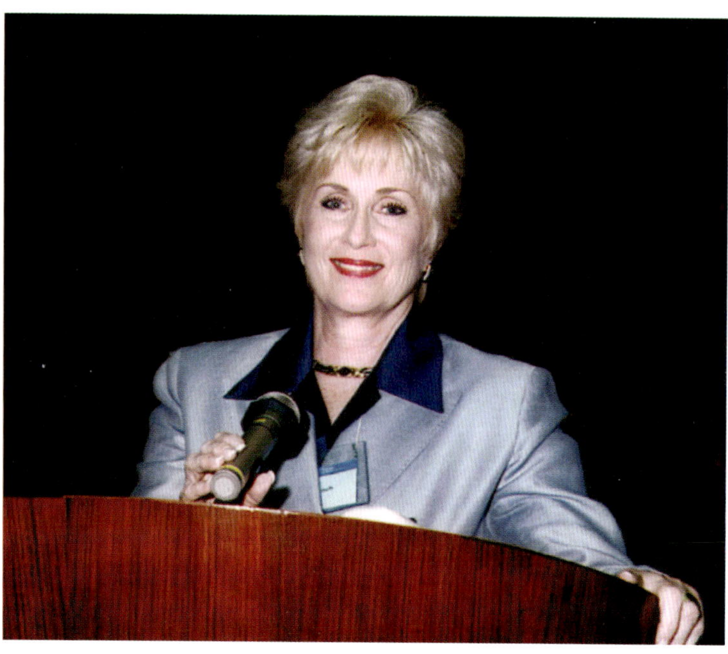

Virginia Lynch, 2018.

When asked about her greatest challenge in the advancement of forensic nursing, she noted the lack of educational opportunities for specializations in both graduate and undergraduate nursing curricula. Additionally, she stated that health care organizations and community agencies had not fully appreciated the potential value of forensic nursing to client services, resulting in insufficient funding for forensic support services and related staff positions. She believes that strong legislative mandates, health care regulation, and advocacy are needed to foster further growth and development of forensic nursing. The demand for the services of nurses with forensic expertise is great as we confront clinical issues related to global violence (Lynch, personal communication, 2018).

Defining the Role of the Nurse as an Oncology Clinical Nurse Specialist:

An Interview with MiKaela Olsen, BSN 1989

MiKaela Olsen was introduced to the profession of nursing by her cousin, who had earned a bachelor of science in nursing (BSN) from Creighton University in Omaha, Nebraska, and who died suddenly of a brain aneurysm at the age of forty-two. Olsen now practices every day in her honor. It was Olsen's mother, however, who thought she had a "natural instinct" to care for the sick, as Olsen also participated in her grandfather's care when he was dying of prostate cancer.

After talking to a counselor in high school, Olsen enrolled in the Army ROTC and pursued her nursing education at Harris College of Nursing (HCN). She credits the "excellent clinical instructors" at HCN with providing a strong foundation and notes that her rotation in pediatric oncology at Cook Children's Hospital was a major influence in her clinical career focus. She also cites the discipline, respect, hard work, and opportunities provided by the ROTC at TCU as major influences in her career. Between her junior and senior year, Olsen received training through the ROTC at Brooke Army Medical Center, where she worked in the emergency room. After graduating with her BSN from TCU and being commissioned a second lieutenant in the US Army, Olsen arrived at her first duty assignment in Ft. Lewis, Washington. At Madigan Army Hospital, Olsen worked on a busy oncology unit. It was there that she was introduced to a clinical nurse specialist (CNS) who "loved teaching" and became her mentor. To further prepare for her career, Olsen obtained a dual master's degree as a nurse practitioner and clinical nurse specialist from the University of California, San Francisco.

Olsen currently practices as a hematology and oncology CNS at the Sidney Kimmel Comprehensive Cancer Center at the Johns Hopkins Hospital (JHH) in Baltimore, Maryland. In this role, she functions in multiple capacities inherent in CNS responsibilities: (1) educator, (2) consultant, (3) clinician, and (4) expert in evidence-based practice. Olsen is in charge of clinical operations for ambulatory oncology services with additional responsibilities across the JHH health system. Olsen serves as

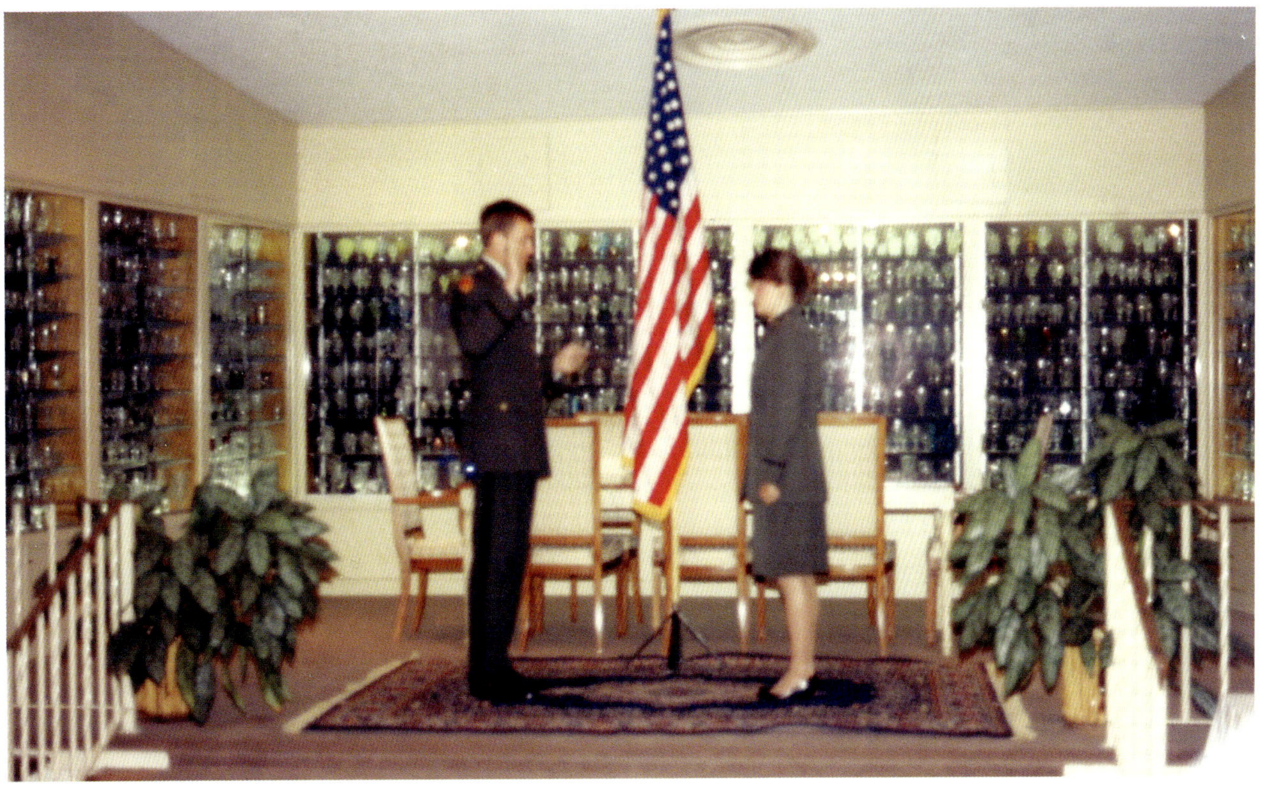

MiKaela Olsen, commissioned at TCU, 1989.

adjunct faculty for the Johns Hopkins School of Nursing and is a faculty associate at the University of Maryland School of Nursing. She is the manager of the peripherally inserted central line catheter (PICC) team for the department of oncology, the chair of the Johns Hopkins Hospital Venous Access Device Committee, and the chair of the Central Line-Associated Bloodstream Infection (CLABSI) Reduction Subcommittee. Olsen is coeditor of the *ONS Safe Handling of Hazardous Drugs Guidelines* (2018) and coeditor for the *Chemotherapy and Biotherapy Guidelines and Recommendations for Practice* (2014). She is the lead editor for the first edition of *Chemotherapy and Immunotherapy Guidelines and Recommendations for Practice,* published in 2018 by the Oncology Nursing Society. She served on the American Society of Clinical Oncology and ONS Chemotherapy Safety Standards Workgroup in 2016. She is the lead editor of the book *Hematologic Malignancies in Adults,* the first nursing textbook published to guide nurses in the care of hematologic malignancy patients. In addition to these books, Olsen has published and extensively presented on the topic of ventricular assist device evidence-based practice and CLABSI reduction and safe handling of hazardous drugs.

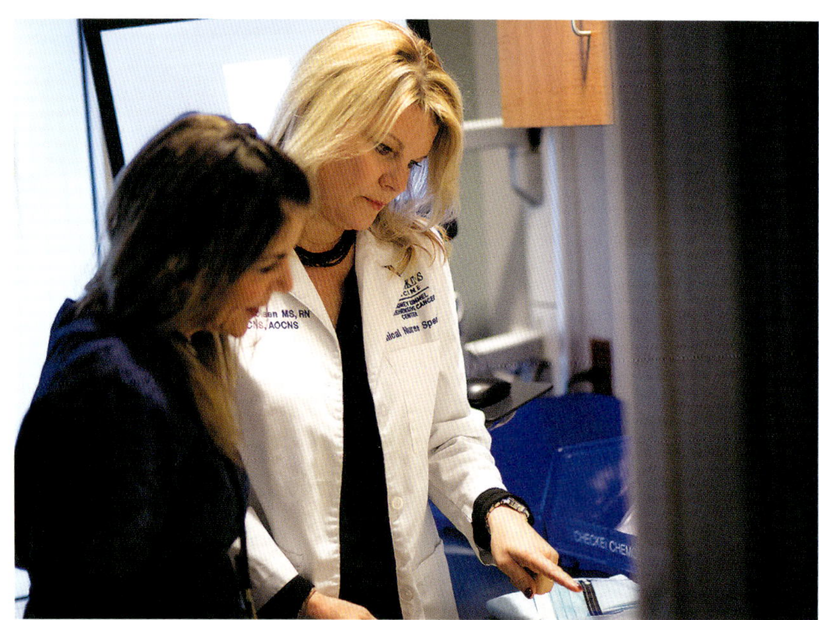

MiKaela Olsen with student.

When asked about the greatest challenges to her work, she quickly responded that the most challenging was convincing people to adopt evidence-based practice. She sees her job as critical to synthesizing evidence and acting as a change agent to implement evidence into practice to improve patient outcomes. Other challenges are the implementation and evaluation of interprofessional activities and policy development. Olsen said the major rewards were "seeing the outcome of the work undertaken and seeing positive patient outcomes" (Olsen, pers. comm., 2018). She also values being able to mentor new graduates.

Olsen completed her doctor of nursing practice (DNP) at the University of Maryland in 2016.

CHALLENGE TWO

Research to Determine What Effects Variables in Nursing Care Have on the Health of People

Context and Trends

In 1983 a report published by the Institute of Medicine (IOM) called for a federal nursing research entity in the mainstream of science. The following year, a task force appointed by the National Institutes of Health (NIH) Director found that "nursing research activities within NIH were relevant to the NIH mission" (National Institute of Nursing Research 2016). The Health Research Extension Act of 1985 (Public Law 99-158) created the National Center for Nursing Research (NCNR) at the NIH. Dr. Ada Sue Hinshaw was appointed as the first director of the NCNR.

The development of Sigma Theta Tau International's (STTI) Ten-Year Plan in the 1980s established a vision and focus for professional development nationally and internationally. Further commitment to scholarship was evidenced by the organization's dedication to "practic[ing] and teaching the science of nursing with three themes: knowledge development, dissemination, and utilization" (Sigma Theta Tau International 2016). In 1987 STTI collaborated with the American Nurses Foundation to provide funds for an annual research grant for beginning or experienced nurse researchers who entered a new field of study (Thompson, pers. comm., 2018). In 1989 STTI introduced the Center for Nursing Scholarship, which was part of the ten-year plan.

Research methods have also changed over time. Traditionally, quantitative research had been used to measure the outcomes and effectiveness of nursing interventions, and this continued in the 1980s (Hunt 2015, 23). Grove, Gray, and Burns in *Understanding Nursing Research: Building an Evidence-Based Practice* (2014) reported that while nurse researchers continued to use this method, there was a movement toward using qualitative methods.

Systematic reviews of research studies, the "clinical expert opinion, and inclusion of patient values" have been identified as the "three main tenets of evidence-based practice" (Hunt 2015, 121). Interprofessional research teams have used systematic reviews to determine if the evidence is sufficient to develop a protocol or if additional research is needed (121). While the evidence-based practice movement was traced to the Royal College of Nursing as early as the 1960s, it became increasingly recognized over time (121).

Harris College of Nursing

The Harris College of Nursing faculty reaffirmed the goal of the university to "expect and encourage . . . fruitful creativity and research" (*TCU Faculty and Staff Handbook*

1983–84, 3) and specified additional goals within the college: (1) "foster research activities and quality scholarship among students and peers" and (2) "initiate and participate in educational and clinical nursing research" (*Harris College of Nursing Self-Study Report 1984,* 55–56).

Students were introduced to research, a strand in the curriculum, at the beginning of their program. Early focus was on how nursing research can be applied to patient care; in later courses students had the opportunity to critique published research studies and discuss how they could affect nursing practice. Honors courses required students to identify areas of interest in nursing, analyze and synthesize findings of nursing investigations, and present their work orally to nursing faculty, students, and invited guests.

To assist faculty members in developing their research programs, individual faculty members participated in peer review of research proposals and manuscripts to be submitted for publication (*Harris College of Nursing Self-Study Report 1984,* 23). By 1984, 23 percent of all faculty members were engaged in research activities (129).

ALUMNI EXAMPLES OF RESEARCH

Conducting Research to Determine What Variables in Nursing Care Can Have on the Health of People:

An Interview with Ainslie Taylor Nibert, BSN 1980

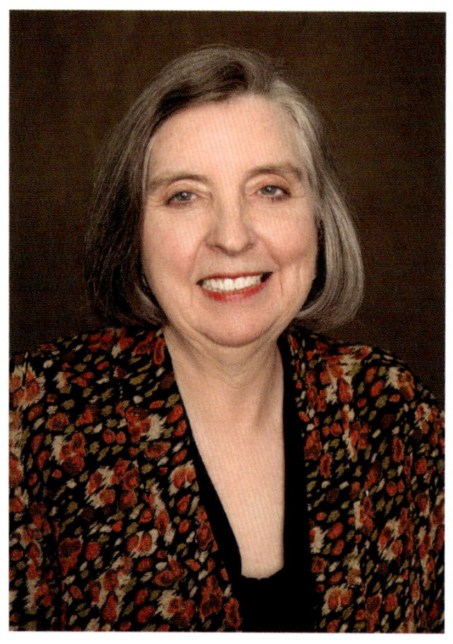

Ainslie Taylor Nibert.

Ainslie Taylor Nibert, a 1980 graduate, currently the associate dean at Texas Woman's University in Houston and an independent health care consultant, had a desire to be a nurse from a very early age.

In a recent interview (November 30, 2017), she talked about her interest in sciences while in high school and as a teenage volunteer at a hospital in Dallas, Texas, where she also noted the caring aspect of nursing. The merging of technology, science, caring, and experiences in critical care influenced her to begin her career as a critical-care nurse. Within a short period, she was identified as a preceptor, and in less than three years she became a unit teacher and head nurse. It was the teaching role that captured her interest and led her to graduate school and a subsequent career in academia.

The pivotal point of Nibert's distinguished career came when she joined Health Education Systems Incorporated

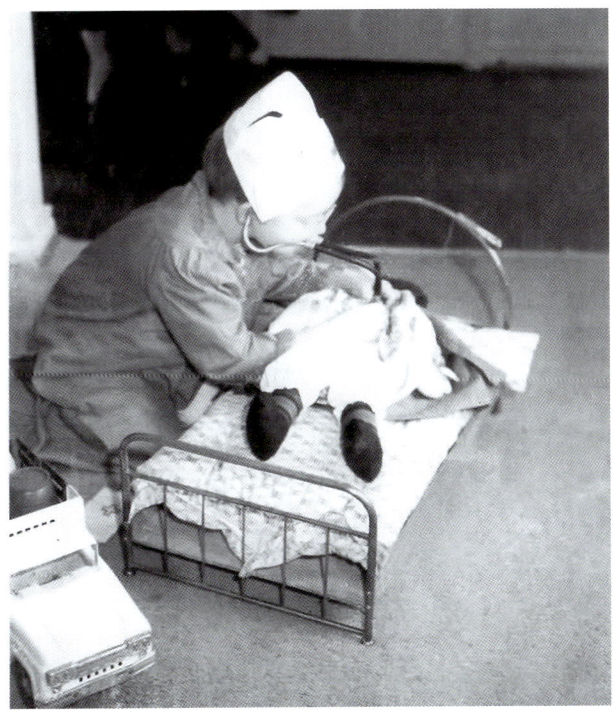

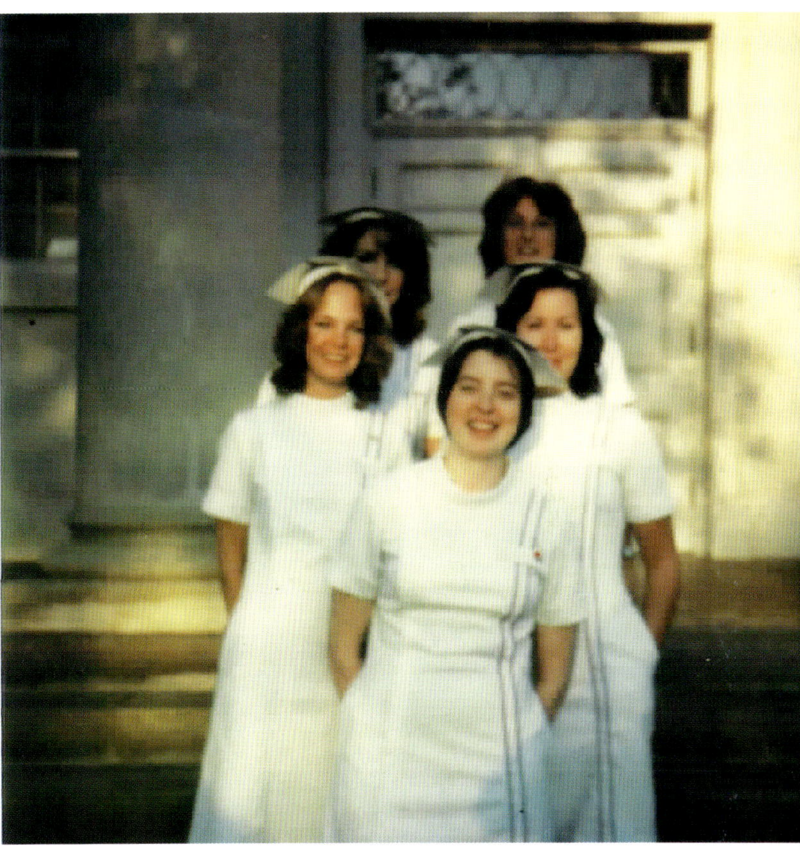

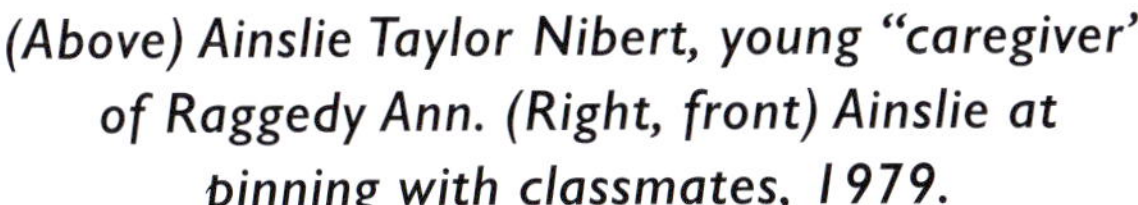

(Above) Ainslie Taylor Nibert, young "caregiver" of Raggedy Ann. (Right, front) Ainslie at pinning with classmates, 1979.

(HESI) as the director of research. There she established the practice of identifying scientifically based research as the foundation for all of the practice and standardized testing products they developed. The creation of psychometrically sound, statistically reliable and valid exams opened the door to evidence-based curricular evaluation and a data-driven approach to assessing total program outcomes. This educational research was used to prepare standardized exams leading to qualified candidates' entry into clinical practice.

During the 1980s Harris College of Nursing responded to national nursing and nursing educational trends through changes in the core curriculum, curricular changes in honors courses, and the addition of electives in which students could increase their knowledge in selected areas. Computer terminals in the skills lab prepared both faculty and students for changes in the emerging technology within the health care system. An increasing number of faculty members returned for advanced degrees that prepared them to conduct and disseminate research for the purpose of positively influencing nursing care and patient outcomes. Graduates, with an increasing diversity in ethnic groups, age, and gender, totaled 840.

Chapter Four

The Nineties

A Decade of Growth

Three deans—Patricia Scearse, Kathy Bond, and Rhonda Keen-Payne—guided faculty members and students through another decade of structural and curricular changes. These changes were needed to move the college forward during a decade increasingly complex with changes in cultural diversity, information technologies, health care systems, and population demographics (Keen 1995, 3). Scearse continued serving as dean until 1995, Bond from 1996 to 1999, and Keen-Payne beginning in 1999.

Harris College of Nursing

According to the 1992 *Harris College of Nursing Self-Study Report to the National League for Nursing,* the specific mission of the Harris College of Nursing (HCN) was "to prepare professional nurses to identify and respond with competence to multiple, complex human health care needs" (Harris College of Nursing Archives). Goals of the HCN were to "(1) prepare graduates who are competent to meet the unique, multiple, and complex human health needs of a global society; (2) promote values and behaviors that encourage respect for diversity, acknowledge human worth and dignity, and support professional nursing practice; and (3) foster an appreciation for the necessity of learning, thinking critically, and continuing to grow personally and professionally." An HCN self-study report from 2000 to the Commission on Collegiate Nursing Education shows that later in the decade, a fourth goal was added: "to contribute to the nursing profession and to society by engaging in scholarship, leadership, and service" (Harris College of Nursing Archives).

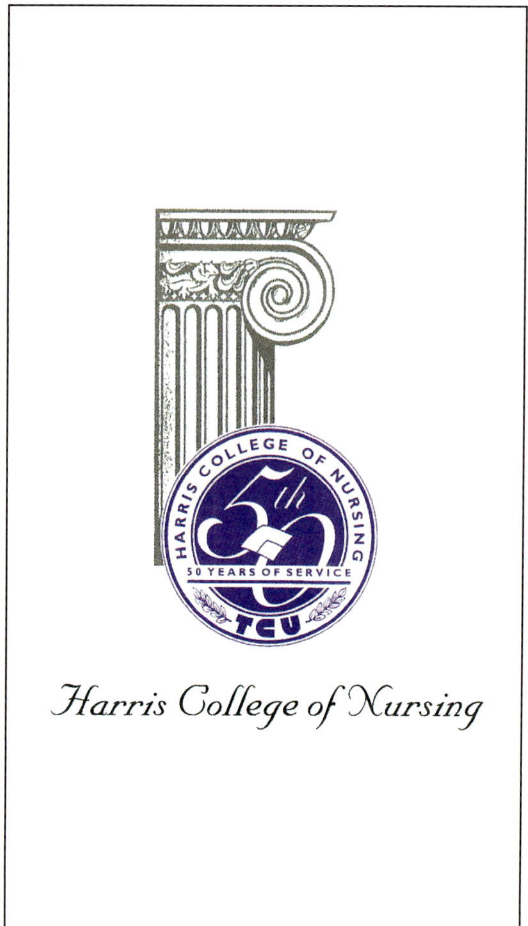

Harris College of Nursing
cordially invites you to celebrate
Fifty Years
of Baccalaureate Nursing Education
at a Gala Dinner
on Friday, April 26, 1996
Grand Ballroom
The Worthington Hotel
Fort Worth, Texas.

Featured speaker
Dr. Patricia Moccia
Chief Executive Officer
National League for Nursing

Presentation of the first
Outstanding Alumnus Award

6:45 p.m. Cash reception
7:30 p.m. Dinner

Complimentary self parking
hotel garage, 200 Main Street

Invitation to the Fiftieth Anniversary Gala.

Fifty Years of TCU Nursing

In 1996, Harris College celebrated fifty years of TCU Nursing. The event offered alumni, faculty, and staff an opportunity to reconnect, participate in a workshop on genetics and in simulation demonstrations, and tour the Annie Richardson Bass Building and campus before the gala celebration in the evening.

Charlotte Pierce, a 1963 graduate, was the mistress of ceremonies for the gala at the Worthington Hotel and announced the first outstanding alumni award given to Jane Hudak, a graduate of the class of 1970. Fort Worth Mayor Bob Bolen joined the guests for the gala and congratulated HCN for its accomplishments and contributions to Fort Worth.

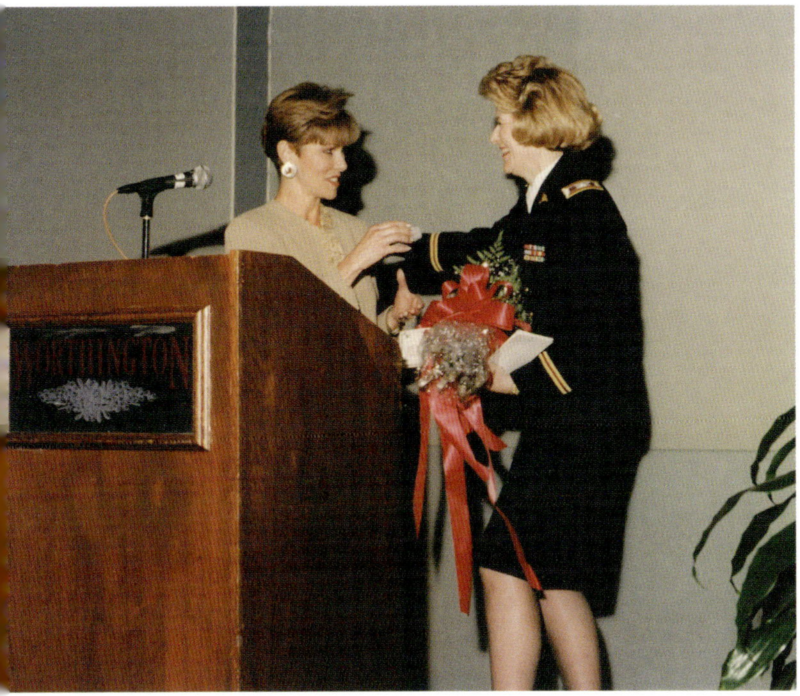

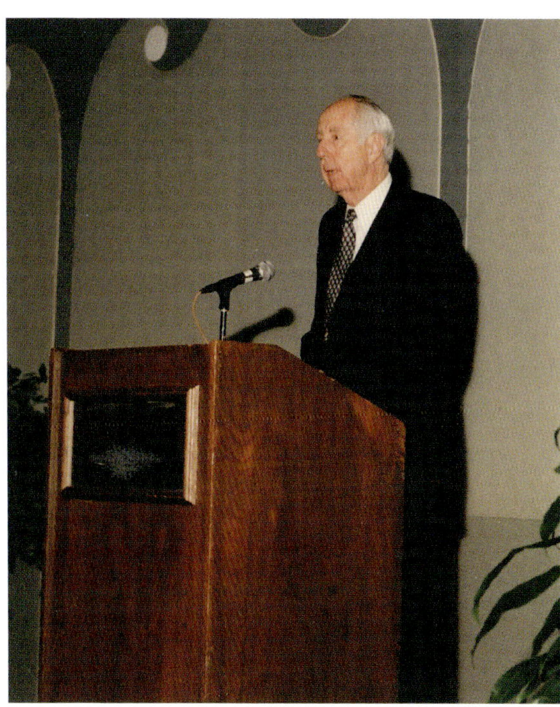

(Left) HCN Alumna President Connie Koehler presenting the Outstanding Alumna Award to Jane Hudak. (Right) Fort Worth Mayor Bob Bolen at the gala, 1996.

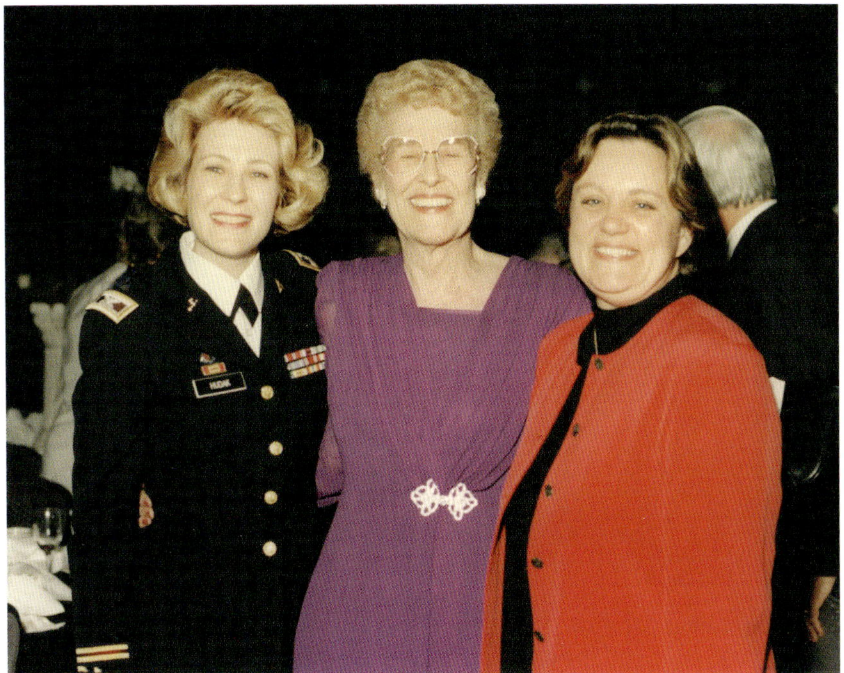

L-R, Jane Hudak, Virginia Jarratt, and Pat Moccia, 1996.

The featured speaker for the evening was Patricia Moccia, chief executive vice president of the National League for Nursing. Moccia, the Green Honors professor for the Harris College, had spoken to the faculty and students the previous day on health care issues in nursing education and practice.

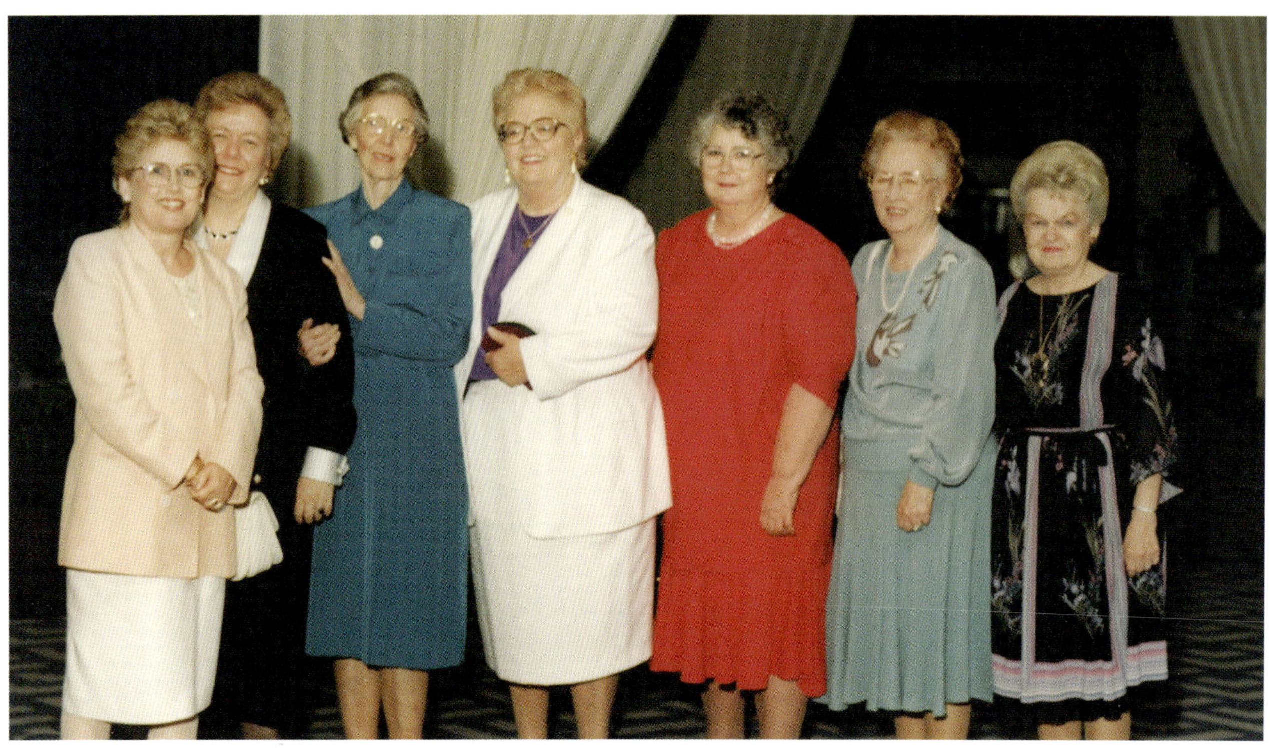

L-R, Betty Shockey, Pat Thompson, Monette Graves, Billie Hightower, Peggy Mayfield, Nell Robinson (Chair of Department of Nutrition), and TCU's Mrs. Klaus, 1996.

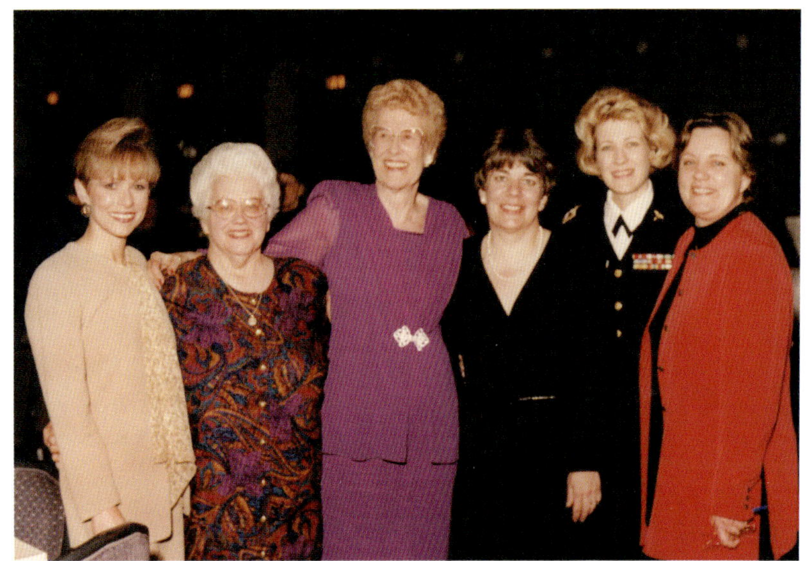

L-R, Connie Koehler, Pat Scearse, Virginia Jarratt, Rhonda Keen-Payne, Jane Hudak, and Pat Moccia, 1996.

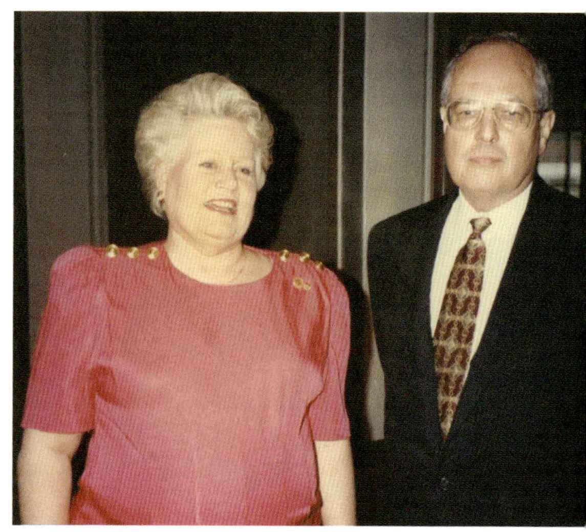

Monica Dewar ('75) and husband, 1996.

CHALLENGE ONE
A Clear Definition of Nursing Roles and Functions

Context and Trends

Incorporation of the total quality management (TQM) system into health care in the early 1990s paved the way for a decade focused on improving the quality of health care services and the value of the patient experience (Andreoli 1992a). In 1990, the Occupational Safety and Health Administration released standards mandating that employers promote and educate employees on the CDC's universal precaution measures to reduce infection transmission (*American Journal of Nursing* 1990). The Patient Self-Determination Act, also enacted in 1990, was instated to encourage patients to actively prepare for future health care decisions in an effort to increase patient involvement in care (Sabatino 2010). Another landmark piece of legislation incorporated into nursing practice in the 1990s was the Health Insurance Portability and Accountability Act (HIPAA). Enacted in 1996, this legislation improved patient confidence in the confidentiality of their data (Bowers 2001).

Implementation of quality improvement measures, however, placed further strain on a nursing population already plagued by a nationwide shortage. To combat this shortage, work by Magnet-recognized hospitals and professional organizations such as the American Nurses Association established and expanded nurse residency programs to attract and retain nurse graduates at health care institutions (American Association of Colleges of Nursing 2002). Developing and perfecting a procedure to delegate care to ancillary personnel, a skill that remains vital in practice even today, was another means of addressing the nursing shortage (Andreoli 1992a). Nurses had to learn how to take care of the ever-increasing number of patients with HIV/AIDS. Although many wanted to refuse to care for these patients, due to fear of infection transmission and the stigma associated with the disease, the situation provided an important reminder that a nurse's responsibility is to provide equal, quality care for all patients, no matter the patients' backgrounds (Downes 1991).

Harris College of Nursing

Early in the 1990s, Dean Scearse noted that the college's organizational structure had changed many times as a result of faculty evaluations regarding efficiency and effectiveness. To efficiently carry out the work of the college, some committees were eliminated and others were combined. For example, in 1991, the bylaws, faculty relations, library, and research committees merged to become the faculty relations committee, and the student relations, honors, social affairs, and recruitment committees merged to become the student relations committee, as HCN reported to the National League for Nursing (Harris College of Nursing Archives). Students had the opportunity to provide input through their participation on the curriculum committee.

In the spring of 1998, Bond introduced the first issue of *Vital Signs,* a semiannual newsletter designed to share the activities at HCN with alumni (Appendix 9).

Focus on Faculty

Faculty recruitment during the decade focused on bringing together a cadre of scholars who were prepared for changes in the curriculum, able to meet promotion and tenure criteria, and clinically skilled and competent to serve as professional role models for nursing students (Scearse 1994, 1). Early in the decade, HCN hired several new faculty members with doctoral preparation in community health nursing and one with doctoral preparation in gerontological nursing. HCN had strong contingents of faculty with expertise in maternal child care and in ethical and cultural aspects of nursing. Some faculty members pursued advanced practice preparation while others were enrolled in continuing education programs on interactive teaching methods and critical thinking. The Lucy Harris Linn Award for Excellence in Teaching was first awarded in 1993.

Faculty members also devoted time to community activities such as health care screenings for a variety of community organizations. Several faculty members served on health-related advisory boards while others served as officers in regional or national nursing organizations. Still others served as legal or clinical consultants to various health care agencies (Scearse 1994, 2). Community agencies receiving faculty assistance included the Juvenile Diabetes Research Foundation, People Helping People, and the Texas Department of State Health Services, according to the *Harris College of Nursing Annual Report* 1996–97 (Harris College of Nursing Archives).

TABLE 3 Lucy Harris Linn Award for Excellence in Teaching

YEAR	NAME
1993	Dr. Mildred Hogstel
1994	Dr. Barbara Johnson
1995	Susan Schulwitz, RN, MS, CNS
1997	Dr. Mary Lou Bond
1998	Dr. Carol Reynolds
2000	Mary C. Robinson, RN, MS

Harris College of Nursing was also well represented through its service to the community and to professional nursing organizations. For example, Marinda Allender served on the editorial board of *Nursing in Pediatrics,* a journal published from 1998 to 2003 by Cook Children's Medical Center of Fort Worth. Carolyn Spence Cagle served on the editorial board of *Advances in Nursing Dimensions.* Linda Curry was appointed as an archival consultant to Sigma Theta Tau International Honor Society of Nursing (STTI). Carol Stephenson was elected the third vice president for the Texas League for Nursing from 1999 to 2001. At the international level, Susan Wilson was a visiting professor at Maua Methodist Hospital School of Nursing in Maua, Kenya, in 1999 and 2000. During that time she visited Jerri Brock Savuto, a 1968 graduate who was serving as a missionary nurse and teaching nursing at Maua Methodist Hospital.

Mildred Hogstel, emeritus professor, was honored in 1997 as the recipient of the Spirituality and Aging Award given by the National Interfaith Coalition on Aging, a unit of the National Council on Aging. Hogstel was honored for helping create the Tarrant County Eldercare/Faith in Action Program, in which churches reach out to the elderly population. In this program she conducted seminars in seventy churches. A specialist in gerontological nursing, Hogstel also won three *American Journal of Nursing* Book of the Year Awards in 1984, 1989, and 1990 (Jones 1997).

Danna Strength collaborated with Hogstel, Curry, and Keen-Payne in developing several chapters in the *Practical Guide to Health Assessment through the Lifespan* in 1992. She also wrote two chapters in the *Manual of Gerontological Nursing* published in 1992. One of these chapters was translated into Italian for publication.

Harris College Students

Harris College of Nursing students in the mid-1990s included traditional students, ROTC scholarship students, transfer students, second degree students, RN students, and licensed vocational nurse students (Keen-Payne 1995). The minority population of the college student body in 1995 ranged between 15 and 19 percent. Annual enrollment was approximately 370 students. Students had diverse backgrounds and varying educational preparation. In the spring of 1999, an HCN student was the recipient of the Tucker Patriotism Award, the top award given by the Air Force ROTC Detachment 845 (Benefield 1999).

Stephanie Evans, president of the TCU chapter of the National Student Nurses' Association (NSNA) during the 1995-1996 academic year, always knew she wanted to be a nurse or a teacher. After reflecting on the choices, she decided that the best way for her to help others in need was to enter nursing school (Stephanie Evans, pers. comm., 2018).

Evans's involvement in the NSNA began when she was asked to participate as a

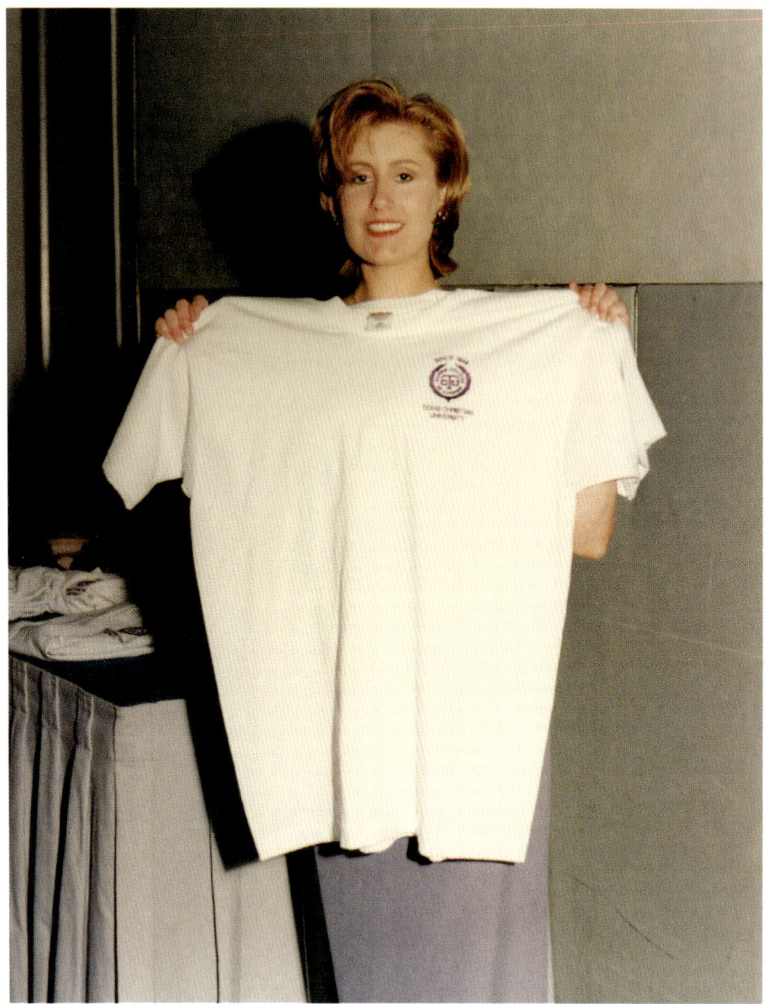

Stephanie Evans as a nursing student, 1996.

sophomore. Along with the officers, she planned events for students and participated in community service activities. She expressed the desire to "give back as much as possible to my community" (Stephanie Evans, pers. comm., 2018). Some of her favorite activities were health fairs in elementary schools, where NSNA members had booths to teach hand washing and dental hygiene. The Harris College NSNA members requested donations to provide items such as toothbrushes and toothpaste to elementary students participating in the health fairs (Stephanie Evans, pers. comm., 2018).

The outgoing president of NSNA asked Evans to run for the office, and Evans accepted the challenge. She found working with faculty and all levels of nursing students to be a rewarding experience. According to Evans, she "LOVED" being an HCN student. She gave the NSNA address at the senior brunch and "remembers including that one day she hoped to return to TCU as a faculty [member] . . . to share her wonderful experiences with other students" (Stephanie Evans, pers. comm., 2018). Her dream came true, and she is now a faculty member in HCN.

Focus on Curriculum

Guided as always by the mission and goals of the college, curriculum revision in the 1990s was further shaped by a commitment to the American Nurses Association Standards of Practice (1986), the Essentials of College and University Education for Professional Nursing developed by the American Association of Colleges of Nursing (1986), and the Essentials of College and University Education for Professional Nursing developed by the American Association of Colleges of Nursing (1986), and the Essential Competencies of Texas Graduates of Educational Programs in Nursing developed by the Board of Nurse Examiners for the State of Texas (1993). In 1998, HCN was granted preliminary accreditation approval by the Commission on Collegiate Nursing Education (CCNE). The program had enjoyed continuous accreditation of the baccalaureate nursing program from the National League for Nursing since 1952.

Goals as recorded in the TCU undergraduate catalog through the 1990s were:

1. To prepare graduates who are competent to meet the unique, complex, and constantly changing nursing needs of society;
2. To support the university's mission and goals;
3. To promote values and behaviors which encourage respect for diversity, acknowledge human worth and dignity, and support professional nursing practice;
4. To foster an appreciation for the necessity of learning and self-growth;
5. To contribute to the nursing profession and to society by engaging in scholarly and service activities.

—TCU 1993–1995, 239; 1995–1997, 252; 1998, 260; 1999, 270

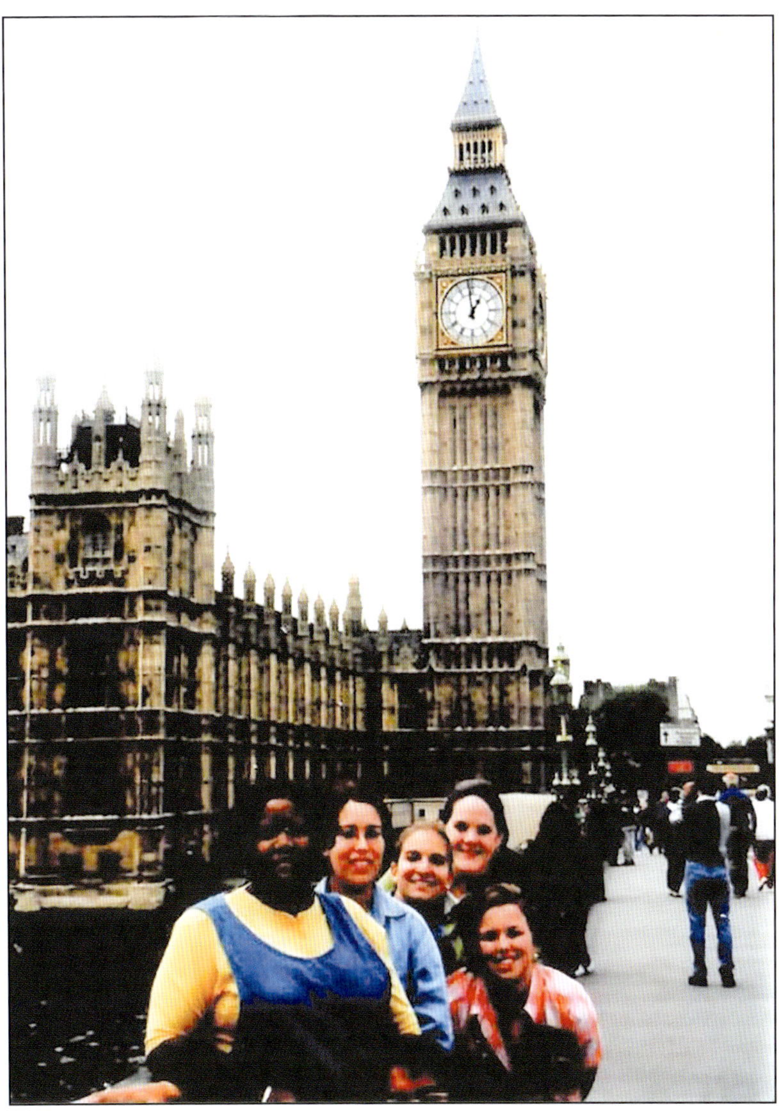

Students in London, 1997.

While retaining the clinical and theoretical components of many nursing courses, the curriculum additionally focused on meeting professional standards in health promotion, acute and chronic illness care, and gerontological nursing, as well as on incorporating concepts from different cultures and ethnicities into acute care in the community settings where students practiced. Nursing theory, nursing research, and statistics were also prioritized to prepare students for expanded roles (Appendix 10).

A study abroad course was offered in London in 1997. Zoranna Jones, who graduated in 1998, reported that she was recruited for the course by Rhonda Keen-Payne when she responded to a question about the history of nursing in a class lecture that focused on nursing history. After some discussion, Keen-Payne told her, "You are going to London!" Although Jones was intrigued by the thought of studying abroad, she wondered how she could do it. The idea was also scary. She persisted, however, and with a TCU scholarship, she found her way to Regent's University London.

Rhonda Keen-Payne gave lectures comparing the United States and English health care systems to the 1997 London group, pointing out that although citizens of England paid high taxes, the health coverage was good. Students learned about the care provided to new mothers and their babies well beyond their time in the hospital. Students also had guided tours to the Florence Nightingale Museum, the Royal College of Nursing, and the Old Operating Theatre Museum. Students later wrote essays and reflections about their experiences as part of the course requirements.

Jones's takeaways from the experience were that there are many ways to do things and that the US way is not the center of the world. While "not happy" during the first week when she found everything "old" and discovered the dorm's communal showers, Jones was "over the shock of everything being different" by the second week. At the end of the third week, she was "ready to stay," having found a passion for diversity and history. When not in class or on field trips, Jones reported spending time in Hyde Park, where she met a young man from Ghana with whom she enjoyed visiting—though she was surprised when he showed up at her dorm with flowers!

Building on the first London course, a second study abroad course was offered in London in 1998, taught by Keen-Payne and Susan Weeks and closely modeled after the course offered the previous year.

ALUMNI EXAMPLES OF CHANGING ROLES

Defining the Role of Associate Director —Brown-Lupton Health Center:

An Interview with Kelle Tillman, BSN 1992; CNS 2013; DNP 2019

Kelle Tillman's interest in nursing started when she read a *Fort Worth Star-Telegram* article in high school about neonatal intensive care units in hospitals. Fascinated by

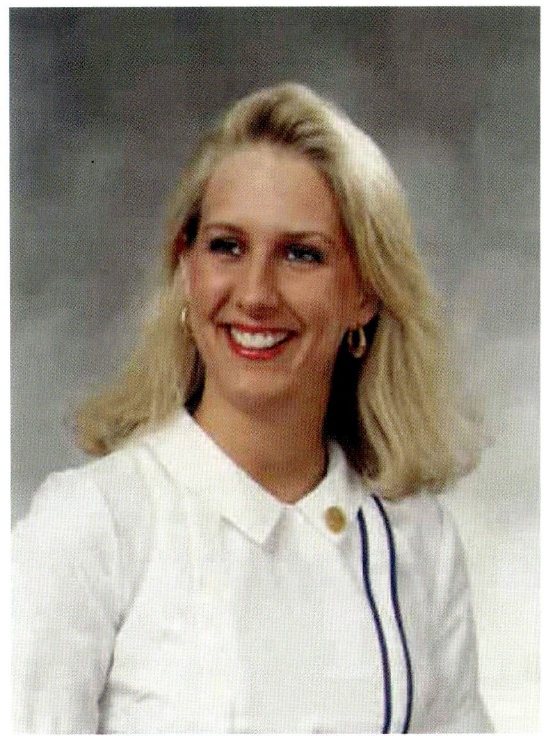

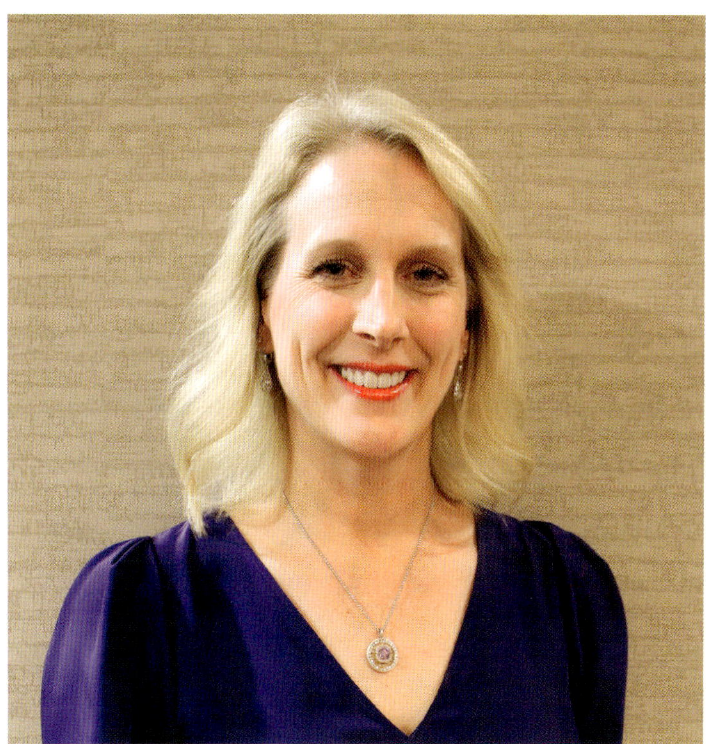

(Left) Kelle Tillman in 1992, BSN. (Right) Kelle in 2020.

the information, she decided to immerse herself in the health care system. Although she was an honors student, Tillman also describes herself as a "rebel," and she announced to her mother that she was going to enter the workplace instead of completing the senior honors courses. Subsequently, she worked with a cardiac surgeon while completing high school.

During her junior year as a nursing student at TCU, Tillman worked as a patient care technician and fell in love with Cook Children's Medical Center in Fort Worth. Upon graduation, she was immediately employed there in the intensive care unit, where she remained for eighteen years.

In 2007, Tillman had a serendipitous encounter at Costco with Marinda Allender, a Harris College faculty member who was Tillman's former instructor and mentor at Cook Children's Medical Center. As they talked, Allender mentioned the TCU Brown-Lupton Health Center was seeking another nurse and asked Tillman if she would consider a career change. The offer was especially appealing because Tillman's schedule at Cook's was rather challenging for a mother with three children at home. She applied and became a member of the health center's team.

During her tenure at the health center, Tillman has filled many roles, particularly the role of caregiver. She has also developed procedures and policy manuals specific to care in the center. One of Tillman's major contributions was preparing the application for accreditation by the Accreditation Association for Ambulatory Health Care, which was approved in 2011. In 2013 she was appointed associate director of the center, which employs a medical director, five physicians, one physician assistant, one nurse practitioner, eight registered nurses, and two licensed vocational nurses.

Major rewards for Tillman are collaborating with colleagues in the Brown-Lupton Health Center and the TCU Counseling and Mental Health Center and seeing the growth and ultimate success of the students they serve. After her own graduation with a doctorate in nursing practice (DNP) in 2019, Tillman hopes to facilitate the full integration of the Brown-Lupton Health Center, the Counseling and Mental Health Center, Wellness Education, and Alcohol and Drug Education into one patient-centered health care facility.

An Interview with Mindi (Ray) Anderson, PhD, ARNP, CPNP-PC, CNE, CHSE-A, ANEF, BSN 1993

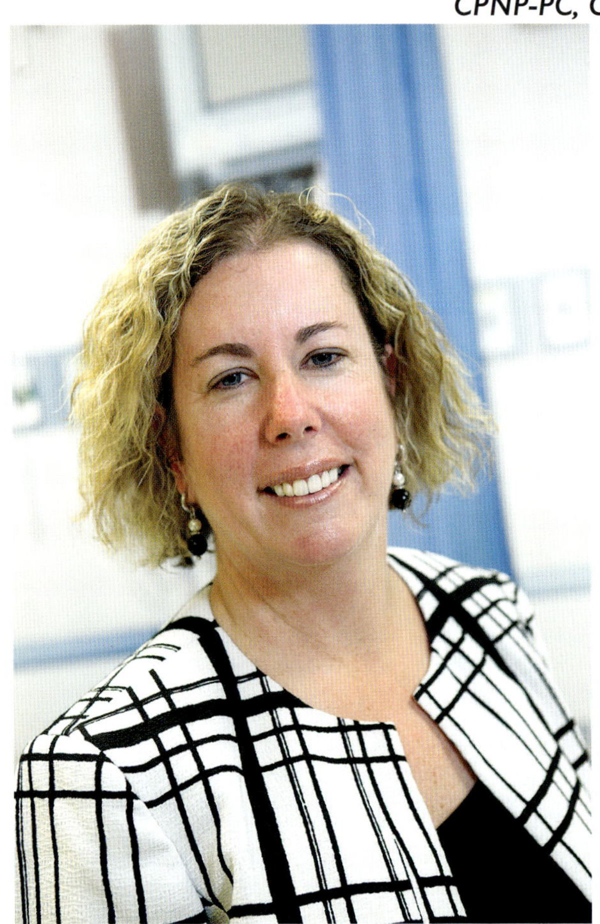

Mindi Anderson.

Mindi Anderson was motivated to be a nurse by her great-aunt Ann Louise Clark, who was a well-known nurse, nurse educator, and textbook author. Anderson stated that, for as long as she could remember, she had always wanted to be a nurse (Mindi Anderson, pers. comm., 2018). At the time of her graduation, she had already developed a passion for pediatrics and teaching. She worked at a children's hospital both prior to and following her graduation, and she soon realized that she also wanted to become a nursing instructor. She returned to school and became a pediatric nurse practitioner with an advanced degree to qualify her for a faculty position.

Anderson acknowledged that she "discovered simulation by accident" early in her career. As she observed how her students reacted to manikin-based simulators and how learning occurred, she was "hooked" (Mindi Anderson, pers. comm., 2018). Simulation became her passion in both teaching and research. She considers Judy LeFlore at the University of Texas at Arlington College of Nursing and Health Innovation to be her mentor in learning the process of research in the simulation field. Anderson also states she was "very lucky" to have had some wonderful teachers at HCN who were passionate about their subjects. She credits Marinda Allender, her pediatric instructor, for spurring her passion for pediatric patient care and being her role model for a caring educator.

Anderson became an associate professor at the University of Central Florida in 2015. She became the program director for an advanced degree and certification in simulation in 2016. She also consults as a nurse scientist at Orlando Health. In addition to these roles, she has been very active in professional organizations. She is a fellow in the American Academy of Nursing and the National League for Nursing Academy of Nurse Education. She is associate editor of the *Simulation & Gaming* journal and is on the editorial review board for *Simulation in Healthcare: The Journal of the Society for Simulation in Healthcare.* In her many roles, Anderson has also developed a passion for traveling and presenting her work to colleagues throughout the world. One of her fondest experiences thus far has been as a Fulbright Specialist in Thailand, helping faculty develop skills in the use of simulation.

When asked about the major challenge in her work, "doing all things" (teaching, research, and service) topped Anderson's list. Her greatest reward has been seeing students' "aha" moments when they learn something new. Her scholarly development through research and publication has also been rewarding. Anderson feels her research with colleagues has helped develop best practices in nursing and health care education. She hopes to make an impact on students both while they are in school and in their future careers.

CHALLENGE TWO
Research to Determine What Effects Variables in Nursing Care Have on the Health of People

Context and Trends

The National Institute of Nursing Research (NINR) achieved institute status at the National Institute of Health (NIH) following the NIH Revitalization Act of 1993. In 1995, Patricia Grady was appointed director of the NINR (National Institute of Nursing Research 2016).

In collaboration with STTI, several professional organizations offered nursing research grants during the 1990s. Examples of research grants included awards by the American Association of Critical-Care Nurses (1992), the Oncology Nursing Foundation (1994), the Emergency Nurses Association (1994), and the Association of periOperative Registered Nurses (1997) (Thompson, pers. comm., 2018).

Three other research awards were also established in 1999, all sponsored by STTI: the Rosemary Berkel Crisp Research Award, the Doris Bloch Research Award, and the Virginia Henderson Clinical Research Grant made possible by the Virginia Henderson Clinical Research Endowment Fund (Thompson, pers. comm., 2018).

Friends of TCU Endow Lectureship in Nursing

W.F. "Tex" and Pauline Curry Rankin have long-standing ties both to Texas Christian University and to nursing. Through the years, the Rankins have proved themselves generous friends of Texas Christian University, establishing scholarships in nursing, pre-medical studies and geology in the 1980s. More recently, they have affirmed their connection to TCU and to Harris College of Nursing through endowing the W.F. "Tex" and Pauline Rankin Professorship in Nursing and the W.F. "Tex" and Pauline Rankin Lectureship in Nursing.

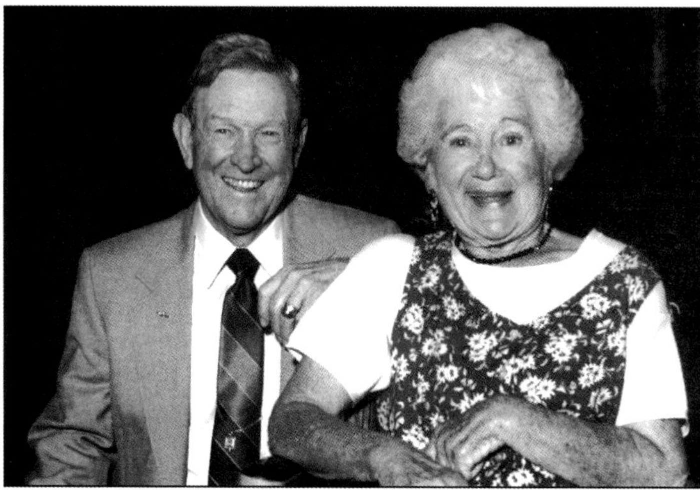

Tex and Polly Rankin.

A 1940 graduate of TCU with a degree in geology, Col. Warner F. "Tex" Rankin, Jr., married Lt. Pauline Curry in 1944. Polly had been one of the 25 flight nurses attached to the 803rd Medical Air Evacuation Squadron in Burma during World War II. As a flight nurse, she was awarded the Air Medal, three Battle Stars and a Distinguished Unit Citation for her tour of October 1943 to October 1944. "In the history of nursing, the actions of these flight nurses in the China-Burma-India theater during World War II were stirringly significant," said Harris College of Nursing Professor and Alumni Rhonda Keen-Payne. "I talk about Polly in my class on the history of nursing. Students and faculty members find her so inspiring." Tex distinguished himself in the war as well, flying 189 combat missions and earning two Distinguished Flying Crosses, two Air Medals, three Battle Stars and a Distinguished Unit Citation.

After the war, Polly became an airline hostess, a job then open only to registered nurses. Tex worked at the Air Force Flight Test Division, flying more than 40 models of aircraft. After his military service, Tex went to Harvard Business School, earning an MBA with high distinction. He also served the Air Force in Europe and at the Pentagon. As Systems Program Director for the C-5A jet transport, he earned the Legion of Merit. At his Air Force retirement in 1970, he was awarded the Oak Leaf Cluster to the Legion of Merit. Tex worked for many years for USPA & IRA insurance.

Tex and Polly have developed a variety of avocational interests. A baseball letterman when he was at TCU, Tex is now an avid golfer. In their earlier years, the Rankins were bridge enthusiasts, and Tex continues to be a top-rate bridge player. They have two sons, Michael Scott and Patrick.

Harris College of Nursing will host the Inaugural Rankin Lectureship in Nursing activities this spring in celebration of National Nurses Week, May 5-7, 1998. The following is a preliminary schedule of events:

Tuesday, May 5, 1998 2-4 p.m. Bass Living Room
Ice Cream Sundaes and Poster Session. The HCN Archives Room will also be available for viewing historical HCN memorabilia. Hosted by the HCN Student Nurses Association

Wednesday, May 6, 1998 4-6 p.m. Dee Jay Kelly Alumni Center
Reception hosted by the TCU Sigma Theta Tau Beta Alpha Chapter and the HCN Alumni Association. A presentation will be made to introduce software programs for tracking financial, clinical pathway and staffing data in relation to patient outcomes.

Thursday, May 7, 1998 Brown-Lupton Student Center Ballroom Reception and keynote speaker Dr. Susan Horne to discuss clinical outcomes research

Look for more information in your mailbox soon or contact Dr. Linda Curry at (817) 257-7496.

Harris College of Nursing

The W. F. "Tex" and Pauline Curry Rankin Professorship

A gift from W. F. "Tex" and Pauline Curry Rankin established an endowed HCN professorship that funds research studies. Pauline Curry Rankin was a flight nurse in Burma during World War II, while Colonel Tex Rankin was a decorated military pilot. The couple married in 1944, and Pauline Curry Rankin's passion for nursing inspired them to become generous benefactors of Harris College.

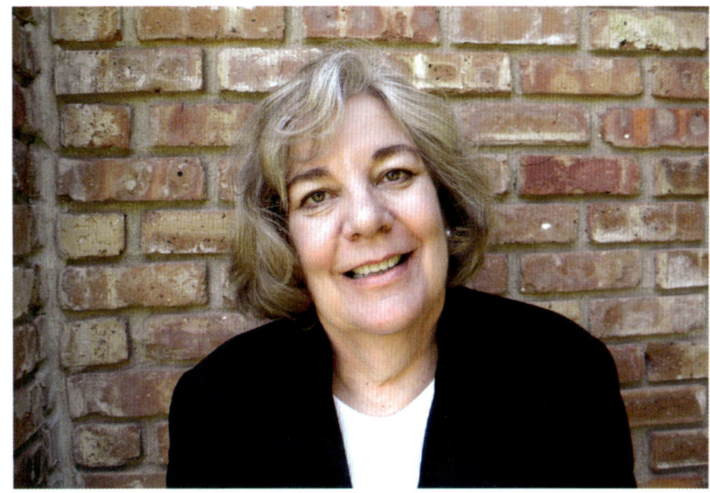

(Above) Rhonda Keen-Payne, Endowed Rankin Professor, 2015. (Below) Andrea and Tex Rankin, 2012.

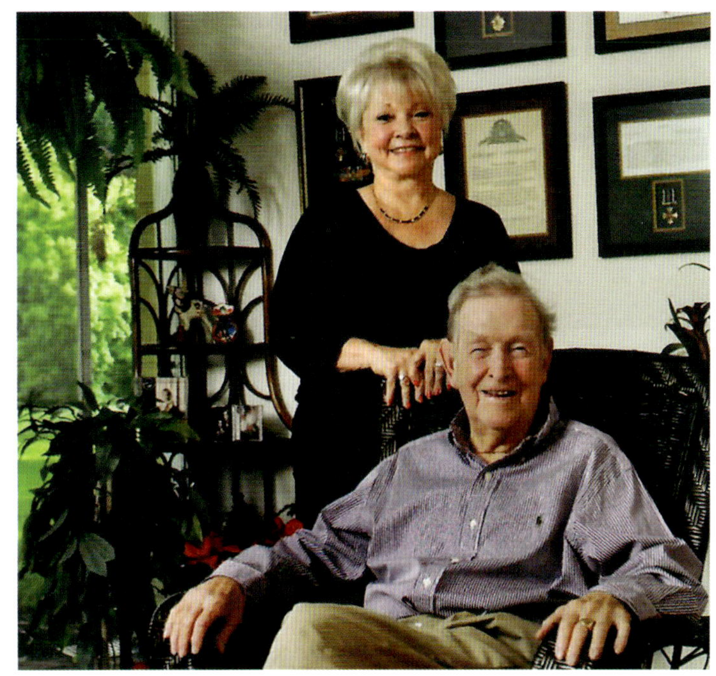

Rhonda Keen-Payne has held the professorship since it was created in 1997. Her research has focused on historical nursing, specifically on the 1918 influenza epidemic in the context of World War I and the Progressive Era, which was a time of reform in women's rights and the birth of nursing as a profession. In 1999, she published "We Must Have Nurses: Spanish Influenza in America, 1918–19" (Keen-Payne 1999). She was also a guest lecturer to doctoral students at Texas Woman's University between 1988 and 2005, on topics that focused on feminism and history in nursing.

The Rankins also provided funds in 1998 for the W. F. "Tex" and Pauline Curry Rankin Lectureship in Nursing, which has brought renowned speakers to the TCU campus. Speakers and topics of national and international interest are found in Appendix 11.

Today, Keen-Payne remains in touch with Andrea Rankin, Tex Rankin's second wife, who currently lives in New Mexico. Andrea Rankin continues to express support for the ongoing work related to the annual lectureship held at TCU.

Focus on Scholarship

Faculty engagement in scholarship increased significantly during the decade. Dean Scearse reported in her 1993–94 annual report that five refereed articles, ten book chapters, and nine non-refereed articles had been published by nine different faculty members. The 1996–97 annual report stated that faculty generated more than forty articles, monographs, book chapters, and books, of which the majority were in refereed journals. In the final annual report of the decade, HCN reported that the goal of achieving twelve refereed publications, the goal for the 1999 academic year, had been met (Harris College of Nursing Archives).

Between 1996 and 1998, the Beta Alpha chapter of STTI awarded four research grants. The Hogstel Gerontological Nursing Research Award was given to six researchers for a variety of studies. Examples of studies conducted were "Self-Management of Advanced Osteoporosis" (Gail Davis), "Coping Behaviors of Urinary Incontinent Adults: Instrument Development," (Laura Talbot), and "Post-Hip Fracture Status in Older Women" (Linda Curry).

ALUMNI EXAMPLES OF RESEARCH

Defining the Role of the Nurse Researcher:

An Interview with Shelby Garner, BSN 1993

Shelby Garner credits her mother, who took up nursing as a second career, as her primary inspiration for entering the nursing profession. She described her mother's excitement for learning new things as leading her to the nurse educator role, which Shelby assumed after practicing nursing in critical care and cardiac specialty home health for ten years (Shelby Garner, pers. comm., 2018).

Garner recalls that in her first research class at TCU in 1992, one of her faculty, Rhonda Keen-Payne, spoke about the importance of moving nursing from a skill-based position to a profession that entailed critical thinking and clinical decision-making. Learning about how nursing research was imperative to establishing and sustaining nursing as a scientific discipline and essential in promoting positive patient outcomes was the "spark that fueled [her] passion for both teaching and research" (Shelby Garner, pers. comm., 2018).

Today, as a nurse educator and researcher, Garner has a passion for mentoring students through the research process. She has supported student research presentations at local, national, and international forums such as the National Conference on Undergraduate Research. Her own research involves nurse migration, building health care capacity in low- and middle-income countries, and developing

USAID
Baptist
BAYLOR
WELCOME
INAUGURATION OF
SIMULATION EDUCATION
& RESEARCH CENTRE
11TH OF JULY, 2017
ASHA BLOCK

ATION EDUCATI
RESEARCH CEN

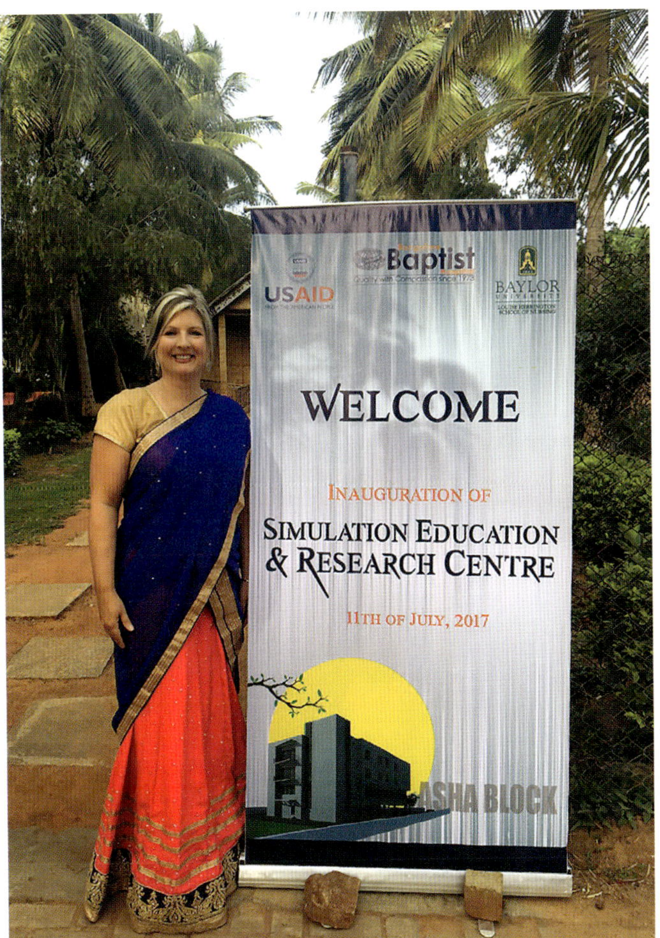

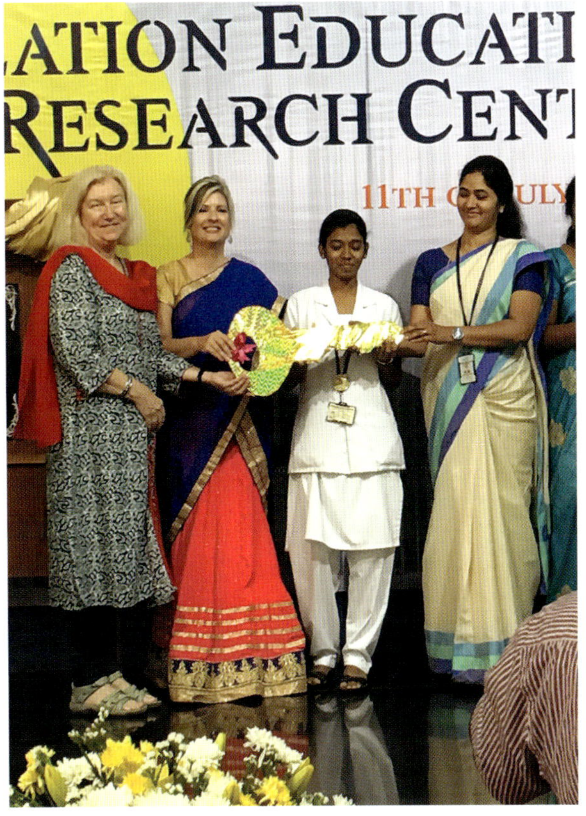

(Left) Shelby Garner by the Simulation Lab sign, 2017. (Above) Shelby with colleagues at the Research Center.

teaching and learning models that transcend cultural boundaries (Shelby Garner, pers. comm., 2018). She has an ongoing research pursuit and partners with colleagues at Bangalore Baptist Hospital and the Rebekah Ann Naylor School of Nursing in Bangalore, India. Her collaborative research seeks to empower health professionals in India to use the latest health care technologies to improve patient care. She and her partners in India have received $652,800 to build the Simulation Education and Research Centre for Nursing Excellence in Bangalore, which will provide a center for health care students and professionals to perfect clinical skills and improve clinical decision-making. She was awarded a 2016–18 Fulbright-Nehru Academic and Professional Excellence Fellowship Flex Grant to study the impact of simulation in nursing education on teaching.

"Collaborating with nurses in India to improve educational and patient outcomes through research has been the highlight of my career," Garner said. She pointed out that the time it takes to build a reciprocal relationship with a global partner presents

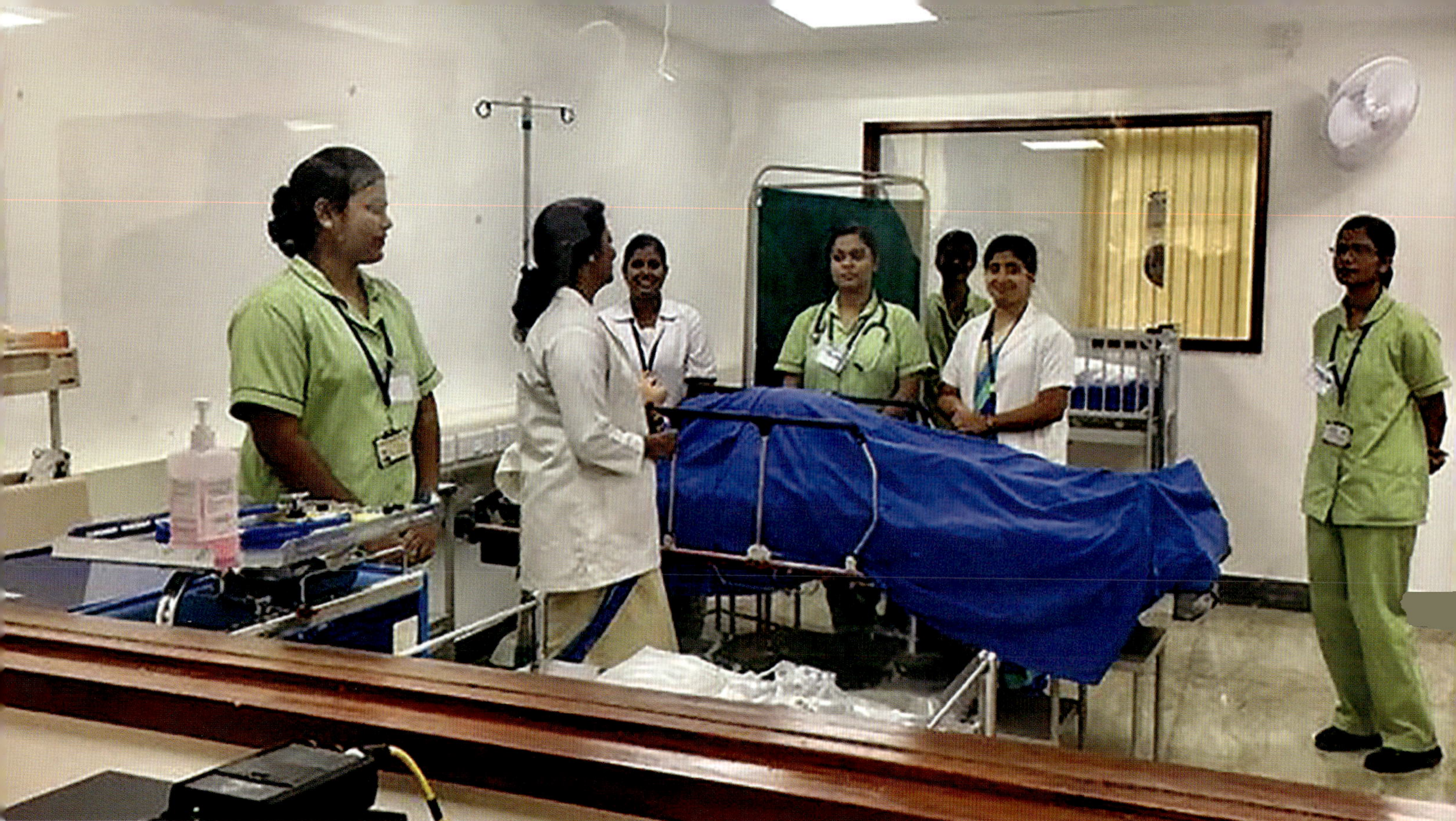

Shelby Garner in Simulation Lab, 2017.

challenges, but sometimes overcoming these makes the outcomes more rewarding. Rewards include "a front row seat to the advancement of the nursing profession as nursing leaders have emerged through collaborative research" (Shelby Garner, pers. comm., 2018).

In summary, as Harris College of Nursing celebrated fifty years, faculty and students continued to respond to the many continuing changes in nursing, nursing education, and the health care system, and they were increasingly recognized at the local and national levels. The TCU Student Nurses Association provided opportunities for its members to engage in activities that prepared them for future professional roles. Curricular foci included expanded content on professional standards in health promotion, on acute and chronic illnesses, and on gerontology. Nursing theory, research, and statistics were emphasized to prepare students for expanded responsibilities. Faculty provided a model for students by increasing their scholarship. The first study abroad course in London was offered, setting the stage for future students to experience nursing in the country of the "founder of modern nursing." At HCN during the 1990s, 998 individuals received their degree.

Chapter Five

The 2000s

Decade of Change

In the summer of 2000, Harris College of Nursing was renamed Harris School of Nursing (HSN) as one of several organizational changes within the university. HSN and the university departments of Communication Sciences and Disorders, Kinesiology, and Social Work combined to form the new college: the College of Health and Human Sciences, with Rhonda Keen-Payne as the dean. At the same time, plans to launch a School of Nurse Anesthesia began in response to a national call for increased programming in that field, according to a 2000 HSN report to the Commission on Collegiate Nursing Education (Harris College of Nursing Archives). In 2005, the College of Health and Human Sciences became the Harris College of Nursing & Health Sciences (HCNHS), maintaining the name of the original funding donor, Charles Harris. The nursing department became known as TCU Nursing. Paulette Burns, who had been the director of the nursing program, became dean of the college in 2006.

TCU and the Commission on the Future of TCU

As an important resource in 2000 for planning and feedback at TCU, the Commission on the Future of TCU was composed of seventeen task forces and included one that focused on the future direction of the College of Health and Human Sciences. As explained in the HSN self-study report for the Commission on Collegiate Nursing in 2000, the goals of this task force were to:

1. Unify the new college,
2. Prepare graduates for professional positions and further education,

3. Contribute to the knowledge of the disciplines through research and writing,

4. Provide professional and educational services to the community.

—*Harris College of Nursing Archives*

The task force discussed general trends in health care and practice, made recommendations to review and revise college curricula as needed to meet professional standards, and identified individual and common research interests to develop priorities for a college research program. It recommended the establishment of an organization to facilitate research through an institute led by a director or associate dean. The task force also prioritized ongoing development and maintenance of community relationships for a heightened awareness of the college in the community. Activities related to the recommendations are described later in this and subsequent chapters.

Board of Visitors

The Harris College of Nursing & Health Sciences (HCNHS) Board of Visitors was chartered in 2008 as a volunteer body established by Dean Paulette Burns to foster a high level of excellence in HCNHS. Membership consisted of local and national leaders who were committed to the mission of the college. Responsibilities included (1) providing advice and counsel on key issues affecting the college, such as new and existing programs and new initiatives, and (2) serving as a link to the community by connecting the priorities of the college to specific individuals within the broader health care and philanthropic community. Members served as ambassadors of the college with the purpose of strengthening the image and visibility of the college beyond the university. They also advocated for the college by providing resources and gifts to meet the short- and long-term goals of the college and assisted in fund development to advance and expand the educational programs and facilities of the college (Board of Visitors 2008).

Focus on the Development of Centers

The Center for Evidence-Based Practice and Research was established in 2006 as a "point of connection between nursing faculty members and the clinical agencies where student practicum experiences occur" (Weeks, Marshall, and Burns 2009, 27). Motivated by the increasing focus on evidence-based practice and research and the pursuit of Magnet status by area hospitals, HCNHS recognized that nursing faculty could provide expertise in these areas to local hospitals. Alyce Schultz, an internationally known expert, visited the TCU campus in 2007 and spoke to faculty and nurses from five area hospitals.

In 2008, the Evidence-Based Practice Fellowship was inaugurated in order to prepare health professionals across disciplines to increase the evidence-based practice in their institutions. Participants in the competitive yearlong fellowship attended class one day each month and designed a project that had the potential to support practice improvements.

The Center for Oncology Education and Research (COER) was established in 2007, in part through a gift from UT Southwestern Moncrief Center Foundation. Under the leadership of COER Director Suzy Lockwood, TCU Nursing was identified by the American Association of Colleges of Nursing (AACN) as the only baccalaureate program in the United States that offered an oncology track. Originally, funding was given toward the development of a baccalaureate track providing didactic and clinical experiences that could encourage students to choose oncology as a career. Following national recognition by AACN with the 2011 Innovations in Professional Nursing Education Award, the goal of COER was expanded.

The goal of COER was to provide opportunities for interdisciplinary, collaborative learning and research between university faculty, students, and community partners regarding cancer care and survivorship concerns. Survivorship-focused research done through COER has been conducted and presented at many national and international professional meetings. Support for students' honor projects has also been an important focus of COER.

COER also sponsors the annual Cowtown Oncology Nursing Symposium, which has been attended by nurses throughout Texas and the United States. Along with giving participants a taste of Cowtown, the symposium features a nationally known speaker.

Responding to demographic shifts in the United States, the Center for Healthy Aging (CHA) was launched in 2007 to support healthy aging initiatives with an emphasis on older adults, their families, and their caregivers. The vision for CHA was to promote, celebrate, and value healthy aging and good quality of life for older adults. Initial funding for CHA was provided by a grant submitted by Dennis Cheek to the TCU Vision in Action program. As an interdisciplinary project, CHA committees and the board included representatives from all departments within the HCNHS.

In September 2007, CHA, in collaboration with the HCNHS Department of Social Work, sponsored a program entitled "Spirituality and End of Life Care: Compassionate Response to Essential Needs." Betty Kramer, a professor of social work at the University of Wisconsin-Madison, presented her research on male caregivers, caregiving gains, and transitions in the caregiving career (Texas Christian University 2007).

During National Gerontological Nursing Week of the same year, HCNHS and CHA held a second program on "Understanding the Older Adult: Holistic Approach to Care." Speakers included a geriatric nurse practitioner, a physician, a social worker, a professor of pastoral theology, and an attorney who specialized in the aging community.

Under the direction of Linda Curry, activities included educational opportunities, resources for the elderly, and activities for TCU and local communities. An extensive list of useful websites and community contacts with a focus on the elderly was available through CHA. During the 2008–09 academic year, CHA provided continuing education credits for eleven interdisciplinary events within Tarrant County with up-to-date information on healthy aging. CHA also established a relationship with the Fort Worth Public Library to display information relevant to Tarrant County elder care services.

In 2009, the functions of CHA were distributed among other units within HCNHS, due to a lack of continued external funding and internal funding that ended in May 2009 (Harris College of Nursing 2009).

Sixtieth Anniversary Celebration

In 2006, the College of Nursing celebrated its sixtieth anniversary. Dean Paulette Burns spoke at the gala on "Connecting to the Past . . . Creating the Future." She began by commenting on the pleasure of being a part of "an outstanding college of nursing with such a legacy of forward-thinking leaders" (Harris College of Nursing Archives). She noted that both a nursing shortage and a nursing faculty shortage occurred at a time of health care crisis, when access to quality, safe, and affordable health care was not available to the forty million people who did not have health insurance.

Burns also described a paradigm shift in education occurring at all levels, as distance education became a respected methodology. The "Creating the Future" section of her speech included comments on new programs, new teaching methodologies, a focus on leadership, and the creation and maintenance of partnerships with clinical agencies, provider networks, international sites, and colleagues in related disciplines.

In closing, Burns acknowledged the legacy of the forerunners: Harris, who "sold his Hereford cattle to help create an endowment for the college"; Chancellor McGruder Ellis Sadler, who "had the courage to transition a hospital diploma program to a university program before it was fashionable to do so"; and Lucy Harris, who had the "strength of character and persistence to make us the first accredited baccalaureate program in the state of Texas—WOW!" (Harris College of Nursing Archives).

In Burns's closing remarks, she commented:

> TCU is a place of community, a place you can belong, a place to call home. It is a place where you sit and talk with faculty one on one, develop lifetime personal relationships, and experience what it feels like to be a valued part of a

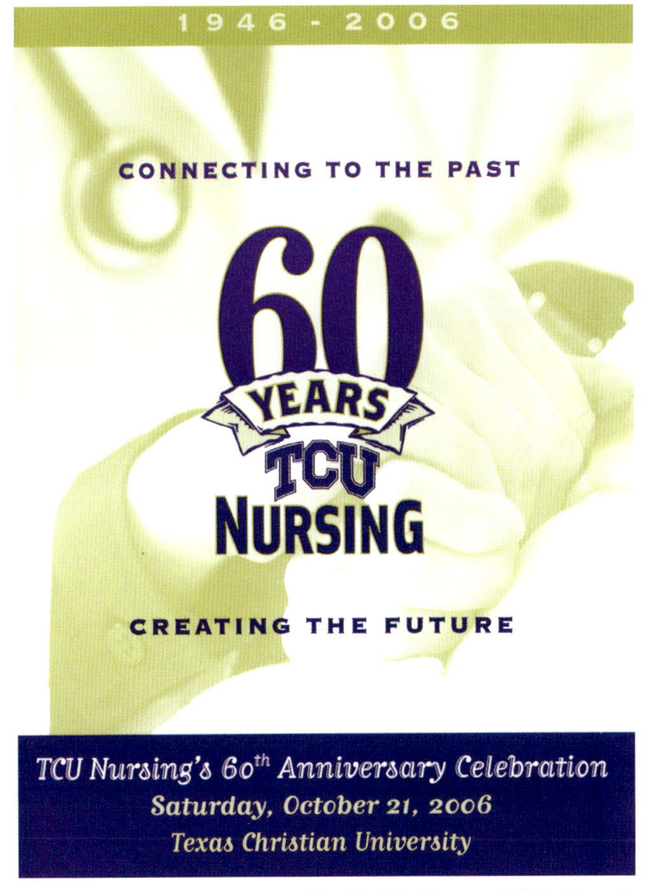

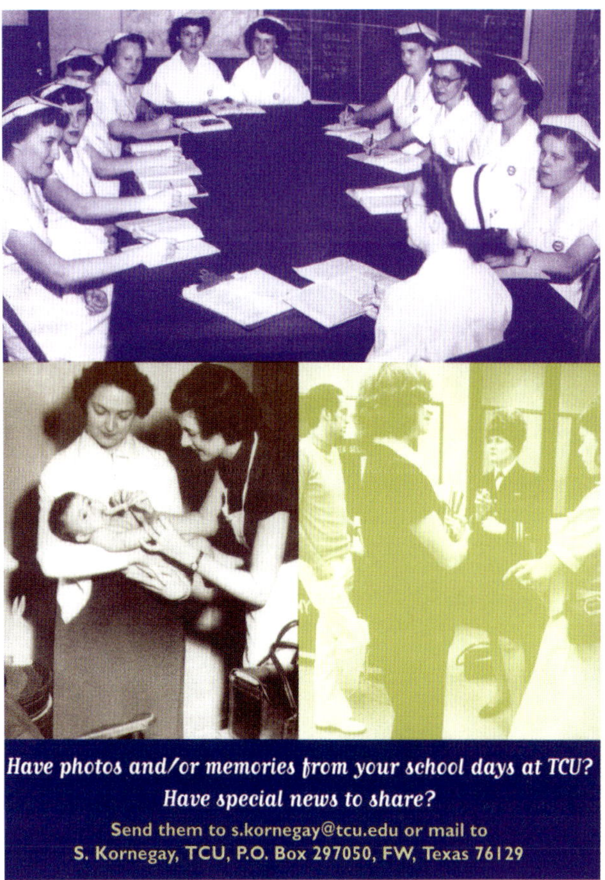

(Left) 60 Years: TCU Nursing. (Right) Historical pictures.

tolerant, inclusive community. So, I ask you to think of the future and how you will carry these values from our past and our present into the future—the value of **striving for excellence,** not just by getting by; the value of **caring deeply;** and the value of **creating and sustaining,** not just being a collection of individuals. I hope the vision of learning, leadership, and legacy will light the path to the future."

— *Dean Paulette Burns; Harris College of Nursing Archives*

CHALLENGE ONE
A Clear Definition of Nursing Roles and Functions

Context and Trends

The Institute of Medicine (IOM) significantly shaped health care in the 2000s with the release of two reports: *To Err is Human: Building a Safer Health System* in 1999 and *Crossing the Quality Chasm: A New Health System for the 21st Century* in 2001. The 1999 report brought to light the impact of medical errors on both the cost of health care and the loss of human lives, and recommended systemic improvements to reduce incidences of individual errors (Quigley 2003). In the 2001 report, the IOM expanded on this topic by noting that medical errors were simply part of a larger problem in health care: quality. Noting the impact of the rapid growth of technology, the chronic conditions of the aging population, and uncoordinated care on the quality of the patient experience, the IOM recommended multiple means to better facilitate the development of a health system which promotes health care that is safe, effective, patient-centered, timely, efficient, and equitable (Institute of Medicine 2001). These ideas were further emphasized by the release of the first National Patient Safety Goals in 2002 by the Joint Commission on Accreditation of Healthcare Organizations to begin promoting a "culture of safety" in health care (Quigley 2003).

While patient safety has always been a priority for nurses, little research had been done to connect the impact of nurses on patient outcomes until the release of the 2004 IOM report, *Keeping Patients Safe: Transforming the Work Environment of Nurses*. This report noted that nurses are key to improving the patient safety problem in health care (Long 2004). The result of the 1999, 2001, and 2004 IOM reports was the development of multiple means for protecting nurses as a way to protect patients. These measures included the Needlestick Safety and Prevention Act of 2001, which sought to reduce needlestick injuries, and the American Nurses Association's "Handle with Care" campaign to prevent musculoskeletal injuries in nurses (Foley 2004; Trossman 2004). However, neither of these improvements engaged the root of the problem in both nursing and health care: the inadequate nursing staff-to-patient ratio. With baby boomers rapidly leaving the workforce and an insufficient number of nursing students to fill their vacancies, significant measures would need to be taken in future decades to relieve this impending nursing crisis (Long 2004).

Harris School of Nursing

The TCU mission statement was revised in July 1999, and after endorsing the values identified by TCU, HSN revised its mission and philosophy in January 2000. Core values included "academic achievement, personal freedom and integrity, the dignity and respect of the individual, and a heritage of inclusiveness, tolerance, and service." The specific mission of HSN was "to prepare professional nurses to identify and respond with competence to multiple, complex human health care needs" (*Harris School of Nursing Self-Study Report 2000*).

The organization of the HSN changed with the formation of the College of Health and Human Sciences (CHHS) in 2000. According to HSN's 2000 *Self-Study Report to the Commission on Collegiate Nursing Education,* the director of HSN reported to the dean of CHHS, managed the school, and served as a liaison between HSN and CHHS (Harris College of Nursing Archives). Faculty committees, which reported to the faculty at regularly scheduled meetings, included curriculum, advisory, faculty relations, peer review, and student relations committees. A school advisory committee also reported to the director. Students served as non-voting members on the curriculum, faculty relations, and student relations committees to provide input and a student perspective. In response to the restructuring, the dean established a college student cabinet in 2000 to inform the dean of student responses, concerns, and suggestions. Members included students from various levels who were elected by students or appointed by the school director. In 2008, the positions of associate dean and director of undergraduate programs were created.

The faculty of HSN in 2000 was composed of twenty-three full-time and six part-time faculty members, all academically and professionally prepared for their academic roles. In addition to the required minimal preparation at the master's degree level, fifteen faculty members were certified in a variety of areas: critical care, emergency care, gerontology, medical-surgical, pulmonary, pediatrics, psychiatric, women's health, hospice, oncology obstetric in-patient, childbirth education, and staff development.

In 2005, Dean Burns was selected by the Robert Wood Johnson Foundation as an Executive Nurse Fellow (2005–08). The program is a three-year advanced leadership program for nurses. A cohort of twenty nurses is selected each year to participate in the fellowship. Burns's project focused on helping nurses expand their clinical and organizational skills to match growing health care needs. The outcome of her project resulted in the expansion of connections with national leaders in nursing and health care and laid the groundwork for the development of the doctor of nursing practice (DNP) program at TCU.

During this decade, three HSN nursing faculty members—Susan Wilson (2000), Susan Weeks (2002), and Patricia Bradley (2004)—were honored as nominees for the Chancellor's Award for Distinguished Teaching. Three faculty—Dennis Cheek (2005), Linda Curry (2006), and Jo Nell Wells (2009)—were also honored as nominees for the Chancellor's Award for Distinguished Research or Creative Activity.

The Deans' Teaching Award was given to Susan Wilson in 2001. Recipients of this award are characterized by a dedication to teaching and innovative strategies that enhance the quality of student outcomes. The Deans' Research Award, which is given in recognition of high-quality research and creative activity over a period of a year, was presented to four nursing faculty members in the 2000s. Nursing faculty recipients were Susan Wilson (2001), Jo Nell Wells (2004), Charles Walker (2006), and Dennis Cheek (2009).

Characteristics and Activities of Students

The composition of the HSN baccalaureate students in the fall of 2000 was 80.6 percent Caucasian, 7.4 percent African American, 4.9 percent Hispanic, 1.8 percent Asian, 0.04 percent American Indian, and 4.6 percent other. Females made up 94.4 percent of the student body and 5.6 percent were male.

In 2007 the ACE Program (Academic Excellence) was established in response to difficulties some students were experiencing with completing the program. Zoranna Jones, who was in charge of advising, brainstormed with Marinda Allender, director of undergraduate nursing, and then she presented several ideas to Dean Burns. Together, they developed a program that proactively provided students with tools to be successful. The services included academic advising, counseling, tutoring, referral to campus resources, and faculty mentoring (Marinda Allender, pers. comm., 2018).

Curriculum

Harris School of Nursing's curriculum prepared baccalaureate graduates to function competently as generalists in a wide variety of practice environments. HSN identified three major roles for nurses based on AACN's definition of professional nurses prepared for the twenty-first century: providers of care; designers, managers, and coordinators of care; and members of the profession. Based on the mission and goals of HSN, the curriculum continued to emphasize the themes of communication, critical thinking, research, management, professionalism, teaching and learning, processes, and values. These themes, integrated into the content of selected courses, provided the basis for the nursing roles and functions assumed by graduates when they entered the workforce. The traditional track, composed of 124 semester hours, provided learning experiences in all major clinical areas in a variety of agencies throughout the Dallas–Fort Worth area (Appendix 12).

The accelerated track, which began in 2004, was designed for students who held non-nursing degrees, preparing them for professional practice through a sixteen-month program also composed of 124 semester hours. However, coursework and clinical times were arranged to maximize experiences in an intense fifty-eight credit hours taken through four straight semesters: summer, fall, spring, summer. The accelerated track built on a broad foundation of liberal arts and included a professional nursing residency in a student's last semester. The degree plan remained the same until 2015 (Appendix 13).

The purpose of the accelerated track was to retain non-nursing college graduates and propel them into professional nursing practice without compromising educational standards. Two clinical partnerships—with Baylor Scott & White All Saints Medical Center and John Peter Smith Health Network in Fort Worth—were initially developed to provide clinical experiences for these students. The project was initially funded by the Texas Higher Education Coordinating Board. Charles Walker was the principal investigator and Suzy Lockwood was the codirector.

The study abroad program, "Global Perspectives in Health: London," was offered in 2000, 2002, 2004, 2008, and 2010, with Susan Weeks and Diane Hawley coordinating the activities. This course was open to all majors with no prerequisites to enroll, a policy that had the benefit of students from other majors interacting with nursing students and demonstrating other ways to think about health and health care. This program welcomed students from education, political science, pre-health, nutrition, business, and radio-TV-film. Housing for both students and faculty members transitioned to London flats with kitchen facilities, which allowed the students to economize on food. The primary pedagogical change was a move from formal lectures to extensive field study. Purposeful content was delivered to the students through readings, discussions, and an elaborate pretest to prepare them for their trip before they even set foot on foreign soil. The intent of this strategy was to give students sufficient background to enjoy their learning abroad. Often, students would comment that they did not realize how and what they were learning until they were encouraged to write a midcourse essay. The reflections discussed in these essays demonstrated the considerable learning that was taking place.

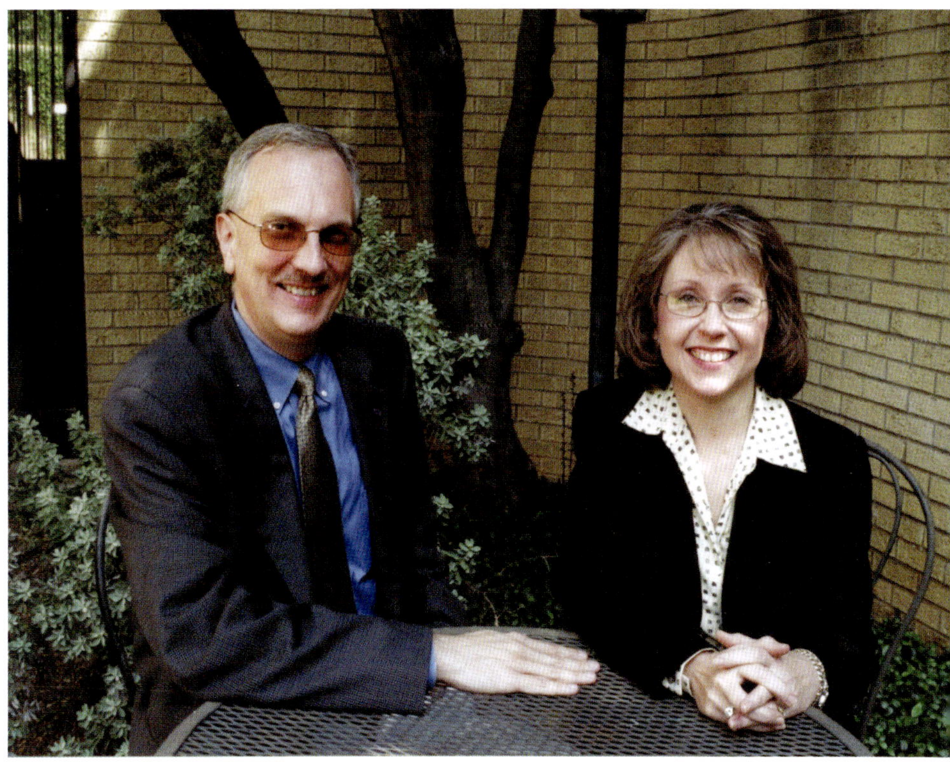

Charles Walker and Suzy Lockwood, founders of the Accelerated BSN Degree Program at TCU, 2004.

Observations of British culture and health care in London functioned as learning laboratories that demonstrated various concepts relating to health and health care from both historical and contemporary perspectives. For example, health concepts having to do with housing, water purity, and sanitation were examined while touring the Tower of London. A favorite memory for many students was thinking

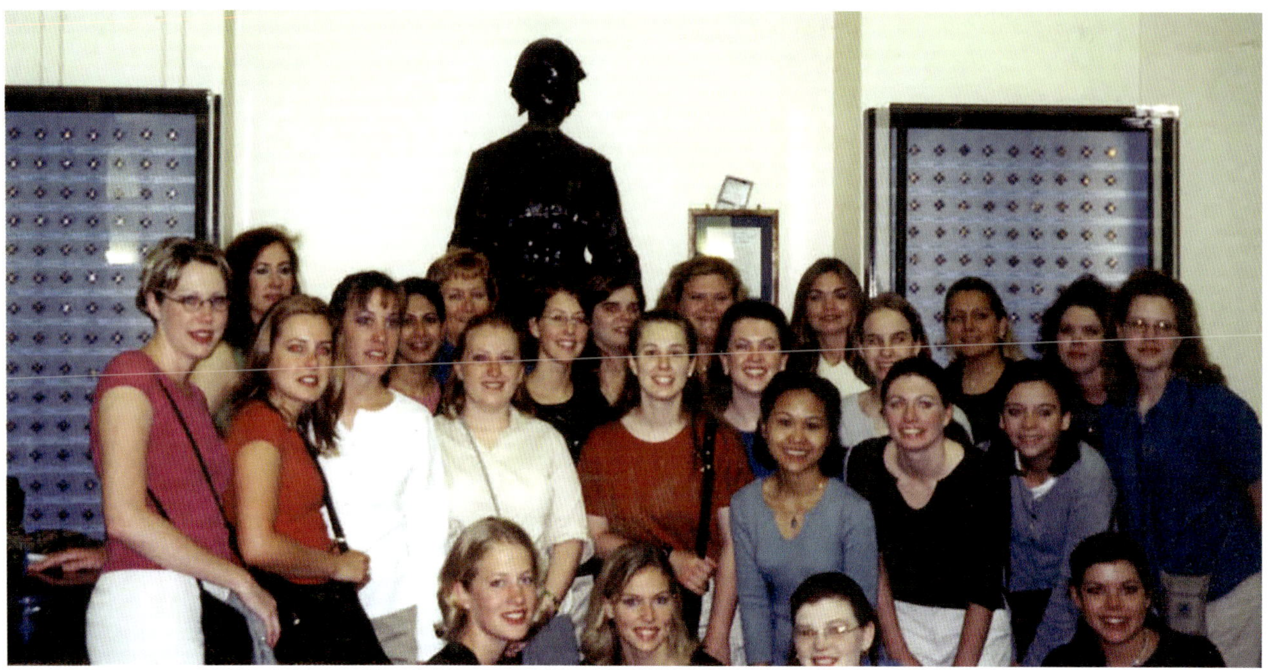

Students at St. Thomas' Hospital in London, Florence Nightingale Chapel, 2002.

about social justice based on who had their heads removed inside the tower versus outside the tower, and which historical figures had some element of choice in the manner of their beheading. Another learning laboratory was St. Paul's Cathedral, which was heavily bombed during World War II. While touring the cathedral, students learned of the unique relationships that formed between the London aristocrats and commoners while they sheltered together in the city's underground spaces during bombing raids. This shared experience led to a greater sense of collective unity, which can be seen in the formation of the British National Health Service in 1948. Additionally, students learned the origin of the British term "loo," referring to the restroom. It derived from the cry of "gardyloo," from the French "regardez l'eau," meaning "watch out for the water"—a phrase shouted by medieval servants as they emptied chamber pots out of upstairs windows into the street.

Beginning in 2000, the final evaluative exercise for each course was a group debate. A common question was, "What methods of health care rationing are used by the United States and the United Kingdom, and which method is preferable?" Students came to understand that all societies must ration health care in some manner. The United Kingdom system often rations care by individuals having to wait for treatment, while the United States often rations care by the ability of individuals to pay.

In London, students had the opportunity to visit the Florence Nightingale Museum, St Thomas' Hospital, and University College Hospital. Tours of cultural sites such as Westminster Abbey, St. Paul's Cathedral, the Museum of London, and theaters also provided immersion into English culture.

An elective in forensic nursing was offered by Debbie Schmidt in 2007 and 2008. This course introduced students to forensic nursing and prepared them to recognize and manage forensic patients in the health care setting and in the community at large. Students learned the history of forensic nursing, how to identify victims of violence, the psychosocial and legal aspects of forensic nursing, the focus of trauma and death investigations, and how to prepare for mass disasters. Students engaged in demonstrations of forensic practices, case studies, class discussions, and field trips to forensic facilities. Guest lecturers included a sexual assault nurse examiner, crime scene investigator, legal nurse consultant, and Federal Bureau of Prisons nurse manager.

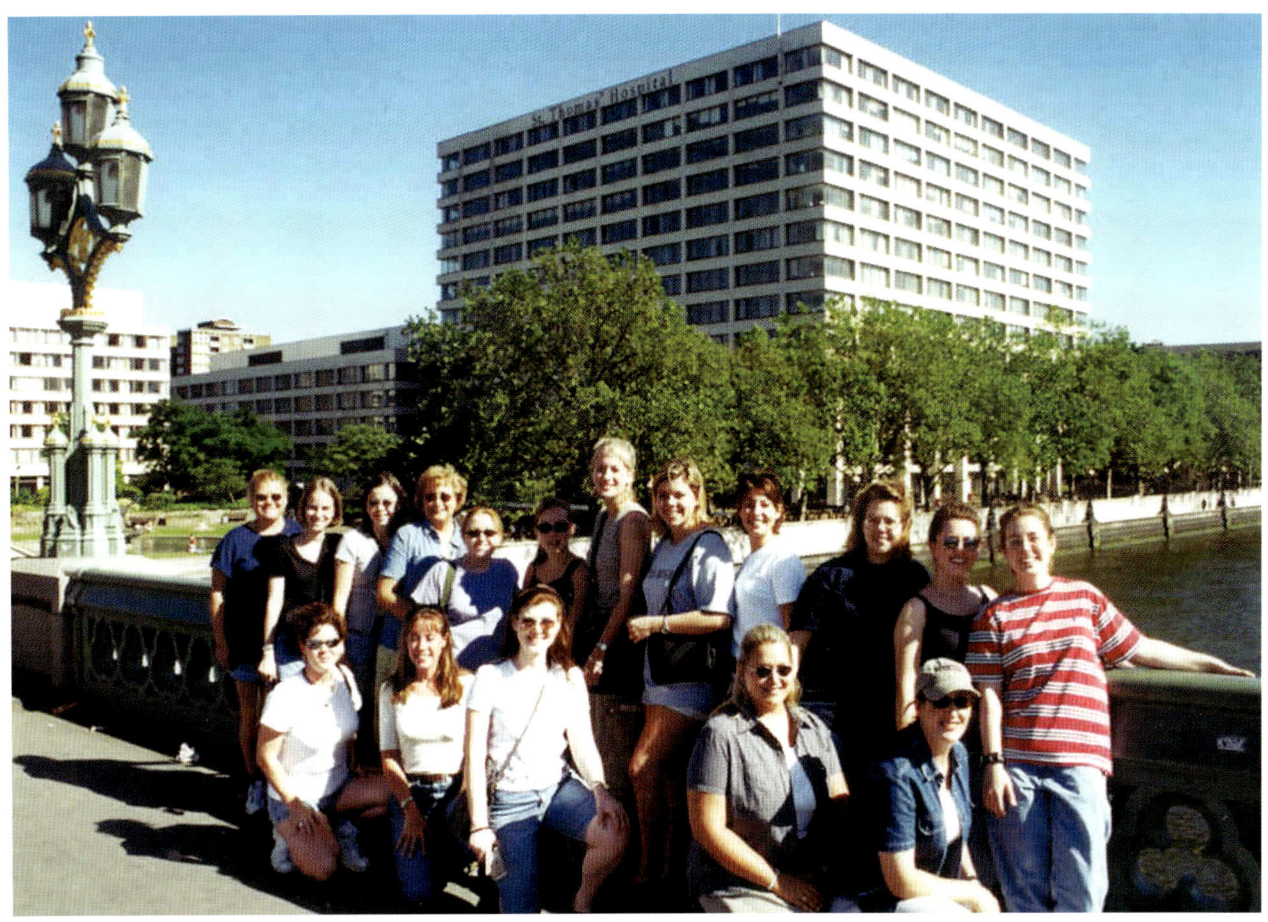

Students in front of St. Thomas' Hospital, London.

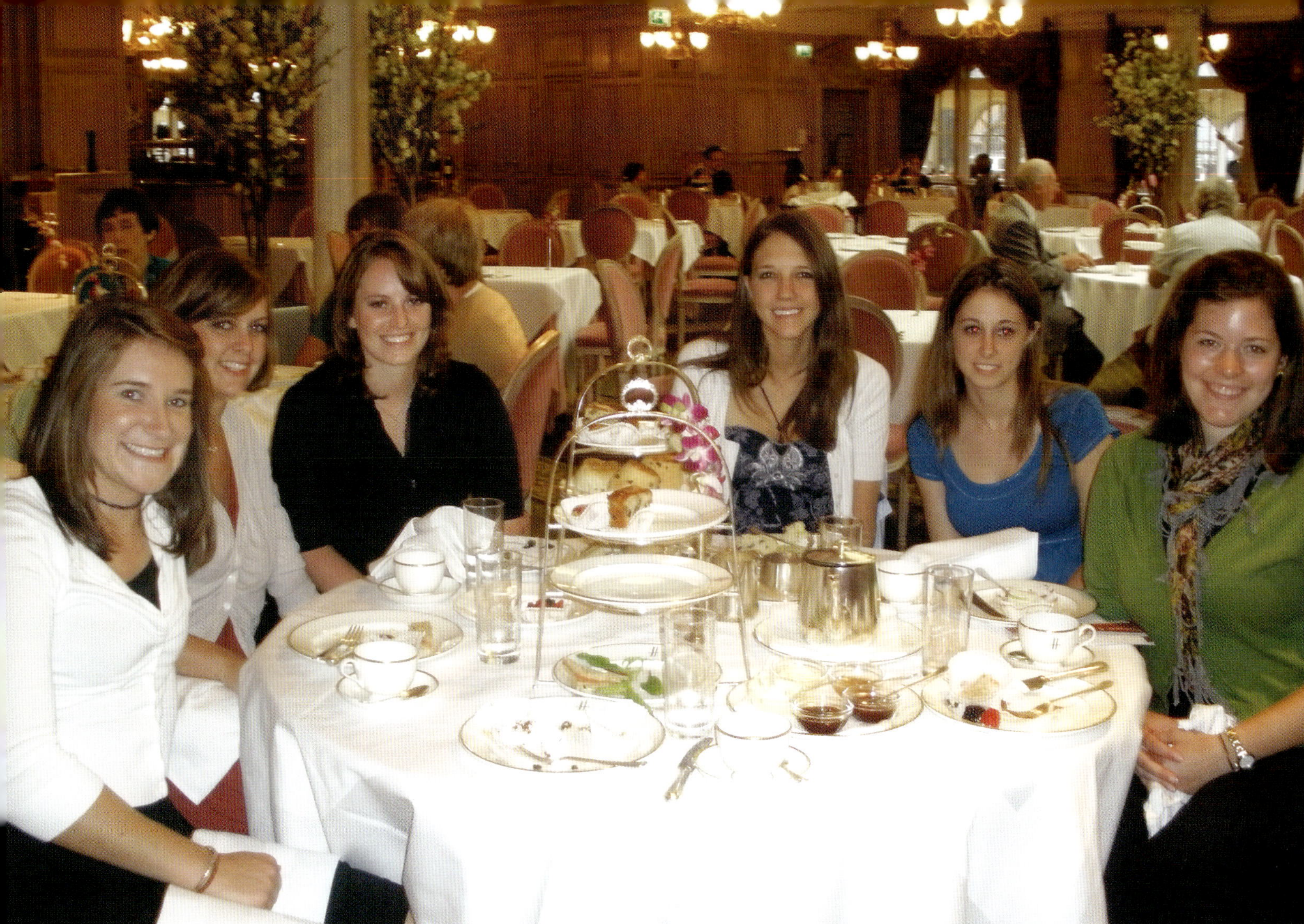

Students at High Tea, Harrods in London, 2008.

Students considered this course helpful and educational. One student reported in the course evaluations that "viewing the autopsy was the best part; getting to see the human anatomy like that was amazing and very educational." Another stated, "The strength of the course was being able to listen to those in the fields of practice that we are learning about. Actually seeing faces to go along with the job descriptions was very helpful."

Graduate Programs

The master of science in nursing (MSN) program began in 2001 and currently has three tracks from which students may choose: nurse administration and leadership, clinical nurse leadership, and nurse education. The original program prepared students to become clinical nurse specialists in medical-surgical nursing.

The nurse administration and leadership track prepares the graduate with knowledge, skills, and abilities to manage and lead nursing units or departments at the highest level to assure quality patient outcomes. Accreditation was granted for the MSN program by the Texas Board of Nursing in 2001. The Commission on Collegiate Nursing Education voluntary accreditation was granted in 2003 (Burns 2003).

The clinical nurse leader (CNL) is an "advanced generalist" who supervises the care of a group of patients, evaluates their risks and outcomes, and coordinates their care with other health care professionals. The CNL role focuses on evidence-based practice, safety, quality, risk reduction, and cost containment. With the development of the CNL track, an academic partnership with Texas Health Resources was created to enhance the care delivery system, which includes twenty-seven acute care and short-stay hospitals (Clark and Weeks 2017). Reflecting upon the successes of the partnership, administrators noted enhanced patient outcomes, high CNL job satisfaction, presentations, and publications as significant outcomes (Clark and Baker 2014).

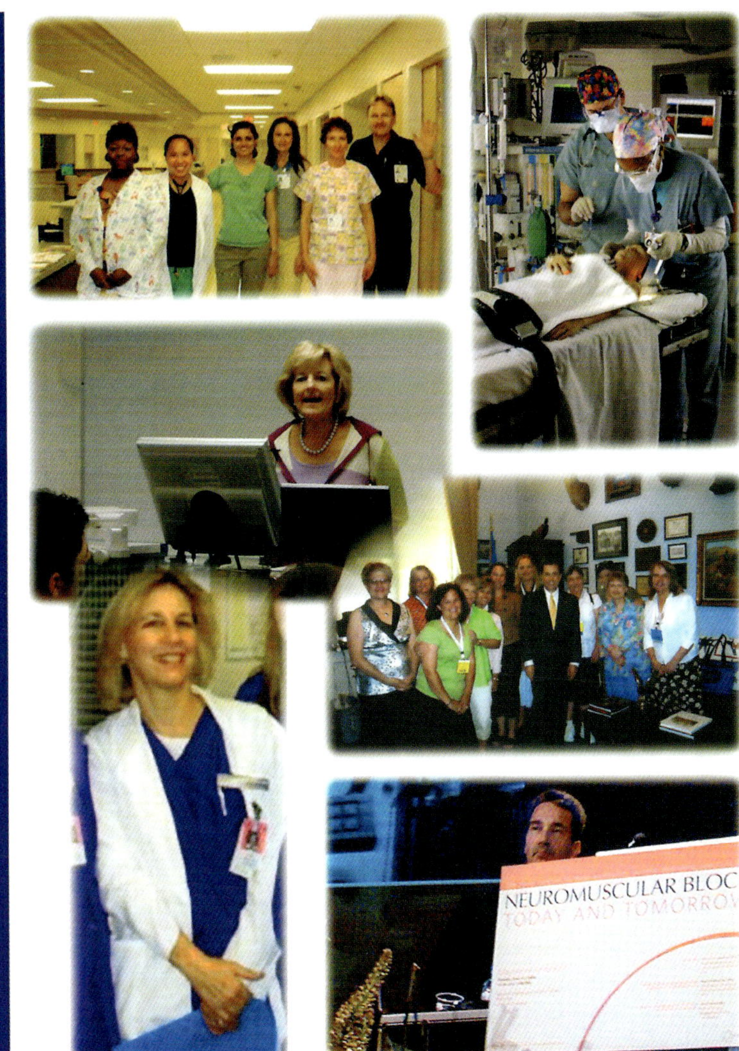

Inaugural 2009 DNP Program Graduates.

The nurse educator is a teacher, scholar, and collaborator who is responsible for the scholarship of teaching, discovery, application, and integration. These educators may practice in academia, staff development, or community settings where they assume leadership in curriculum, instruction, and evaluation. The first class of seven

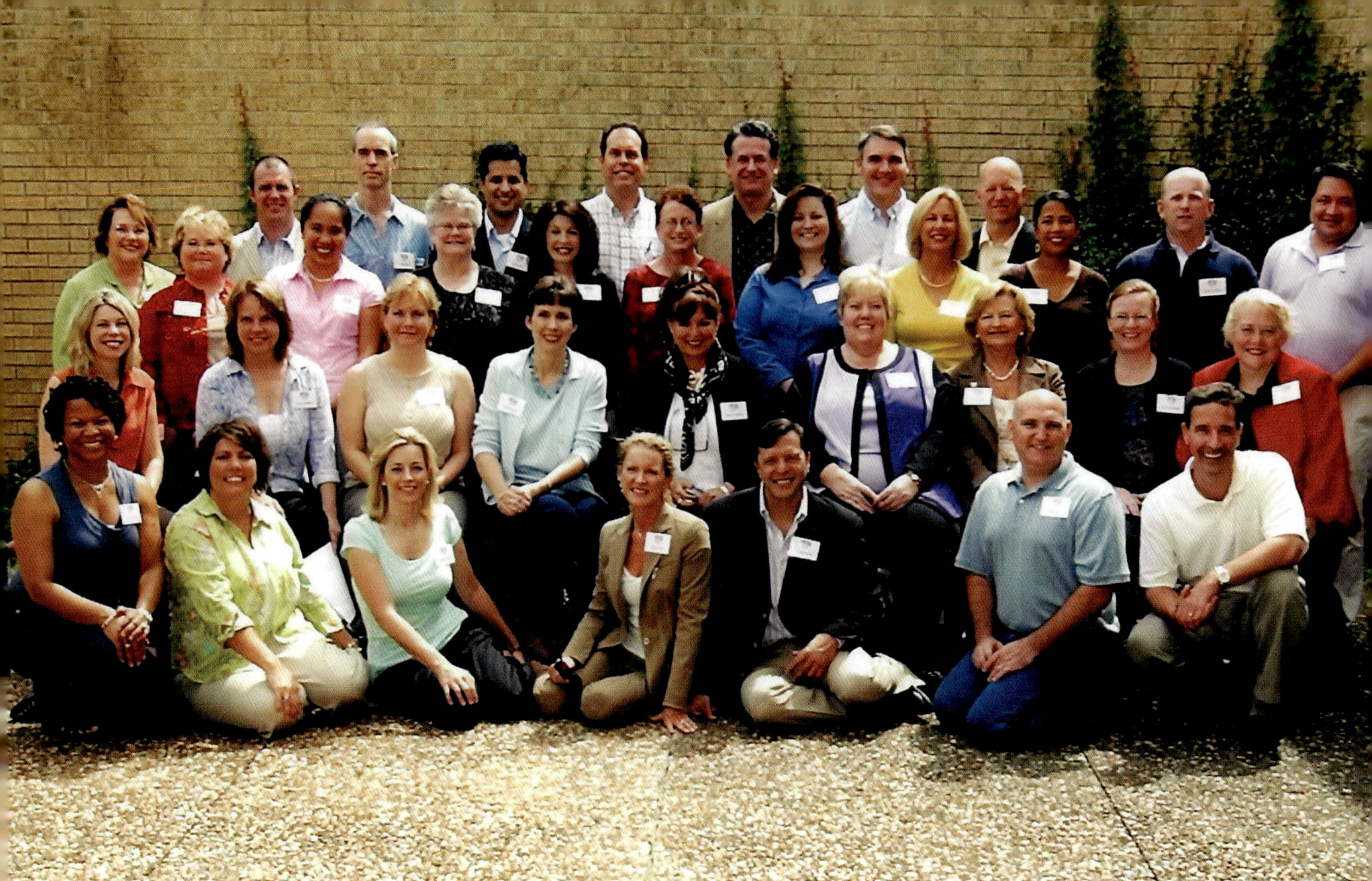

First DNP graduates.

MSN students graduated in 2004, as reported by Burns in the HSN annual report for 2003–04 (Harris College of Nursing Archives).

In 2007, the post-master's DNP program began by opening admission to advanced practice registered nurses (APRNs). Nurse administrators and executives were subsequently admitted to this program in 2009 (Baker, pers. comm., 2018). The DNP program prepares individuals to lead efforts in solving complex health care issues and developing new health care opportunities. Graduates of the DNP program are prepared for clinical leadership in a variety of settings: health care facilities, government agencies, and educational settings. The DNP program responds to the Institute of Medicine's call for schools of nursing to double the number of nurses with a doctorate (PhD or DNP) by 2020. The program is also in line with TCU's mission: "Learning to Change the World." DNP students at TCU are charged with "Making a Difference in Healthcare" (TCU 2017-2018 Graduate Catalog). The program is accredited by the Commission on Collegiate Nursing Education.

Selected Activities of DNP Graduates

Graduates from the DNP program have served in a variety of roles since completing their studies at TCU. Mindy Whitten (2009) has served on the health care reform committee for the state of Oklahoma. Mark Welliver (2009) is coeditor of *Drug/Drug Interactions,* which was published in 2016. He also was appointed director of research for Sunbelt Anesthesia Services. Juan Quintana (2009), the president of Sleepy Anesthesia, served as president of the Texas Association of Nurse Anesthetists from 2005 to 2006. In 2010, Quintana became the first certified registered nurse anesthetist to serve on the Medicare Evidence Development and Coverage Advisory Committee, an independent body that provides the Medicare agency guidance and expert advice on the science and technology affecting health care delivery.

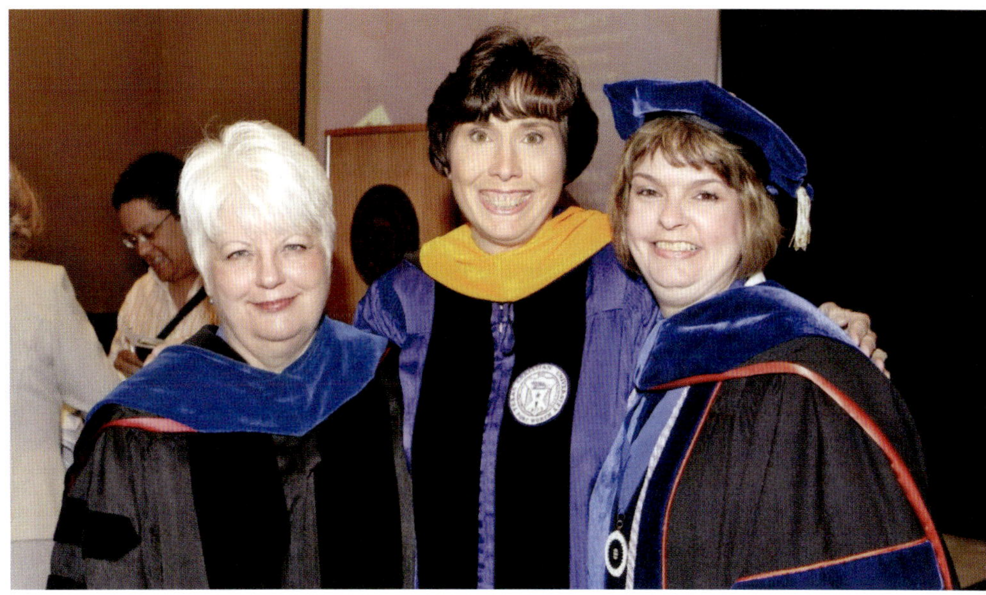

L-R, Paulette Burns, Susan Weeks, and Kathy Baker at 2009 graduation.

Robin Christian (2009) was the founding director of the Joanna Briggs Institute Collaborating Center at the University of Mississippi Medical Center. Suzanne Staebler (2010) was selected the 2011 recipient of the Distinguished Service in Neonatal Nursing Award by the National Association of Neonatal Nurses. Mae Centeno (2010) was featured on the evening news with Katie Couric, where she discussed "Turning Heart Failure into Heart Success," which covered work at Baylor University Medical Center to reduce heart failure readmissions.

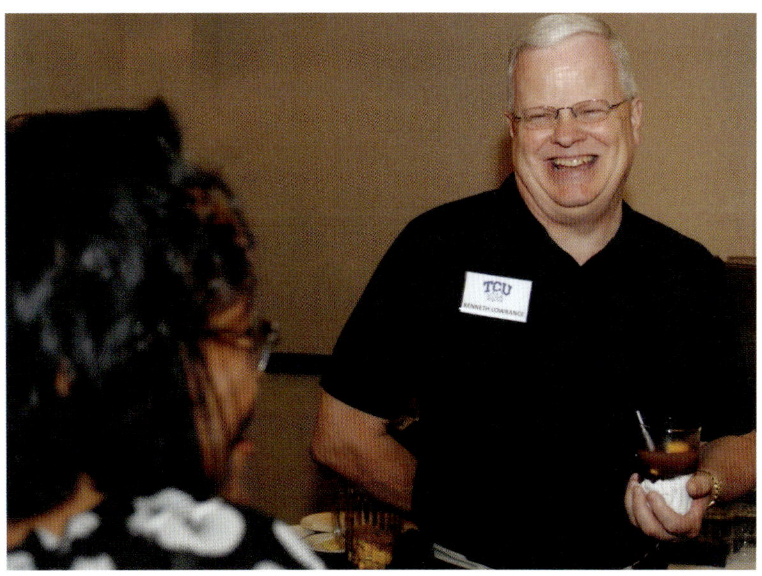

Kenneth Lowrance as student, 2009.

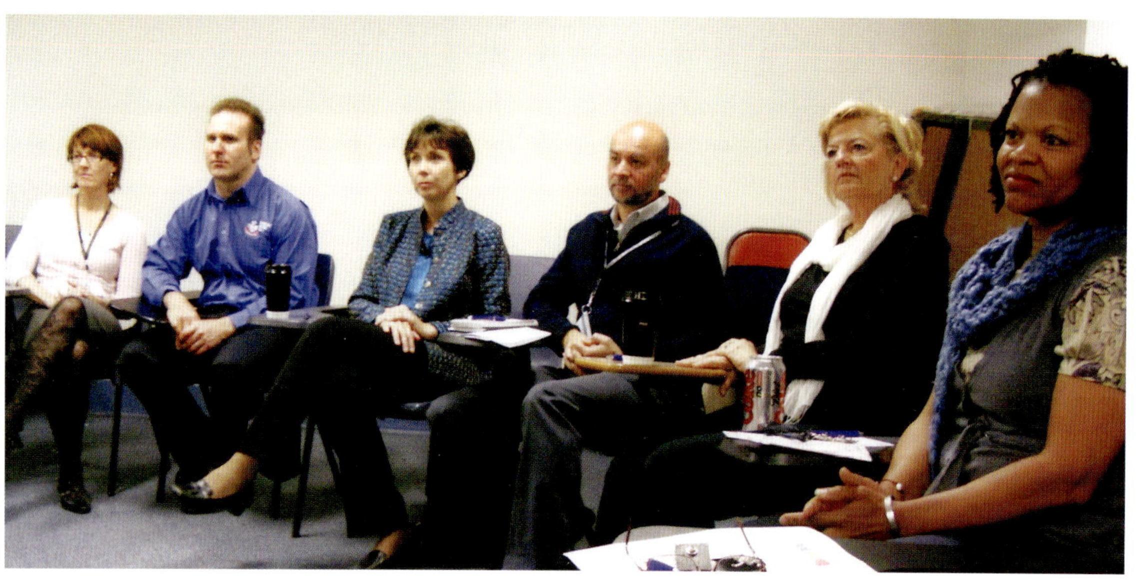

(Above) Discussion with students about Joanna Briggs Institute, 2008.

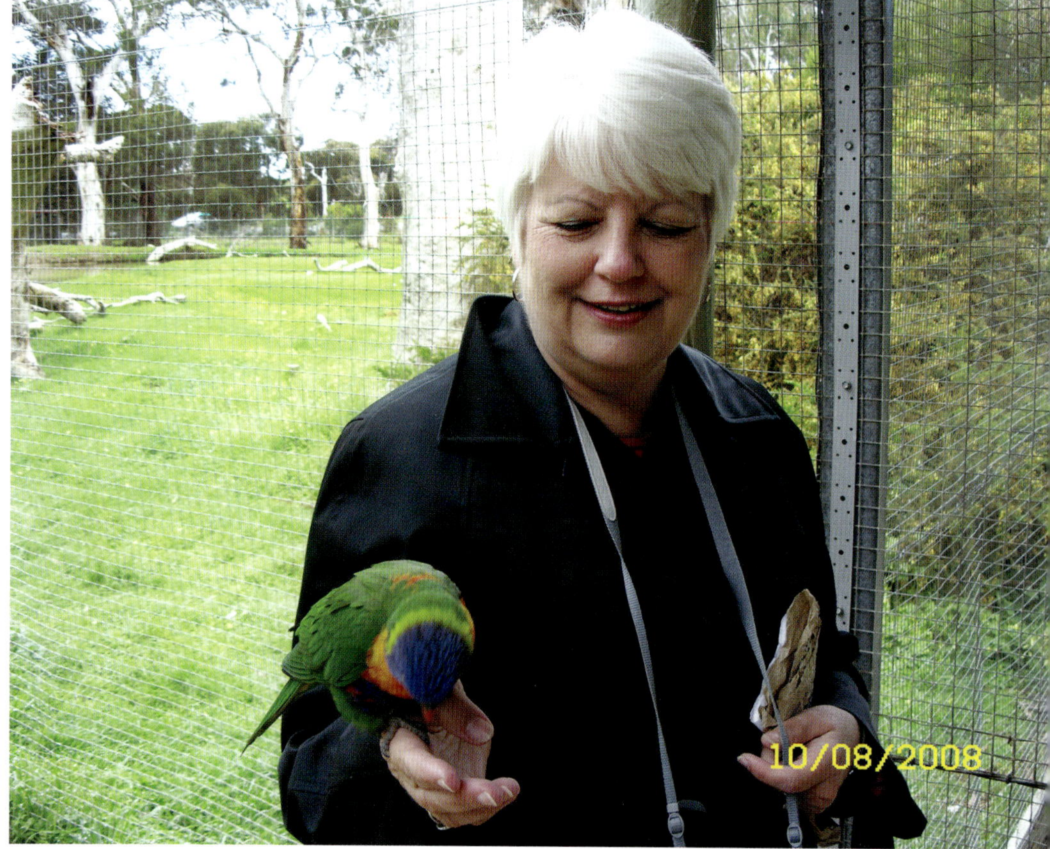

(Right) Paulette Burns in Australia with parrot during participation in JBI program, 2008.

ALUMNI EXAMPLES OF CHANGING ROLES

Defining the Role of the Nurse as a Nurse Educator and Researcher:

An Interview with Danielle Walker, BSN 2003 (TCU)

Motivated by the desire to help people, Danielle Walker initially thought she wanted to be a doctor. After volunteering at a local children's hospital and working with a hematologist during the first few summers of college, she observed that frequently doctors did not have as much time to spend with patients as she wanted to spend (Danielle Walker, pers. comm., 2018). The doctors' focus was on the disease instead of the person. As an avid reader, Walker also explored nursing through the works of Clara Barton, the founder of the American Red Cross, and Louisa May Alcott, an author and nurse. Learning about contemporary nursing from her parents' friends, who were nurses, was also influential in her decision to become a nurse.

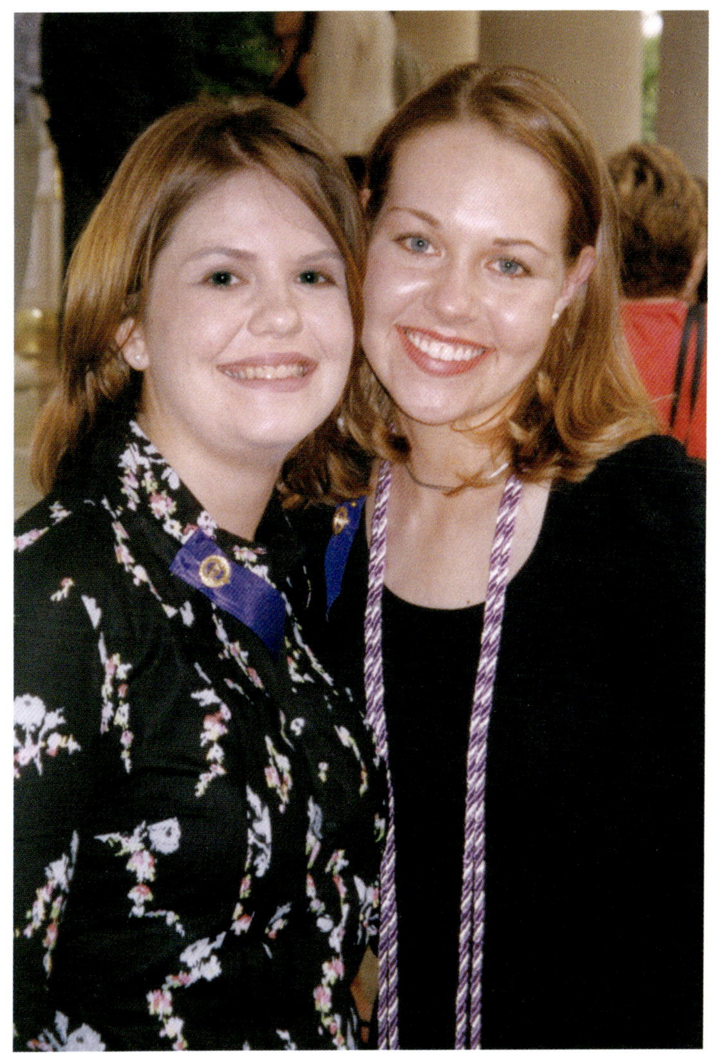

Danielle Walker and Melissa Leahy, 2003.

Based on her student experiences in maternity nursing, Walker knew that after graduation she wanted to work in labor and delivery. After working for three years in Parkland Hospital's Labor and Delivery Triage department and working a few more years in an operating room setting, she pursued a master's degree in nursing education. Originally, her desire was to focus on midwifery, but advanced practice nursing degrees were in transition. Parkland was transitioning to a master's level program, and no other midwifery program existed within geographical reach. After reflection, Walker realized a favorite part of her day was helping patients take care of themselves. Additionally, she began advocating for and empowering other nurses to provide

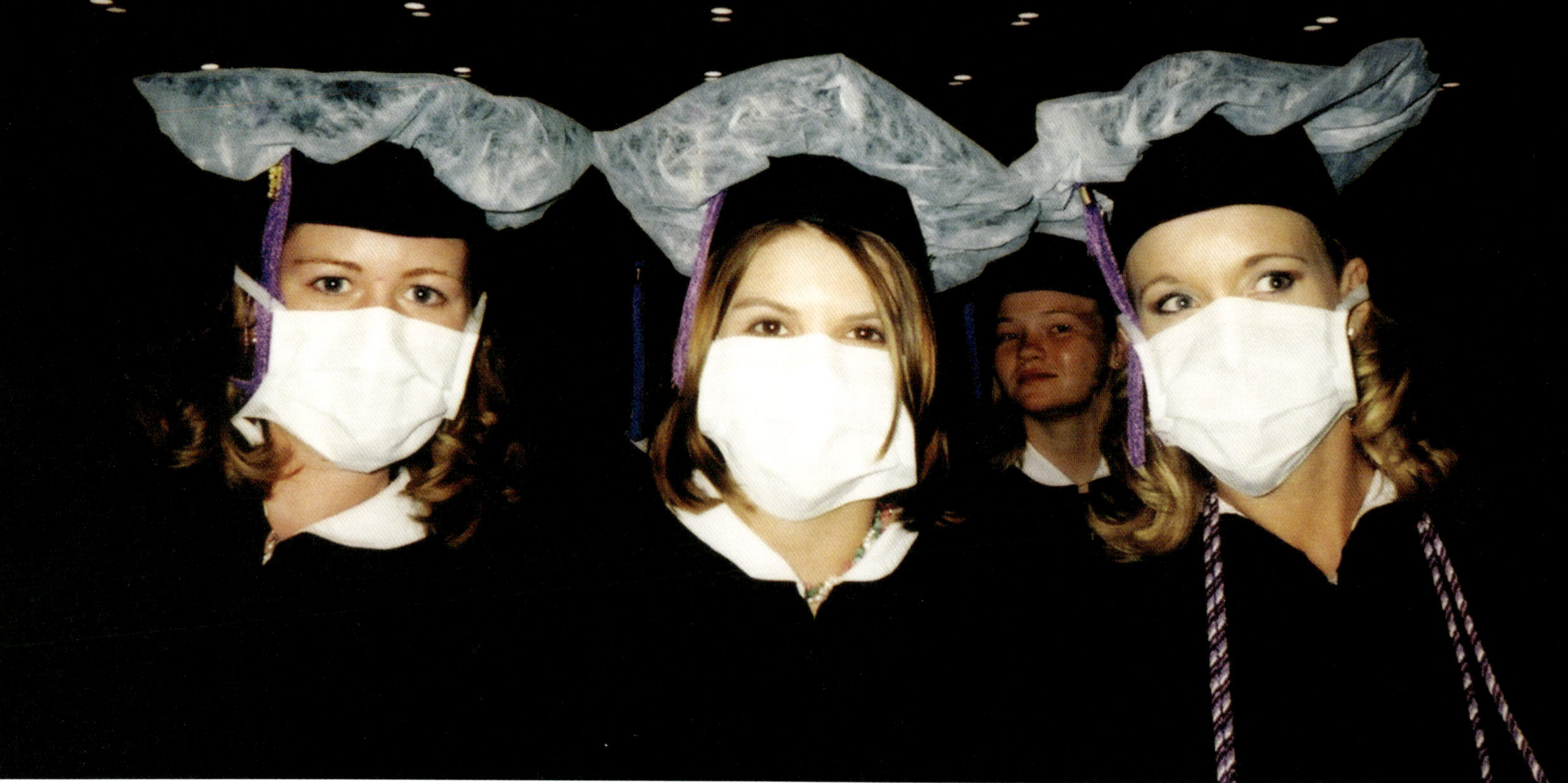

Danielle Walker and classmates at graduation, 2003.

safe and effective nursing care. This led Walker to pursue a master's degree in nursing education from Texas Woman's University in 2009 and ultimately a PhD in nursing education from the University of Texas Medical Branch at Galveston.

"Why do we teach this in a certain way?" "How can we make it better?" "How does this teaching method lead to better nursing care and health outcomes?" (Danielle Walker, pers. comm., 2018). These questions became the impetus for Walker's focus on nursing education research.

Walker currently teaches both public health courses and a course called Member of the Healthcare Team, which explores health care systems in the United States and around the world. In these courses, she uses a variety of pedagogies emphasizing service learning, reflective practice, and experiential learning. When asked about the challenges of conducting nursing education research, Walker notes that while she had been supported in her work at TCU, the science of nursing education research is still developing in the larger academic nursing community. Her current project, the development of a Health Literacy Knowledge and Experiences Survey, will provide a reliable and valid tool to assess the knowledge and experience of nursing students and practicing nurses. Having a tool that can assess gaps in knowledge and experience is the first step in improving health literacy proficiency (Danielle Walker, pers. comm., 2018).

Defining the Role of the Nurse as a Foreign Service Medical Provider:

An Interview with Dr. Deborah Edwards, DNP 2009

Deborah Edwards credits her mother, who was "empathetic, a patient advocate, a teacher, a motivator, a leader, and a team player" for being the motivating factor for Edwards to become a nurse (Deborah Edwards, pers. comm., 2018). With a desire to remain close to patient care, she selected the family nurse practitioner role, which "defined her as a professional" (Deborah Edwards, pers. comm., 2018). She then pursued a DNP and credits her capstone project with providing her with new insights into research. Combined with activities of the Joanna Briggs Institute, her days as a DNP student solidified for her the importance of evidence-based research. She also acknowledges that the study abroad program in Adelaide, Australia, enlightened her worldview of culture and health care.

Although Edwards and her family were not directly impacted by losses of family members, homes, or jobs following Hurricane Katrina, the displacement of various Veteran Affairs Hospital Clinics in Louisiana influenced her move to North Carolina, where a physician she worked with recruited her for the Department of State Foreign Service.

As a Foreign Service Medical Provider, Edwards assumed the role of a primary

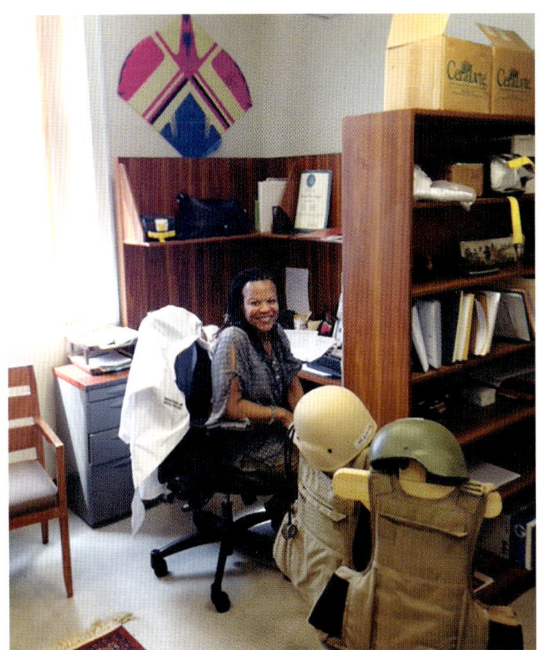

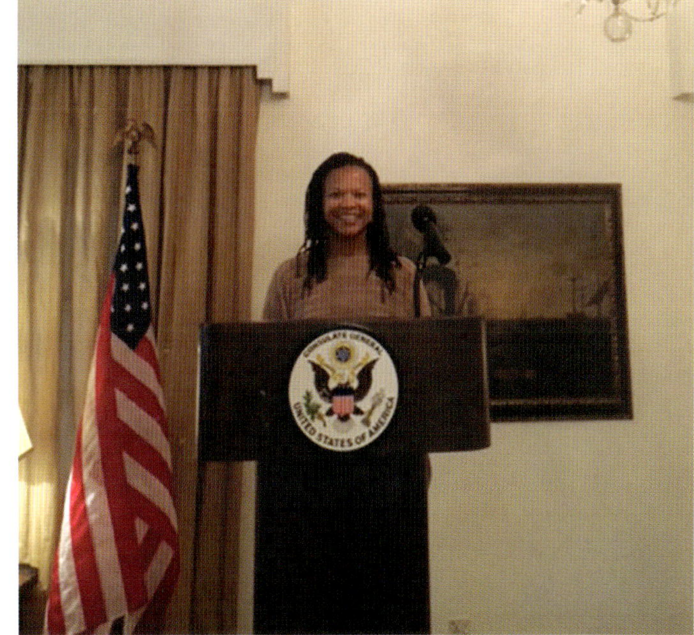

(Left) Deborah Edwards at work in office in Karachi, 2009.
(Right) A presentation by Deborah Edwards, 2009.

care provider for Foreign Service officers and their families on directed assignments to embassies and consulates outside of the United States. Currently, she serves in Karachi, Pakistan. Foreign Service Medical Providers are considered US diplomats in the Foreign Service "with the overall mission of promoting peace, supporting prosperity, and protecting American citizens while advancing the interests of the US abroad." There are currently 127 Medical Providers serving in the 270 consulates and embassies throughout the world (Deborah Edwards, pers. comm., 2018).

Noting both the challenges and rewards of the role, Edwards points out that some of the US embassies and consulates are in spartan and difficult environments. In many developing countries, Medical Providers are faced with complicated medical situations on an ongoing basis. These can range from "complicated and emergent cardiac events to serious infectious disease cases like malaria or dengue" (Deborah Edwards, pers. comm., 2018).

Rewards of the role are many, including having the opportunity to work in embassies, consulates, and other diplomatic missions around the world; experiencing various cultures and customs firsthand; and knowing that the work has an impact upon the world (Deborah Edwards, pers. comm., 2018).

Defining the Role of a Nurse Officer with the Indian Health Service:

An Interview with Traci Murray, BSN 2009 (TCU)

Traci Murray's motivation to become a nurse grew out of her enjoyment of the sciences coupled with her passion to help others (Traci Murray, pers. comm., 2018). While a student, she found community/public health nursing to be a unique area of nursing that she found both interesting and challenging.

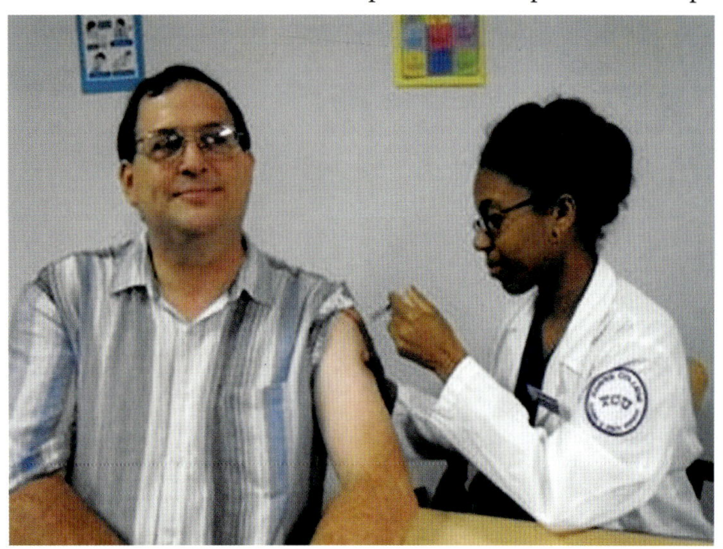

Traci Murray giving Dr. Cheek a flu vaccination, 2009.

Murray was introduced to the US Public Health Service (USPHS) Commissioned Corps as a student, when Capt. James Dickens spoke to her class about opportunities for nurses. Several years later, she accepted a public health training opportunity with the CDC and there met her mentor, Cdr. Anita Pullani, who was a USPHS officer. Pullani encouraged her to apply to USPHS. Murray credits Dickens with "planting the seed" and Pullani with "watering it"

(Traci Murray, pers. comm., 2018).

Learning activities at Harris College influenced Murray's current role as she found herself intrigued with the focus on "true primary prevention and population health" (Traci Murray, pers. comm., 2018). Following encouragement from her mentor, Pamela Frable, she applied to the CDC Public Health Associate Program, which she calls a "stepping stone" to a fulfilling career. Her role as a nurse cadet in the Army ROTC at TCU helped her adjust to her role as a nurse officer in USPHS. Involvement in Chi Eta Phi Sorority also helped her develop leadership and communication skills (Traci Murray, pers. comm., 2018).

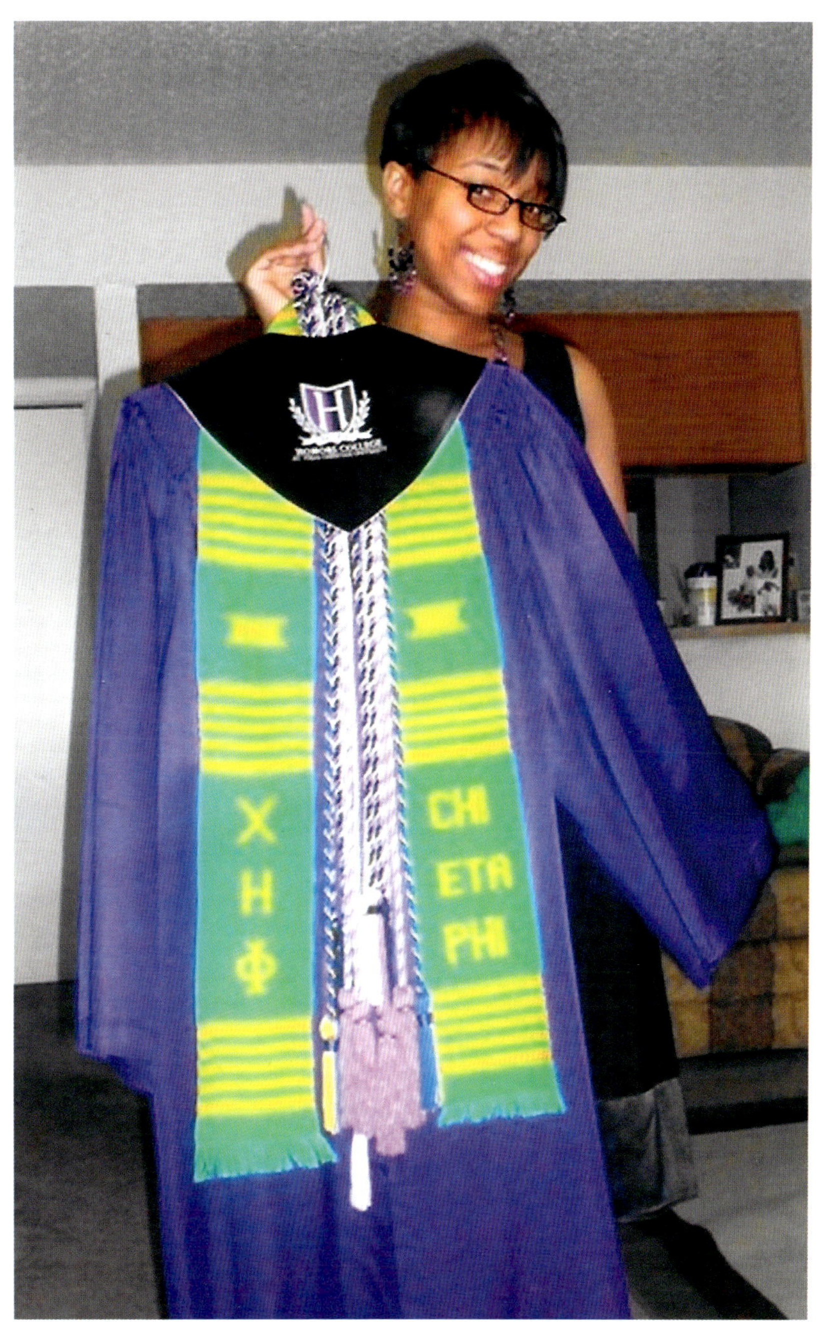

Traci Murray with graduation gown, 2017.

Murray currently serves as a nurse officer with the Indian Health Service (IHS) on the Navajo reservation in Shiprock, New Mexico. She has worked in an outpatient clinic, in nursing education, and in administrative settings. As an officer, she is committed to maintaining professional and physical fitness "to ensure I am ready to deploy with the corps for any public health emergency" (Traci Murray, pers. comm., 2018). She remains active in Chi Eta Phi Sorority and other professional organizations.

The major challenges in the IHS are the limited resources available to meet the health care needs of its patient population.

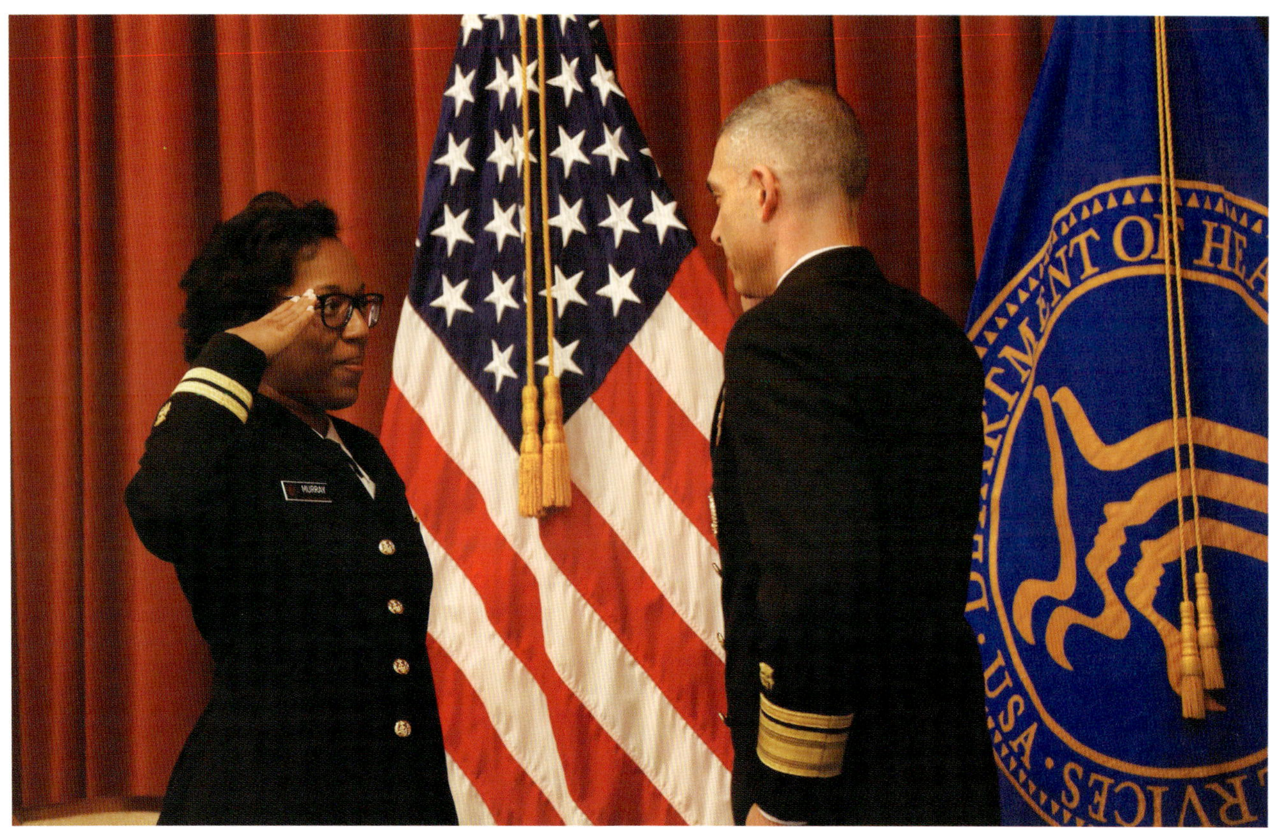

Traci graduating from USPHS's Officer Basic Course in Maryland, 2017.

Facilities and units are significantly short staffed and operate on tight budgets.

Nevertheless she has found her career to be "incredibly rewarding." Looking toward the future, she notes many exciting roles for nurse officers with agencies like the CDC and the US Food and Drug Administration, and she looks forward to opportunities for continued service.

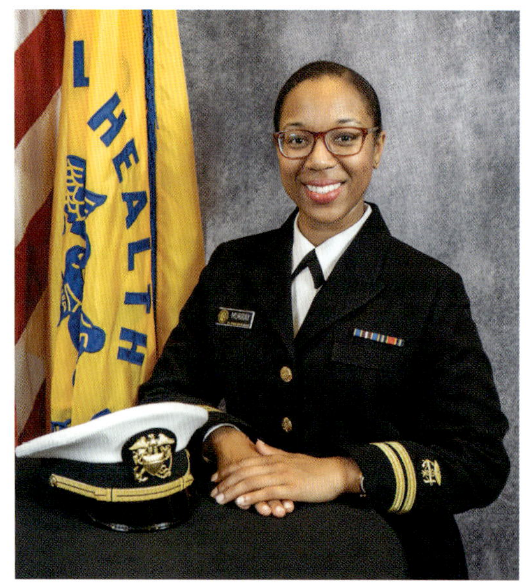

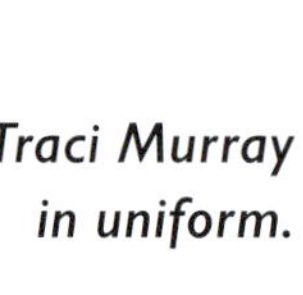

Traci Murray in uniform.

Defining the Role of the Certified Registered Nurse Anesthetist:

An Interview with Juan Quintana, CRNA, DNP 2009

Juan Quintana always knew he wanted to be in health care to help people. After spending eight years as an ICU nurse caring for critically ill patients, he realized he "wanted a stronger role in the care of [his] patients." He chose to become a certified registered nurse anesthetist (CRNA) because he believed that it "emphasized the ability of the health care provider to care for each patient as if they were my family, my mother, my child." He saw the role of the CRNA as one that involved both leadership and patient care on a daily basis and concluded that he had found his niche (Juan Quintana, pers. comm., 2018).

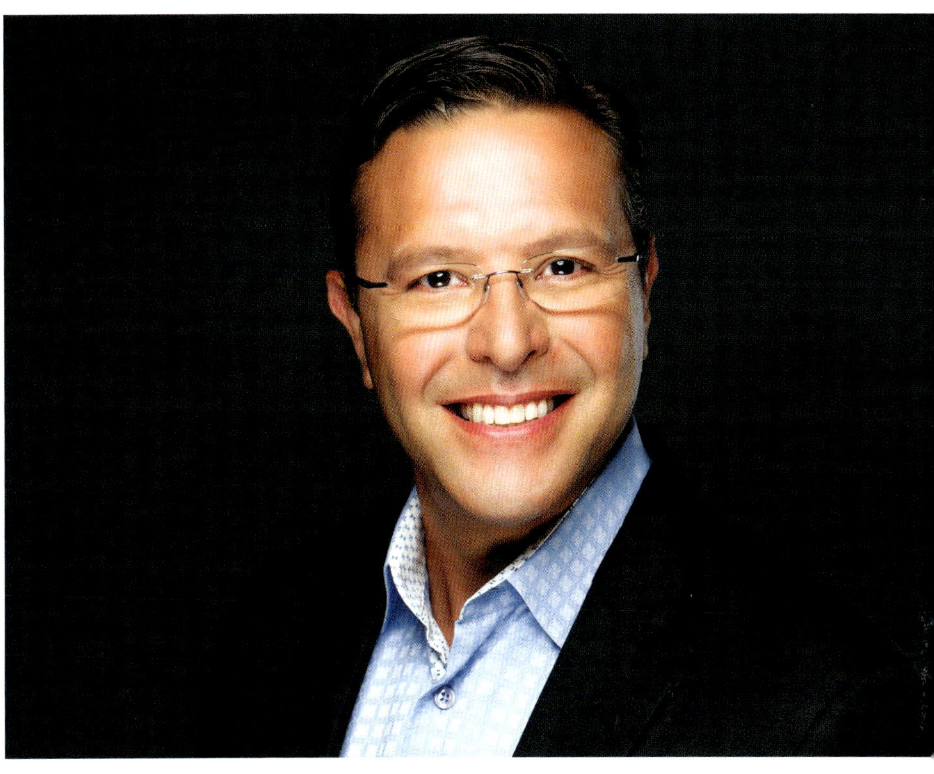

Dr. Juan Quintanta, 2018.

Quintana credited the DNP program with providing opportunities to identify and assume leadership roles at the state level. He realized that with the DNP degree he could move forward to make positive changes at the national level, stating that the faculty members at TCU were instrumental in encouraging all forms of leadership and helping students realize that barriers could become opportunities (Juan Quintana, pers. comm., 2018).

One year after obtaining his master's degree, Quintana founded Sleepy Anesthesia. His goal was to show the health care community that CRNAs could provide outstanding, high-quality health care in a cost-effective manner. The company subsequently diversified to include the Anesthesia Management Company, an anesthesia billing company and turnkey educational company that teaches the business of anesthesia to both graduate students and CRNAs in practice.

Quintana served on the board of the American Association of Nurse Anesthetists and was the association's president from 2015–16. During his tenure as president, the organization and its members struggled for "reimbursement equality at the national level and tr[ied] to gain independent practice of all APRNs/CRNAs at the Veterans Health Administration so that veterans would receive better access to health care services" (Juan Quintana, pers. comm., 2018).

Quintana identified protectionism as the biggest challenge for an APRN in the health care system, where he believed that health care administrators and physician trade organizations were worried that APRNs were trying to take over the system (Juan Quintana, pers. comm., 2018). He continued by saying that APRNs, just like their physician colleagues, educate themselves to improve the health and well-being of patients.

Quintana said the most rewarding aspect of his role was providing outstanding care to patients each and every day by reducing their anxiety, fear, and pain in times of stress. He also acknowledges the privilege of watching CRNAs he taught succeed in their own right. He says that the future of the APRN is brilliant.

CHALLENGE TWO
Research to Determine What Effects Variables in Nursing Care Have on the Health of People

Context and Trends

The Summer Genetics Institute (SGI) was established by the National Institute of Nursing Research (NINR) based at the National Institute of Health (NIH). SGI is a two-month, full-time summer research-training program for faculty, graduate students, and advanced practice nurses (Grady 2016). In 2005–06, nursing celebrated twenty years at NIH and contributed to the NIH Roadmap Initiative to identify and address opportunities and gaps in research. The areas of scientific focus in the strategic plan were determined by identifying areas where "the needs are greatest and for which NINR-supported research could have the largest impact" (Grady 2016, 4). These included symptom science, wellness, self-management, and end-of-life and palliative care.

STTI's collaboration with a variety of professional organizations during the first decade of the 2000s increased the number of research grants available. Eleven grants, with funds provided through shared resources, came from the Western Institute of Nursing (2003), the Hospice and Palliative Nurses Foundation (2003), the Canadian Nurses Foundation (2004), the Association of Nurses in AIDS Care (2004), the Midwest Nursing Research Society (2004), the National League for Nursing (2007), the Alpha Eta Collaborative Research Grant (2008), the Council for the Advancement of Nursing Science (2008), the Southern Nursing Research Society (2008), and the STTI/ATI Educational Assessment Nursing Research Grant (2009). In addition, STTI provided funds for the Doris Bloch Research Award and the Joan K. Stout, RN, Research Grant (Thomas, pers. comm., 2018).

Support for nursing education research was first offered by the National League for Nursing (NLN) in 2000. Funding became available to NLN members to develop, design, and conduct research studies with potential for broad-based significance for future decision-making and policy establishment at both institutional and national levels with the goal of transforming nursing education (National League for Nursing 2008).

Selected Nursing Research Grants

Faculty members' research activities from 2000 to 2010 consisted of both small studies and larger research programs. Programs of research were implemented by teams of faculty members, students, and colleagues outside the school. Jo Nell Wells, Patricia Bradley, and Carolyn Cagle received the first national research award from NINR to the Harris School of Nursing faculty for the study "Mexican American Caregiver Experience" in the 2003–04 academic year. During the following academic year, Lazelle Benefield was funded by NINR to study "Distance Caregiving of Cognitively Impaired Elders Living Alone at Home." Additional funding was received from the Hillcrest Foundation to build and equip Dennis Cheek's nursing research lab.

During the same decade, the Beta Alpha Chapter of Sigma Theta Tau International awarded eight research grants. Additionally, fifteen grants were awarded from Hogstel Gerontological funds to support selected studies. Topics of study included "Complementary Therapies used by Older Adults in Tarrant County" (Kathy Baldwin and Dennis Cheek), "Residential-to-Institutional Relocation Stress" (Charles Walker), and "A Study of Older Adults' Use of Hospice Services in Texas" (Barbara Raudonis).

FACULTY RESEARCH: SELECTED EXAMPLES

Health Concerns of LGBTQ Elders

Beginning in 2002, Charles Walker led an interprofessional (nursing and social work) research team exploring health concerns of LGBTQ elders in long-term care facilities, as this population was unrepresented in the literature. This study led to a second focus in 2014 that addressed the life journeys and health care challenges of older transgender adults and their partners, the "most marginalized and least understood LGBT population" (Charles Walker, pers. comm., 2018). The primary method of data collection was theoretical case studies.

Outcomes revealed the individual life stories of LGBTQ elders and contributed to a broader knowledge base about elder diversity, including such practice improvements as trans-sensitive nursing assessment and interventions. This program of research served to overturn heterosexist biases and transgender stereotypes that could interfere with care ideals and healthy client outcomes. Future research goals include synthesizing theories used in previous work—including lifespan, empowerment, liberation theology, radical feminism, strength-based pedagogy, and narrative inquiry—to explain the experiences of older transgender adults (Charles Walker, pers. comm., 2018).

The Experience of the Mexican American Family Cancer Caregiver

Jo Nell Wells led a research team funded by the NIH and the NINR from 2004 to 2006 to describe the experience of the Mexican American Family Cancer Caregiver (MAFCG). The initial study identified unmet caregiver needs and generated a theoretical basis for further studies. The team's work has served to support family caregivers and thereby indirectly support cancer patients' physical, mental, emotional, social, and psychological needs (Jo Nell Wells, pers. comm., 2018).

The research that started with the foundational NIH/NINR funding has continued with additional funding from the TCU Harris College and the Center for Oncology Education and Research (2015–18). Each project has built on past work to address an unstudied area in cancer care. The team projects have led to the development of evidence-based learning materials, prepared in English and Spanish at a low literacy level, to address targeted needs of MAFCGs. This work seeks to relieve caregiver suffering and improve the lives of cancer patients and their families. It also addresses the need for controlled trial evidence supporting clinical interventions for MAFCGs. Findings from the work are intended to provide the field with objective data in an era of health care cost containment and respond to health care literature that seeks priority evaluation of psychosocial interventions to improve family caregiver outcomes. Further studies on a wider scale are planned in order to give voice to an underserved ethnic minority group that experiences an undue burden of cancer (Jo Nell Wells, pers. comm., 2018). This interdisciplinary team has included TCU faculty (Patricia Bradley, Carolyn Cagle, Tracy Dietz, and Andrea Erwin); *promotoras de salud,* or community health workers (Maria Quintana and Gabriela Hernandez); and numerous TCU nursing students who have served as research assistants.

Faculty Role as Editor-in-Chief: Research-Related Journal

Charles Walker contributed to knowledge dissemination in his role as editor-in-chief of the *Journal of Theory Construction & Testing* from 2003–17. The publication was a niche journal focusing on theory development in nursing and related fields such as kinesiology, education, and philosophy of science. Manuscripts were submitted from countries around the globe, including Canada, Indonesia, Iran, New Zealand, Norway, and South Africa (Charles Walker, pers. comm., 2018).

During Walker's tenure as editor-in-chief, the journal's mission shifted from exclusive attention to the work of nurse theorists and researchers to include articles related to pedagogical theory, abductive logic, and pastoral care. Walker indicates his "greatest professional reward" came from developing novice scholars and showing them how to represent their work and express their findings in the most persuasive way possible (Charles Walker, pers. comm., 2018).

Faculty Role as Editor

Kathy Baker became the editor of *Gastroenterology Nursing*. This journal keeps gastroenterology nurses and associates informed of the latest developments in research, evidenced-based practice techniques, equipment, diagnostics, and therapy. It is the official journal of the Society of Gastroenterology Nursing and Associates and the Canadian Society of Gastroenterology Nurses and Associates (*Gastroenterology Nursing* 2018).

Student Research Activities

Three BSN students participated in the Seventh Annual Harris College of Nursing & Health Sciences Student Research Symposium. One of the three award winners, Kate Lunati, had her manuscript selected for the *Undergraduate Journal of Research and Creativity*.

ALUMNI EXAMPLES OF RESEARCH

Defining the Role of the Nurse Researcher:

An Interview with Jessica Grace Smith, BSN 2008 TCU

Jessica Smith was motivated to pursue nursing because of "reciprocal interactions and synergistic exchanges" she shared with her grandmother, whom she helped care for. Smith states that her grandmother passed down familial wisdom that she benefits from today. From these exchanges, she envisioned nursing as a "dynamic career with meaningful engagement with older adults" and "an avenue to improve their lives as well as enhance my own growth and development as a person" (Jessica Smith, pers. comm., 2018).

Working in the Fort Worth health systems as a student and novice nurse, Smith saw how health systems could have a significant impact on nursing and patient outcomes. She became motivated to study the potential influence of work relationships on work environments and how these might affect patient outcomes.

As a young graduate, Smith saw research as an avenue for making significant contributions to the nursing profession. She "became interested in civility even as she experienced uncivil behaviors as a nurse from other nurses" and found uncivil behaviors "a troubling phenomenon that was interfering with full collaboration in patient care" (Jessica Smith, pers. comm., 2018). Following the completion of her dissertation, entitled "RN Perceptions of Coworker Incivility and Collective Efficacy as Influential to Hospital Structures and Outcomes," she was encouraged by her mentors—Pamela Frable of TCU and Karen Morin of the University of Wisconsin-Milwaukee—to pursue a postdoctoral fellowship. She applied for and accepted a postdoctoral fellowship for 2016 through 2018 at the University of Pennsylvania, under the mentorship of Linda Aiken, Eileen Lake, and Matthew McHugh at the Center for Health Outcomes and Policy Research at the University of Pennsylvania.

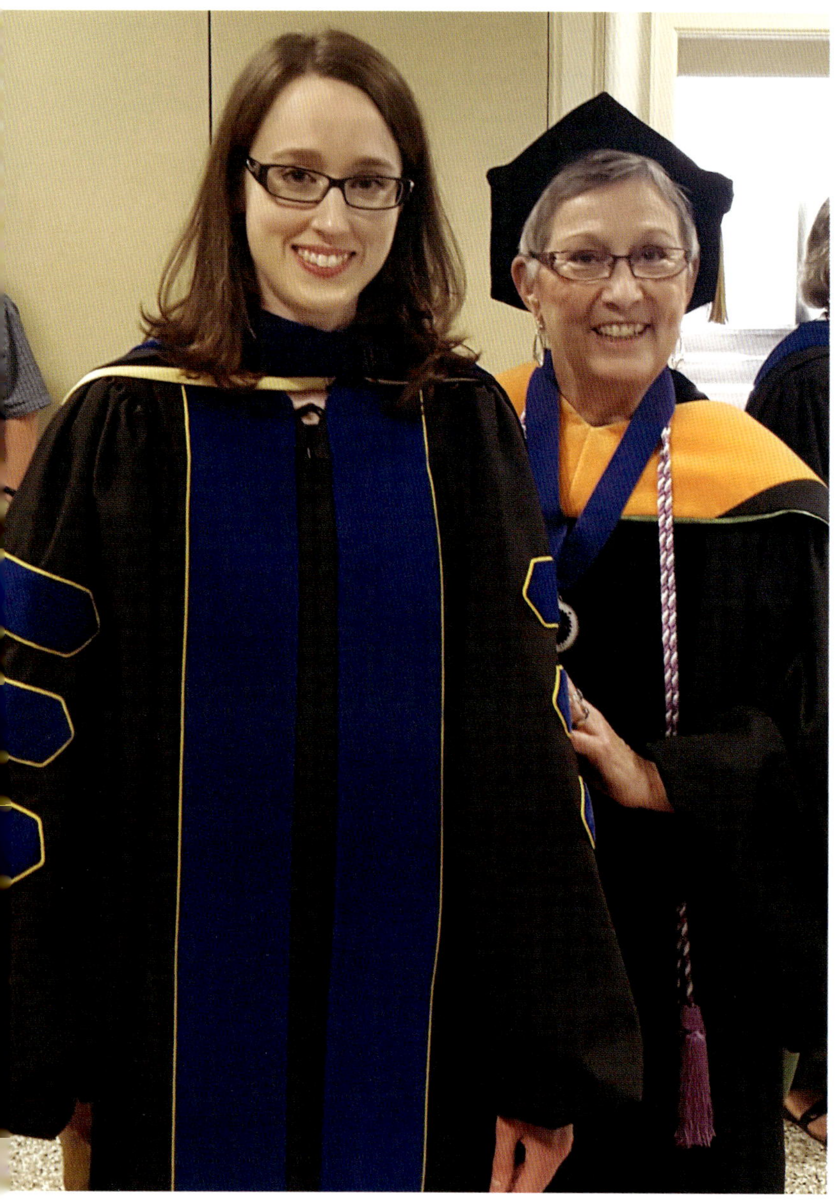
Jessica Grace Smith and Dr. Karen Morin, 2018.

In 2018, Smith published a total of eight manuscripts, five of which support the establishment of better work environments. As an avid researcher, it is her "wholehearted desire to develop and sustain a program of nursing research to extend our understanding of how nursing resources influence nurse and patient outcomes" (Jessica Smith, pers. comm., 2018).

As Smith began her role as a nurse educator at the University of Texas at

Arlington in 2018, it was her aim to be an effective nurse educator and positive role model for students. She further hopes to "dispel common misunderstandings of nursing research and inspire others to see nursing research as a rewarding career path" (Jessica Smith, pers. comm., 2018).

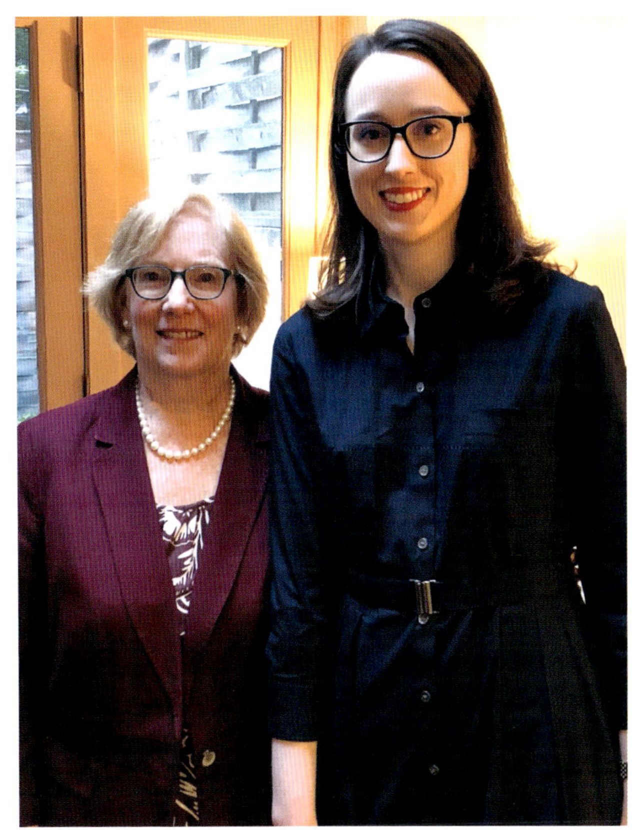

Dr. Linda Aiken and Jessica Grace Smith, 2018.

In summary, in the year 2000, Harris College of Nursing became Harris School of Nursing as a school within the Harris College of Nursing & Health Sciences, along with the addition of Communication Sciences and Disorders, Kinesiology, and Social Work departments to the college, and plans for a School of Nurse Anesthesia. Two centers were established: the Center for Evidence-Based Practice and Research and the Center of Oncology Research and Education. A board of visitors was appointed by Dean Burns in 2008 to assist in fostering a "high level of excellence."

Faculty continued to conduct and disseminate research at local, national, and international levels. An accelerated BSN program was established for individuals with degrees in other disciplines. Study abroad to England and Geneva was available to students of all disciplines in 2000, 2002, 2004, 2008, and 2010. The master of science in nursing (MSN) and the doctor of nursing practice (DNP) graduate programs were established. Graduates of Harris School of Nursing included 906 BSN students, fifty-four MSN students and twenty-three DNP students. The goal of "Connecting to the Past . . . Creating the Future," as celebrated in 2006 at the sixtieth anniversary gala, was still moving forward.

Chapter Six

2010–2018

A Decade of Forward Movement

The 2015 issue of *Harris Magazine* was dedicated to the "doers, dreamers and trailblazers" who helped make the college what it is today—a "vibrant contributor to the health of our community" (Weeks 2015). Stories of students, faculty, and staff members reflect how the college is learning to make a difference in the global community. In 2016, Susan Weeks challenged readers to "take a look . . . and you'll see many points of pride and plenty of reasons to keep moving forward" (Weeks 2016).

The Center for Evidence-Based Practice and Research (CEBPR) was established in Harris College in 2006 as a result of an internal university funding mechanism known as Vision in Action. The CEBPR affiliated with the Joanna Briggs Institute (JBI) in 2009 as a collaborating center, and held an opening ceremony in April 2010 with Anne Wilson from the University of Adelaide as the speaker. JBI is an international not-for-profit research and development unit of the Royal Adelaide Hospital and the University of Adelaide in South Australia. The institute collaborates with international centers to assist in improving health care outcomes throughout the world through the synthesis, transfer, and utilization of evidence identifying feasible, appropriate, meaningful, and effective health care practices. As a collaborating center of the JBI, the TCU CEBPR offers educational programs ranging from short courses on evidence-based practice to the multiday Comprehensive Systematic Review Training.

The addition and renovation of the Annie Richardson Bass Building was dedicated in April of 2015 with a state-of-the-art Health Professions Learning Center that features programmable, high-tech mannequins in realistic practice settings. Housed within the building are Nursing, Social Work, Nurse Anesthesia, and Nutrition. Although the Department of Nutritional Sciences is administratively aligned with TCU's College of Science and Engineering, it is housed with Harris College and participates extensively in the interprofessional education initiatives of Harris College (Susan Weeks, pers. comm., 2018).

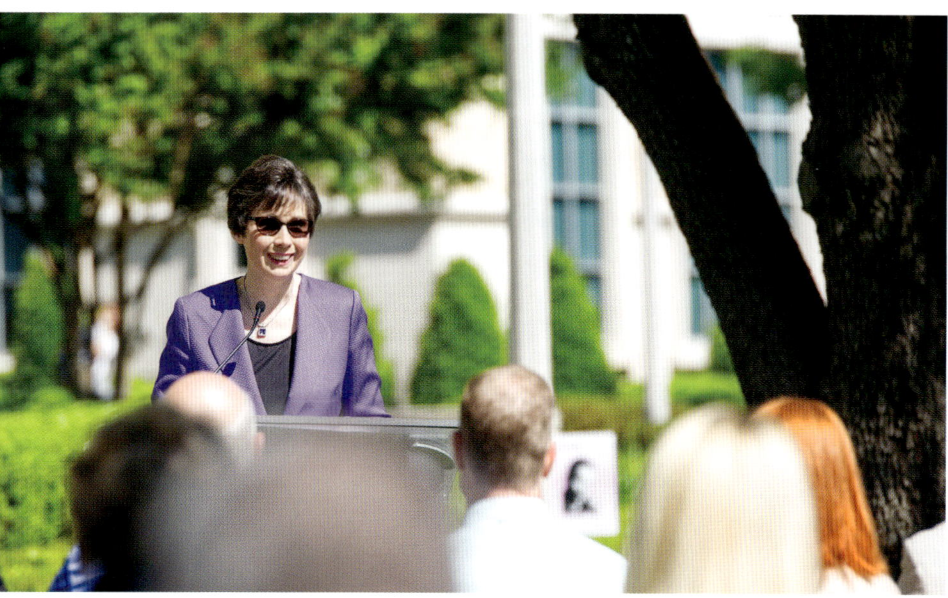

(Above) Susan Weeks speaking at the dedication of the Contemplation Garden, 2018. (Below) Suzy Lockwood at the dedication of the Contemplation Garden.

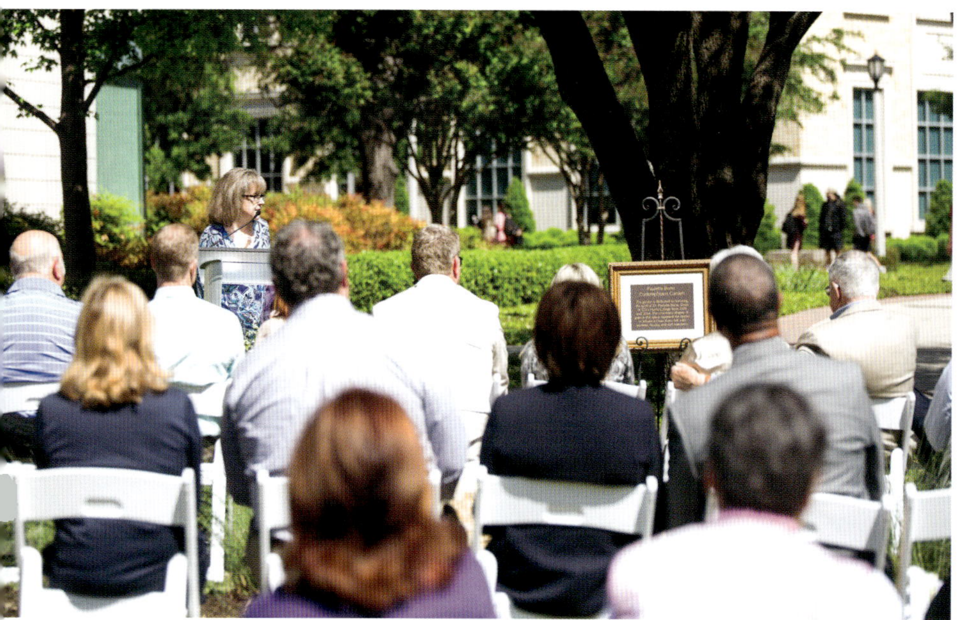

On April 27, 2018, the Paulette Burns Contemplation Garden next to the Annie Richardson Bass Building was dedicated. Burns had advocated for a garden to be part of the Bass Building during its renovation, but the project budget did not accommodate it (Susan Weeks, pers. comm., 2018). Soon after Burns was diagnosed with a terminal illness, Weeks worked with the provost to create a contemplation garden in honor of Burns. Following an announcement at the dedication of the building in 2015, subsequent donations made the garden possible, and the project moved forward.

Speaking at the dedication ceremony, Weeks reflected on the impact Burns had on her as a person and on all of those with whom she came in contact. Professionally, Burns served as president of the Texas Organization of Baccalaureate and Graduate Nursing Education, assumed multiple leadership roles at the American Association of Colleges of Nursing, and was selected as a DFW Great 100 Nurse by the Texas Nurses Association.

In addition to her professional accomplishments, Burns's personal attributes continue to influence the spirit of the college. She was never afraid to have fun, and as "kind as she was, she also was

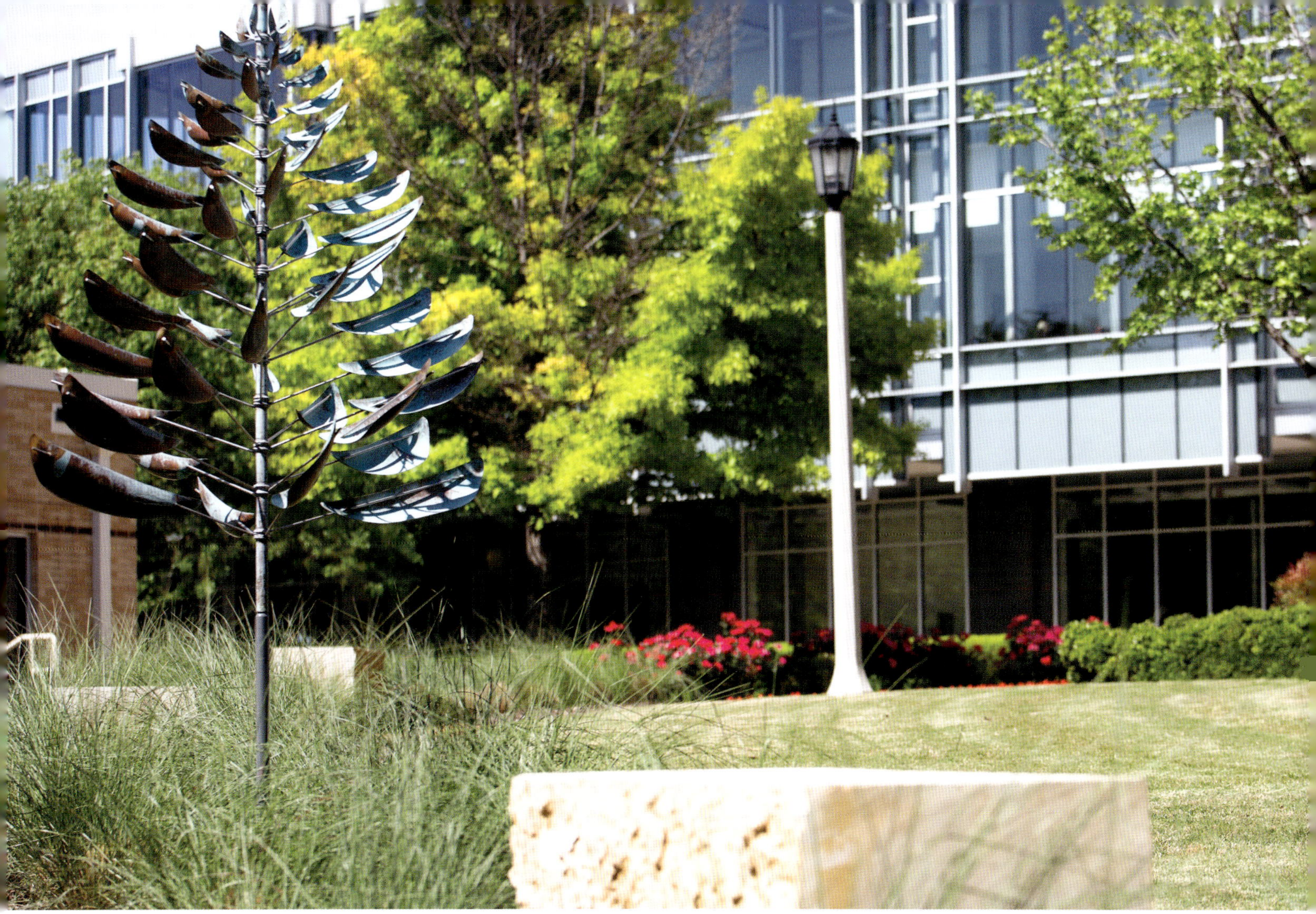

(Above) Wind Tree in Contemplation Garden, 2018.
(Right) Paulette Burns, former Dean for whom the Contemplation Garden is named.

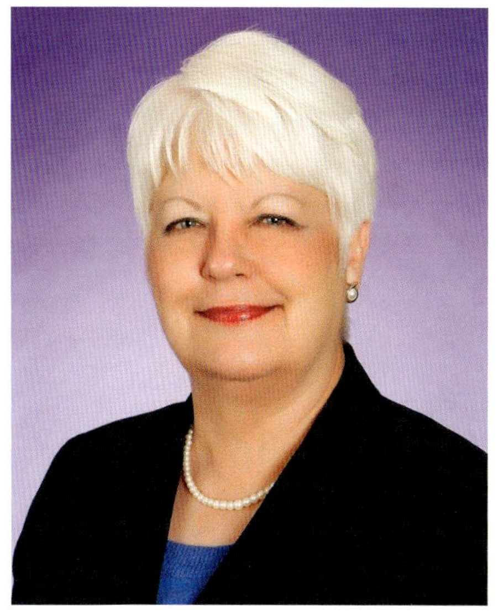

quite competitive . . . and loved a good challenge." She was "always humble and unassuming; never arrogant, and unfailingly kind." As Weeks described Paulette's legacy, she recalled a frequent phrase used to challenge groups she led: "Let's keep talking. Be bold." Weeks, who became the acting dean during Burns's illness and later the permanent dean, noted in closing that the college family had been able to journey forward because of Paulette Burns's insights (Susan Weeks, pers. comm., 2018).

Provost Nowell Donovan noted that the wind sculpture represented the spirit of Burns, who inspired so many, blowing through the garden.

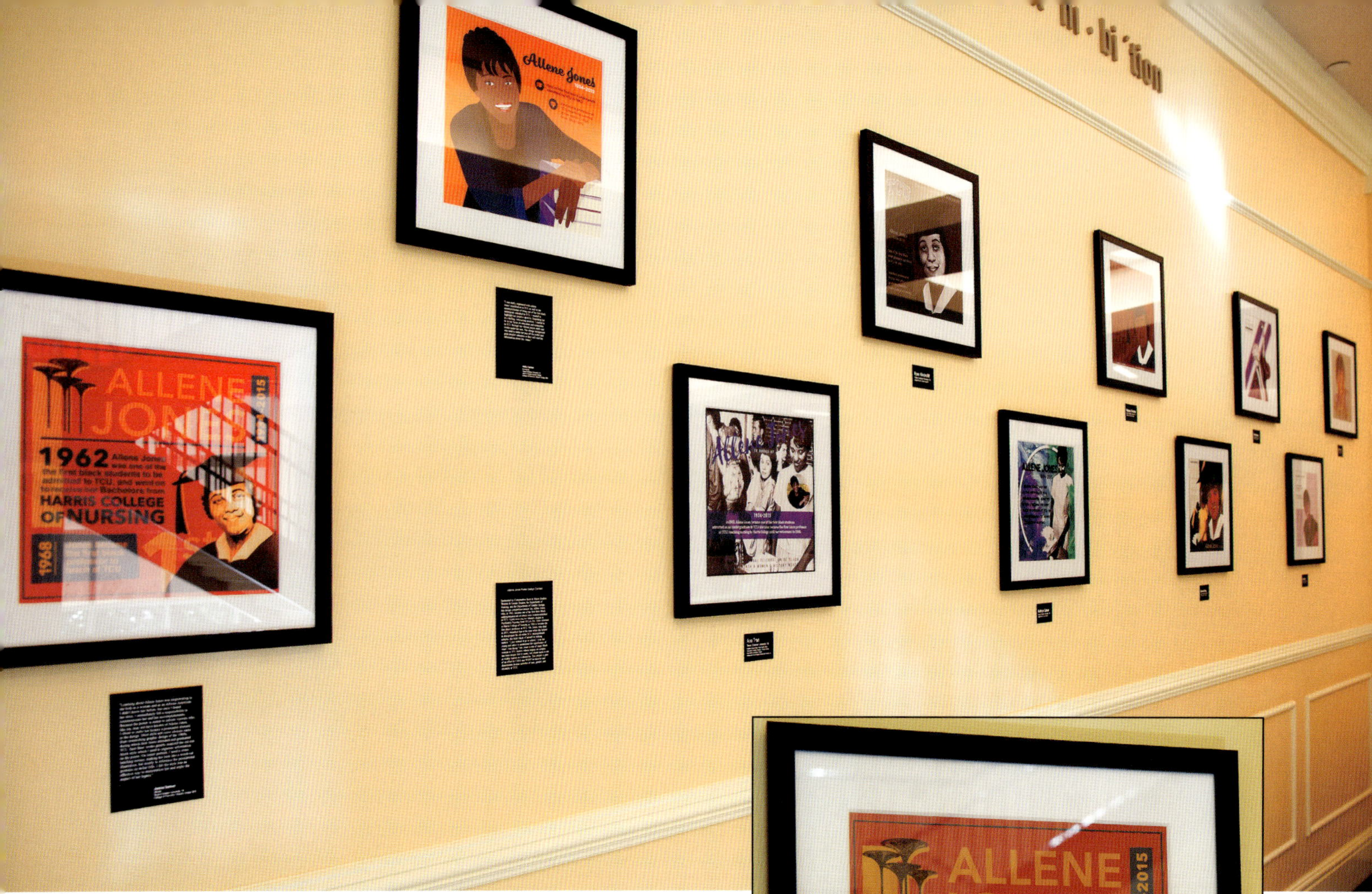

(Above) Allene Jones Poster Contest Display in the University Union, 2018. (Inset, right) Allene Jones, first African American student admitted to Harris College and the first African American professor.

Allene Jones, a graduate of Harris College of Nursing who was the first African American professor at TCU in 1968, was honored by the Departments of Graphic Design, Comparative Race and Ethnic Studies, Women and Gender Studies, and TCU Nursing in the Allene Jones Poster Design Contest. Jones, who came to TCU in 1962 as an undergraduate student, was one of the first three African American undergraduates—all of whom were women. Before her death in 2015, she commented that when she helped to desegregate the all-white TCU undergraduate campus, she didn't think of herself as making history: "She just wanted to go to school . . . and was too young and naïve to understand the

Student Congress Convenes Tonight
See Page 2

The Skiff

TEXAS CHRISTIAN UNIVERSITY ★ ★ ★ ★ FORT WORTH, TEXAS

Texas Integration Expanding Widely
See Page 5

VOL. 61, No. 2 TUESDAY, SEPTEMBER 35, 1962 8 PAGES

Young Pianists Start Contest Preliminaries

After some withdrawals and disqualifications the Van Cliburn International Quadrennial Piano Competition opened yesterday with about 50 of the world's leading young pianists participating in the preliminary elimination performances.

All events are being held in Ed Landreth Auditorium.

Contestants represent 17 countries, including four entries from the Soviet Union.

The United States is represented by 25 contestants, Mexico, Korea, Japan and Argentina 3 each; England, Canada, Brazil, and Uruguay by 2 each; the Bahamas, Belgium, Guatemala, France, Portugal, Switzerland and New Zealand by one.

Semifinals Scheduled

Semifinals are scheduled Oct. 1-3 and the finals, to be played with the Fort Worth Symphony Orchestra, will be the evenings of Oct. 4-5.

On the afternoon of Oct. 7, the $10,000 first winner will present a solo recital and the awards will be made.

Other prizes are $5,000 for second, $1,000 for third, $750 for fourth and $500 for fifth. Cliburn, the Texan for whom the competition is named, will attend and award a $600 prize to the best performance of chamber music among the 12 semifinalists.

Winner Due Contracts

Sponsored by the National Guild of Piano Teachers, the Fort Worth Piano Teachers Forum, the Fort Worth Chamber of Commerce and TCU, the event is planned for each four years.

The first place winner will play a concert in New York's Carnegie Hall and with a number of symphony orchestras in the United States and abroad. A concert management contract with Sol Hurok, internationally known impresario, also is part of the award.

During the preliminary rounds contestants will play seven compositions. Required are Samuel Barber's "Sonata Opus 26" and a commissioned work by American Composer Lee Hoiby, "Com-

will be $5 each and the solo recital by the first place winner will cost $2.

The playing requirements were set up by Cliburn himself. Contestants must play from memory, except for the chamber music, the content of three demanding programs.

Judges for the competition were drawn from performing pianists in Brazil, Mexico, Japan, England, the Soviet Union and the United States. Serge Saxe, president of the Fort Worth Opera Association, is chairman of the judging panel.

Through the week long preliminaries contestants will be identified by number only. Names will not be announced even to the audience.

Mother of Dean Moore Due Burial Wednesday

Funeral services will he held

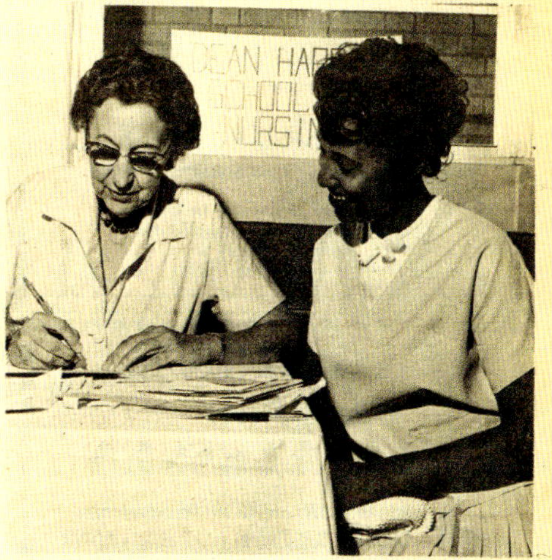

Dean Lucy Harris of Harris College of Nursing enrolls Mrs. Allene Jones, the University's first Negro undergraduate student. (Skiff Photo by Linda Kaye)

Harris College Desegregates As 6,200 Register in the Round

More than 6,200 students signed

ases over last fall by the end of

Brite College probably would add

Dean Harris and Allene Jones in 1962.

significance of what she was doing" (Poster Presentation, 2018). She embodied the concept of "being bold" as coined by Burns some fifty years later.

Centers within the College

Laura Thielke, director of the Health Professions Learning Center (HPLC), commented that "the entire HPLC was created with the future of learning in mind" (Thielke 2015, 16). The center is designed to "look like a clinical facility . . . and provides hands-on-experiences . . . that are essential to cultivating health care professionals who are prepared for the workforce" (Ladisic 2015, 14).

The HPLC spans two floors in the Annie Richardson Bass Building and is composed of four learning spaces. The practice laboratory, basic care laboratory, and acute care simulation area provide initial exposure to patient care equipment and

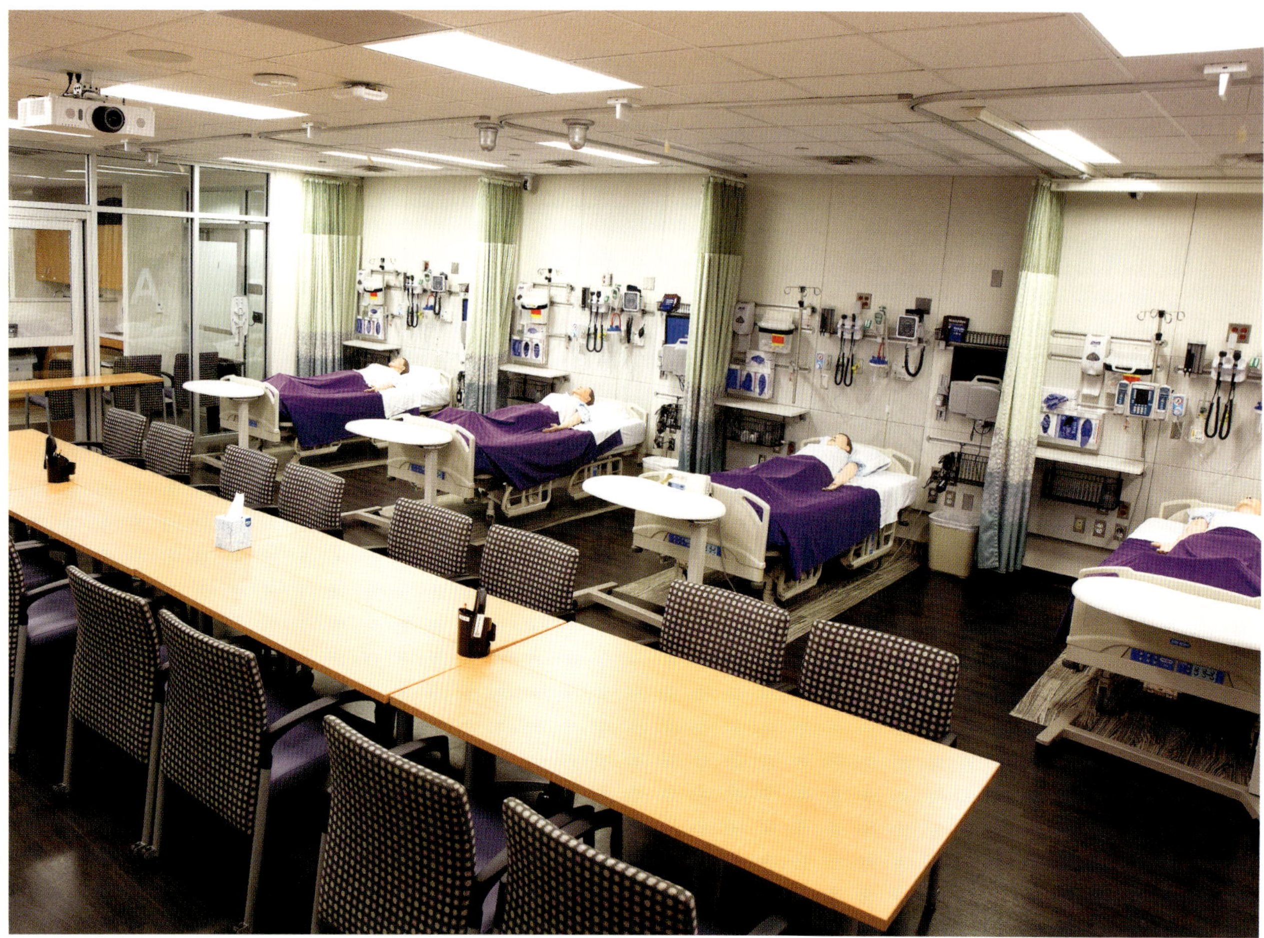

Basic Care Lab with beds, 2018.

technology, such as bedside computers with an electronic health record, automated medication dispensing machines, and "smart" intravenous (IV) pumps. The ambulatory care center features a suite that provides undergraduate and graduate students an opportunity to practice physical assessments and provide care to simulated patients in outpatient clinic and residential settings.

The acute care simulation center's suite is equipped with patient care technology that is used in inpatient hospital settings. High-fidelity mannequins mimic real-life patients with simulator models that represent people of different ages and ethnicities. These mannequins, along with standardized patients (actors), provide students with experiences in adult medical-surgical, emergency, labor and delivery, and pediatric settings.

The basic care lab is designed for students to learn health assessment and safe, fundamental skills. Faculty members provide demonstrations, and students practice skills under supervision using task trainers and mid-fidelity mannequins. The practice lab is a space designed for students to independently practice skills outside of lab, simulation, and clinical courses. With four hospital beds, the area resembles the basic care lab and includes virtual IV haptic devices, which assist students with learning how to start an IV.

Due to the increased use of simulation as a major pedagogical approach within programs that prepare health professionals, the revised baccalaureate nursing curriculum, implemented in fall 2015, included three courses dedicated entirely to high-fidelity simulation. Clinical Reasoning in Simulation I, II, and III courses, taught entirely with simulation during the last three semesters of the program, include scenarios that integrate concepts learned in didactic and clinical courses. The

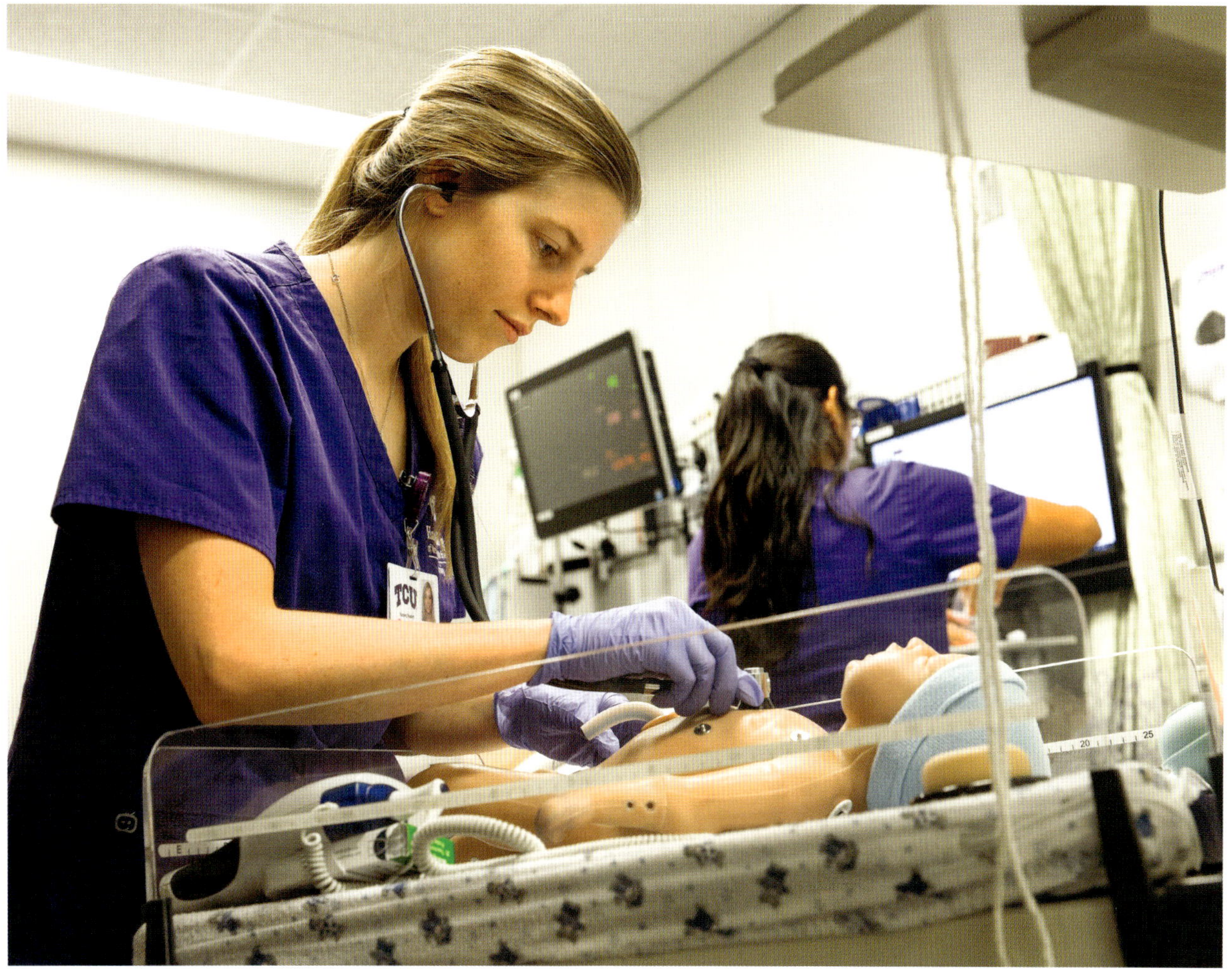

Students in the Acute Care Simulation Area.

center is also used to support interprofessional education, with learning opportunities designed to enhance communication and teamwork among health professionals. In order to promote success for these initiatives, faculty development in simulation was conducted, and five staff positions were added to the HPLC.

According to Thielke (2015), the HPLC "provides evidence of Harris College's dedication to staying on the cutting edge of health sciences innovation" (16). Students have the opportunity to learn from what they did, either correctly or incorrectly, "without fear of harm to a human patient" (16).

The Health Innovation Institute at TCU (HIIAT), led by Executive Director Weeks, was formed in 2016 as an institute that housed four related centers: the Center for Translational Research, the Center for Collaborative Practice, the Center for Oncology Education and Research (described in chapter 5), and Let's inspire innovation 'N Kids (LiiNK). These centers, which previously operated independently of one another, now have a unifying structure which better contributes to the advancement of each center's mission through innovation and collaboration. Two of the centers, the Center for Translational Research and the Center for Collaborative Practice, were formed from different portfolios of activity that had developed within the Center for Evidence-Based Practice and Research (Susan Weeks, pers. comm., 2018).

> The Center for Translational Research, directed by Dru Riddle, bridges the gap between the laboratory bench and the bedside by combining research findings of both, identifying best practices, and helping patients, families, consumers, and practitioners answer questions about how to make health care decisions. The Center for Collaborative Practice, directed by Linda Humphries, assists hospital systems, community health agencies, schools, and acute-care and long-term care agencies in the implementation of evidence-based guidelines into practice settings. The LiiNK Center, directed by Debbie Rhea, bridges the gap between academic and social, emotional, and healthy well-being for children, parents, educators, and administrators. Demonstrated outcomes include the improvement of teacher satisfaction and happiness, the development of healthier students and teachers through unstructured, outdoor play; increased activity; and effective classroom environments.

In addition to activities within the HIIAT, there is significant support within HCNHS for interprofessional education (IPE), which has been defined as "when students from two or more professions learn about, from, and with each other to enable effective collaboration and improve health" (World Health Organization 2010). Students majoring in kinesiology, nursing, nurse anesthesia, social work, and speech-language pathology have opportunities to learn together as part of their academic programs. These experiences occur during multi-institutional case-based activities and interdepartmental experiences.

The Harris Academic Resource Center (HARC) was established in 2012 as an initiative to promote the academic success and foster individual development of all Harris College undergraduate students. Professional advisers are available to meet with first- and second-year undergraduate students and answer questions regarding core, major, and minor requirements; assist students to achieve success; assess academic skills; provide recommendations; and refer students to campus resources as needed. Each semester, the center invites Harris College undergraduate students to stop by and receive a goody bag and breakfast as they prepare for final exams, an event called "Fuel for Finals."

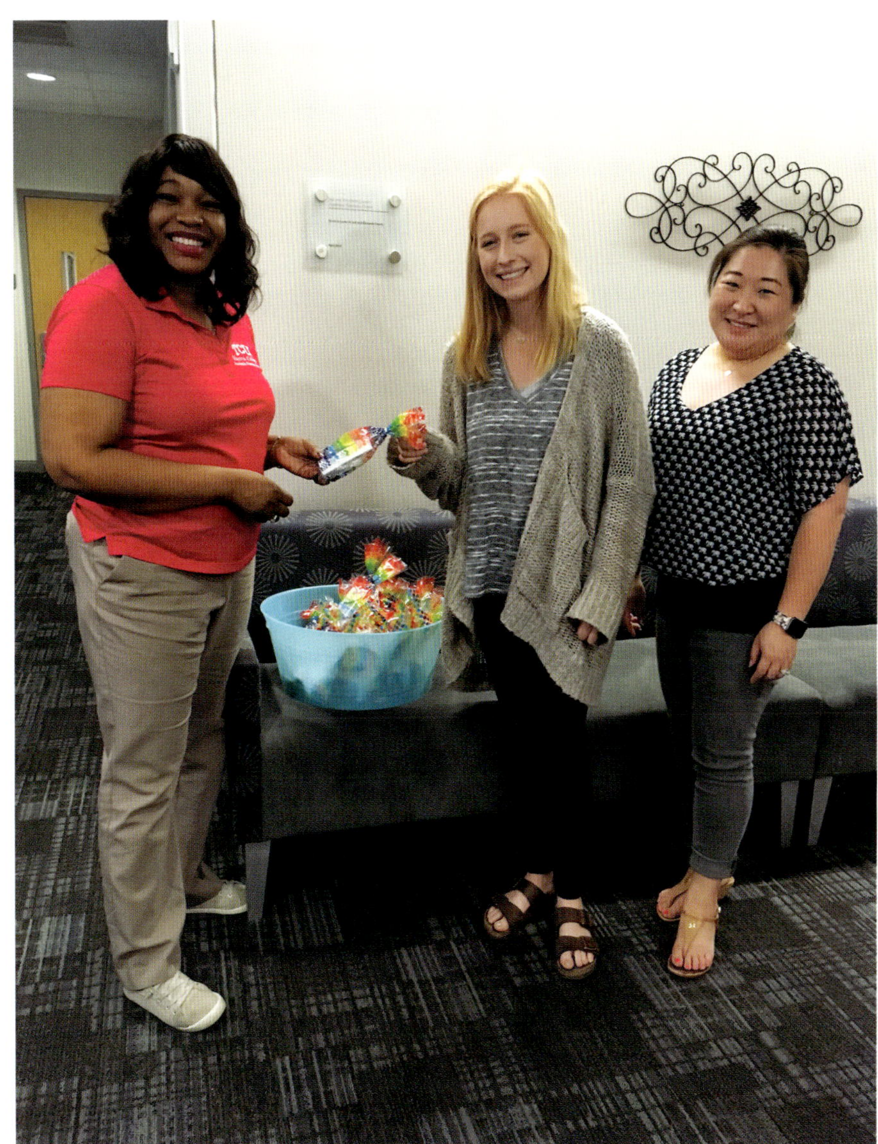

L-R, Zoranna Jones, Makayla Kelly, and Amanda Duvall preparing for finals with help of "Goody Bag," 2018.

Other events include a chili cook-off among the various departments in the fall, followed by a crawfish boil in the spring. These events are heavily attended by students, faculty, and staff of the college (Zoranna Jones, pers. comm., 2018).

The center also provides activities and presentations which focus on health professions, improving academic skills, information about study abroad, information about participation in the Honors College, information about career opportunities, and preparation for graduate study.

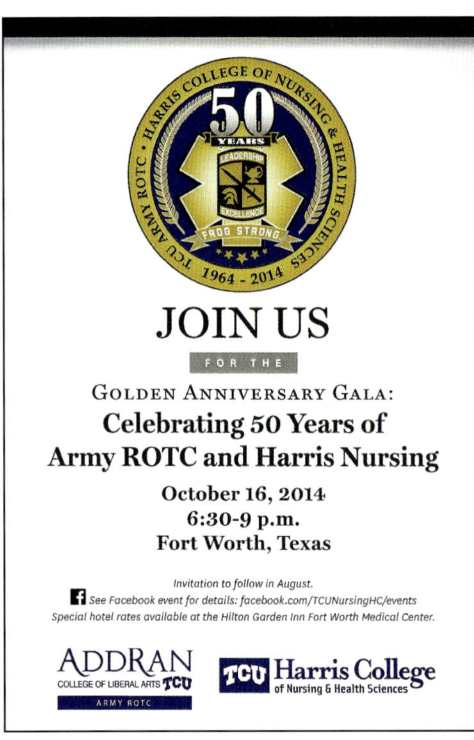

Fiftieth Anniversary of TCU Army ROTC and TCU Nursing.

The Golden Anniversary Gala of Army ROTC and TCU Nursing

The Golden Anniversary Gala: Celebrating 50 Years of Army ROTC and TCU Nursing was held on Thursday, October 16, 2014 at the Hilton Garden Inn, Fort Worth. The event celebrated the long-standing partnership between TCU Nursing and Army ROTC. The speaker for the gala was Colonel Nicole Kerkenbush, MHA, MN, RN-BC, a 1992 TCU alumna, who is currently chief information officer of the US Surgeon General's Office and deputy director of the Solution Delivery Division.

Celebrating Seventy Years

In 2016, TCU Nursing celebrated seventy years with an anniversary gala in the Brown-Lupton University Union Ballroom. Prior to the gala, attendees had the opportunity to tour the nursing building and view a display of TCU Nursing uniforms through the decades.

The evening was celebrated with dinner and dancing to music by Trey and the Tritones. Melissa Sherrod gave a presentation about the history of TCU Nursing, offering historical photos and sharing an observation Lucy Harris made in 1973 that "it is unlikely that any similar undertaking ever got underway with more inherent reasons for failure and fewer chances of success than did the Harris College of Nursing."

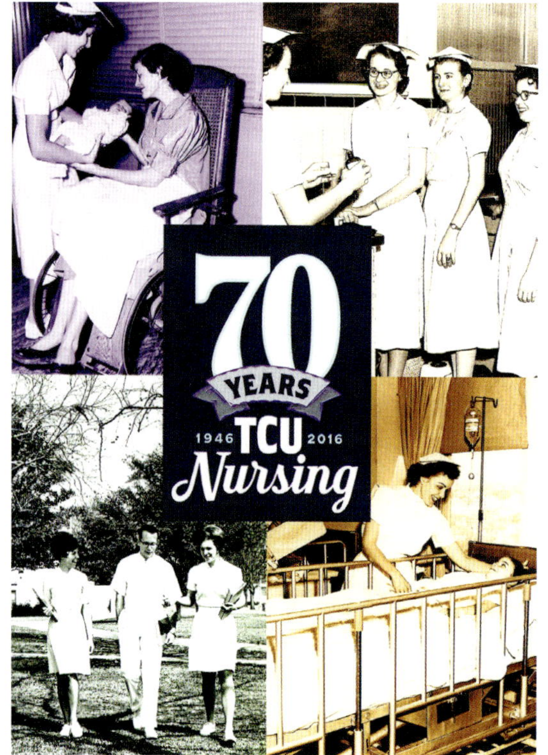

70 Years: TCU Nursing 1946–2016.

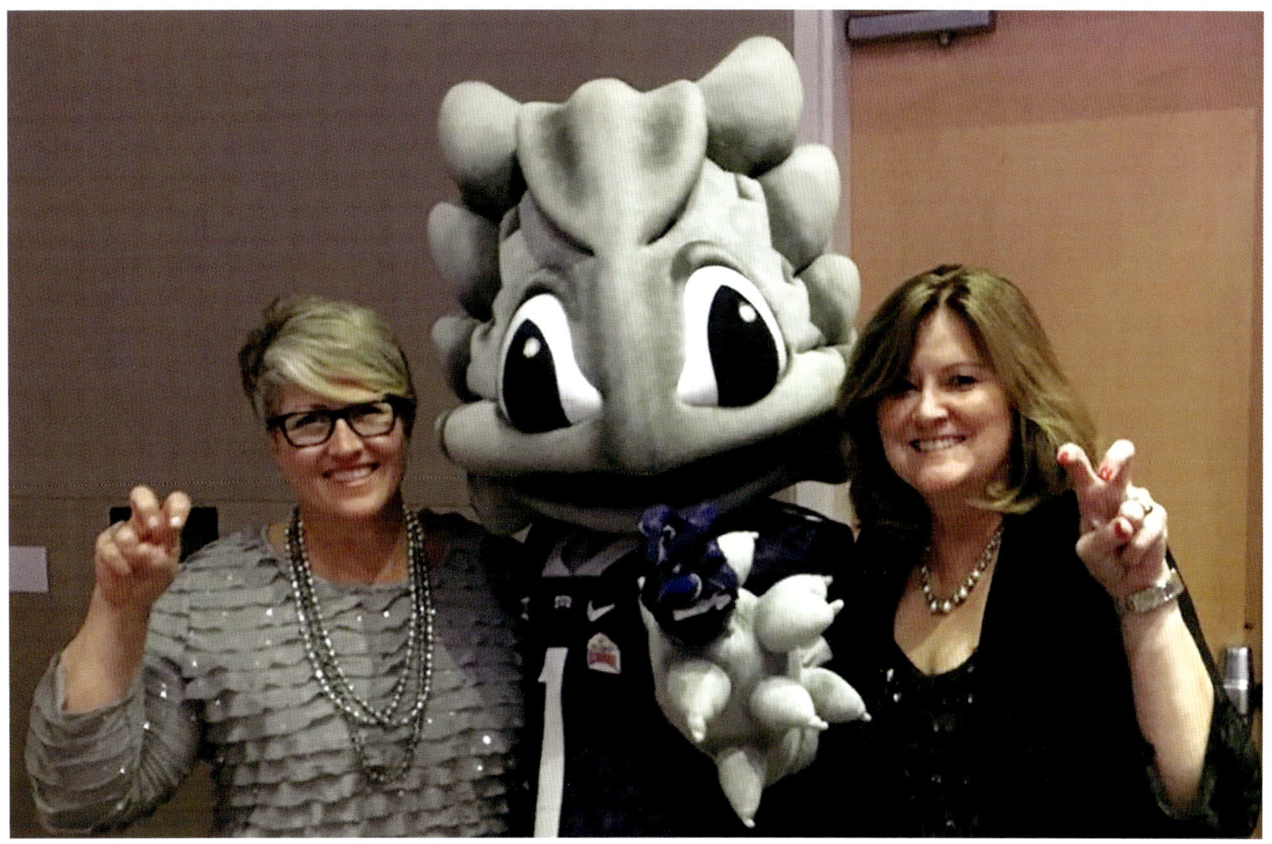

Judy Clark, Cathy Johnson, and SuperFrog, 2016.

CHALLENGE ONE

A Clear Definition of Nursing Roles and Functions

Context and Trends

In 2010, President Barack Obama signed the Patient Protection and Affordable Care Act into law. Widely known for its significant impact on insurance access and reform, the Affordable Care Act has also allowed significant strides to be made in improving care quality and cost. These measures include removing reimbursement to the hospitals for hospital-acquired conditions, focusing the health care budget on prevention and health promotion strategies, and endorsing care continuity with patient-centered medical homes (Salmond and Echevarria 2017). In addition to political means, progress in nursing practices have also allowed for quality improvements in health care. The evidence-based practice (EBP) model is one such improvement. Unlike research models, the EBP model incorporates research evidence on best practice measures with clinical applicability and patient preferences, and results in

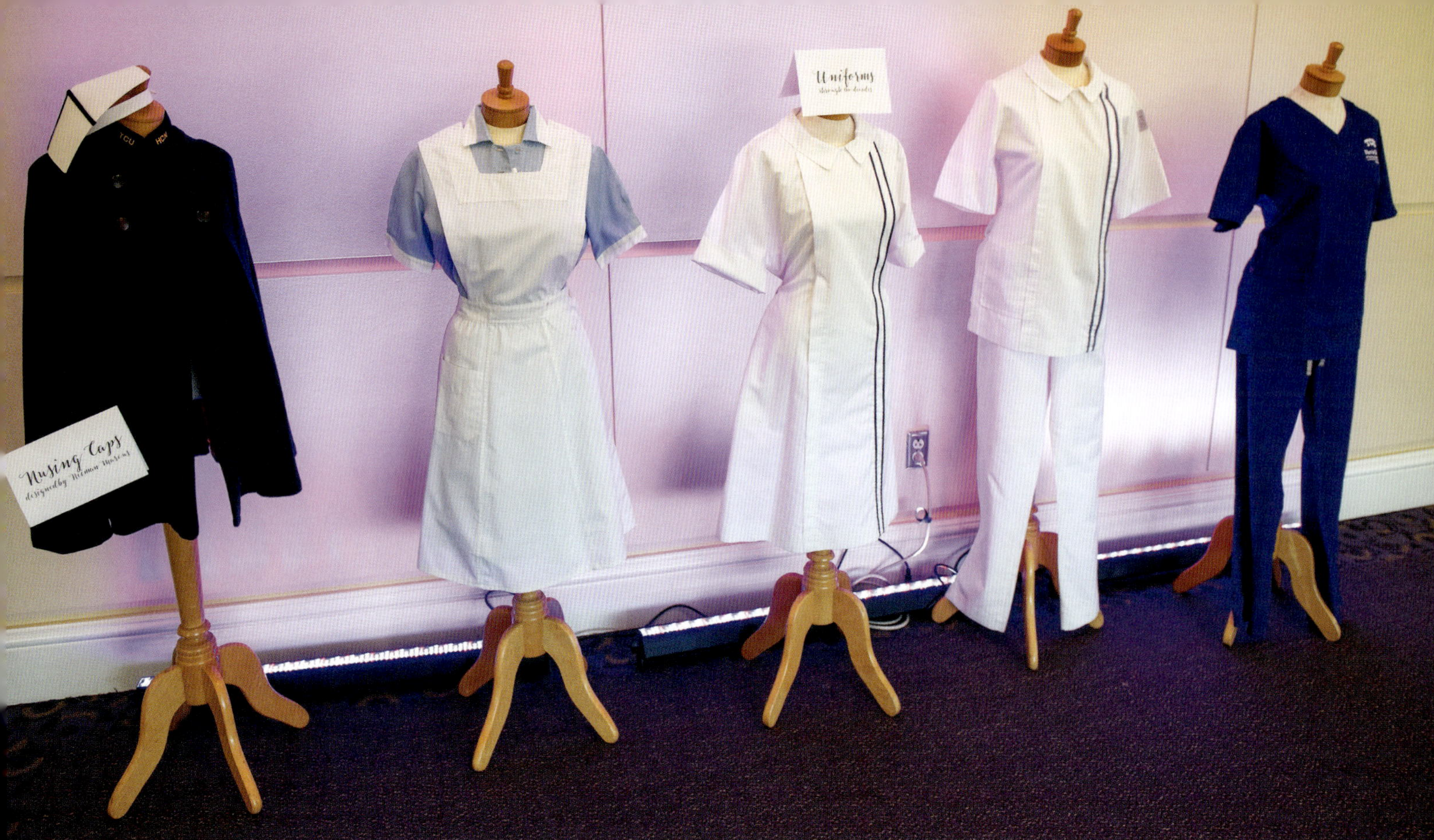

Harris College caps and uniforms displayed at 70th Anniversary Gala.

marked improvement in patient care quality (Stevens 2013). Concurrently, the additions of the Quality and Safety Education for Nurses (QSEN) initiatives and interprofessional education into nursing curriculum have allowed for the preparation of a generation of nurses already poised to provide the highest quality of patient care upon graduation (Dolanksy and Moore 2013; Eggenberger, Sherman, and Keller 2014).

The landmark report—*The Future of Nursing: Leading Change, Advancing Health Care* (2011)—provided guidelines for improvement of the health care system to increase the positive outcomes of patient care. It included four key messages for the future of nursing:

1. Nurses should practice to the full extent of their education and training.

2. Nurses should achieve higher levels of education and training through an improved education system that promotes seamless academic progression.

3. Nurses should be full partners with physicians and other health professionals in redesigning health care in the United States.

4. Effective workforce planning and policy making require better data collection and an improved information infrastructure.

Developments in research and technology have also had a significant impact on health care during this decade. The expansion of the field of genetics and genomics has profoundly improved treatment and disease prevention with more targeted drug therapies and earlier identification of disease-susceptibility genes. In addition, the rise of laparoscopic and robotic surgeries has increased surgical accuracy and reduced recovery times, decreasing costs for both patients and care providers (Huston 2013). Lastly, further technological impact on health care can be found in the widespread implementation of electronic health records (EHRs). The use of EHRs significantly reduces the incidence of medical errors and consequent adverse events, as well as the length of patient hospital stays and seven-day readmission rates (Hessels, Flynn, Cimiotti, Bakken, and Gershon 2015). While these measures are highly beneficial in improving patient outcomes, they can sometimes compromise a nurse's ability to provide compassionate and humane care. In a world focused more on automation and efficiency, it is the duty of nurses to continue to keep care centered on the most important thing: the patient.

In 2016, Melissa Sherrod published "The History of Cesarean Birth from 1900 to 2016," noting that nurses currently struggle with conflicting priorities about the delivery of nursing care during childbirth and the expectations held by attending physicians. In her analysis of this history, she suggests that scientific advances in childbirth, such as the performance of technologically sophisticated interventions once performed only by physicians, can "affect the perception of comfort that nurses traditionally offered" in their roles (Sherrod 2017, 628).

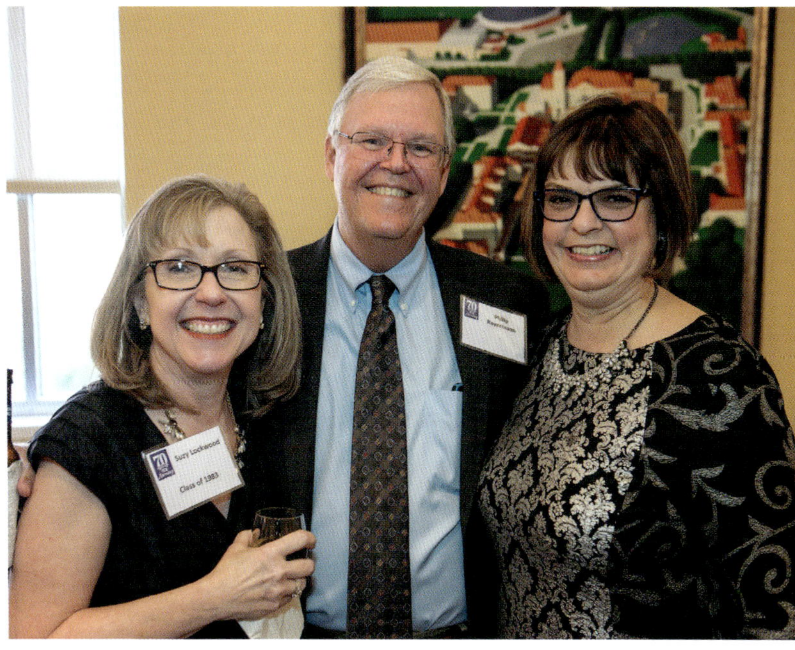

(Above) L-R, Suzy Lockwood, husband Philip, and Kathy Baker. (Below) L-R, Suzy Lockwood, BSN 1983; William and Connie Koehler (Furham), BSN 1975; and Dennis Cheek.

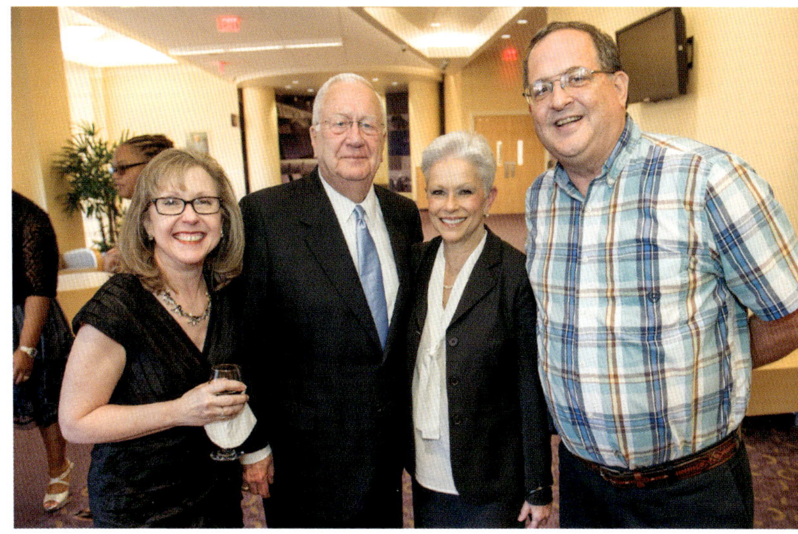

TCU Nursing

Curriculum

The undergraduate curriculum continues to offer two equivalent tracks: a traditional baccalaureate track (TBT) and an accelerated baccalaureate track (ABT). The ABT was designed and implemented to meet the unique needs of students already holding an undergraduate degree who seek rapid entry into professional nursing practice. In 2010, the Commission on Collegiate Nursing Education (CCNE) granted accreditation to the baccalaureate program for a term of ten years.

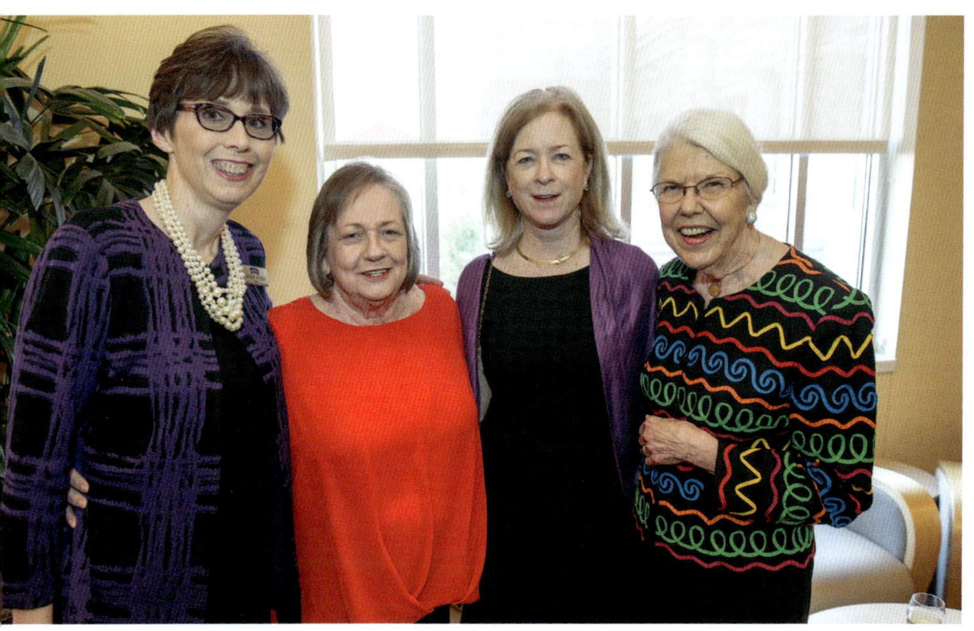

L-R, Susan Weeks, DeVonna Tinney, Marinda Allender, and Gail Davis at the 70th Anniversary Gala.

TCU Nursing earned the American Association of Colleges of Nursing (AACN) Innovations in Professional Nursing Award in the category of small schools without an academic health center during the 2011–12 academic year. This award was in recognition of the outcomes of the baccalaureate nursing emphasis in oncology program. Suzy Lockwood, who submitted the application along with Dean Paulette Burns, accepted the award at the AACN fall meeting.

In 2011, Melissa Sherrod and Diane Hawley planned and implemented a gerontological nursing elective, offered online, with an interdisciplinary practicum. This course was designed to meet the 2010 AACN Recommended Baccalaureate Competencies and Curricular Guidelines for the Nursing Care of Older Adults.

In the 1990s public health nursing faculty facilitated clinical experiences with local health departments in which students made home visits to promote healthy families. By the 2000s, local health departments were changing, and the specialty of public health nursing increasingly focused on establishing partnerships with communities to promote the wellbeing of populations. Public health nursing faculty began designing clinical experiences rooted in service learning, a teaching strategy in which students and partners together identify how to simultaneously meet learning outcome objectives and community needs. Faculty created a community-based, service learning model that focused on working with population aggregates and systems over multiple semesters. Faculty, students, and partners collaborated to develop initiatives that emphasize outcomes evaluation and sustainable change in systems and populations. Strong, continuous faculty involvement fostered service learning partnerships through which successive cohorts of public health nursing students contributed to significant community change over time.

One example of the success of this transdisciplinary learning is the "Safe Routes to Schools" project, which demonstrated how the vision of a public health nurse, Sharon Canclini, resulted in changing existing policies, systems, and environments in two school districts. Safe Routes to Schools interventions insure that children can safely walk or ride bicycles to school. Faculty and students collaborate with the district and its families as well as with Tarrant County and Fort Worth planners, engineers, government officials, and elected representatives. At the ribbon-cutting ceremony marking the successful conclusion of the initial, ten-year Safe Routes effort with the Mansfield ISD, the Eagle Mountain Saginaw ISD invited Canclini and TCU public health nursing to partner in designing and implementing its Safe Routes program.

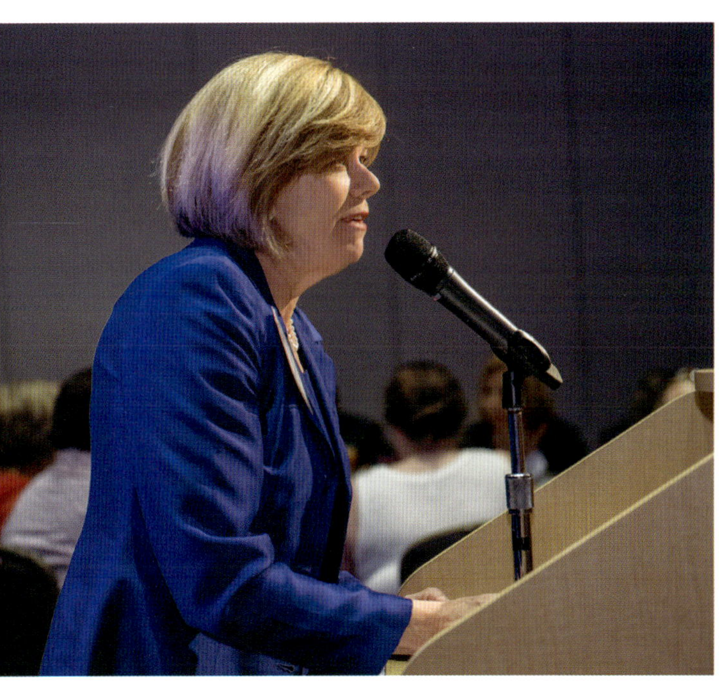

Melissa Sherrod speaking on the history of HCN at the 70th Anniversary Gala.

Another example shows how partnerships between faculty members and school stakeholders in parochial and public schools achieved mutual and meaningful objectives—a hallmark of service learning. Debra McLachlan built a partnership with Nancy Eder, RN, and the Catholic Schools of the Fort Worth Diocese. McLachlan and public health nursing students worked with youth in several elementary and high schools to promote health of students, families, teachers, and staff. In one nutrition intervention, nursing students created guidelines that helped children and their parents make healthy choices at the numerous fast-food restaurants in the community. The nursing students also set up a mock grocery store like the one in the neighborhood, where children could practice how to shop wisely. McLachlan and public health nursing students published an article about another intervention they created, *Emotion Locomotion,* in which elementary school children learned to

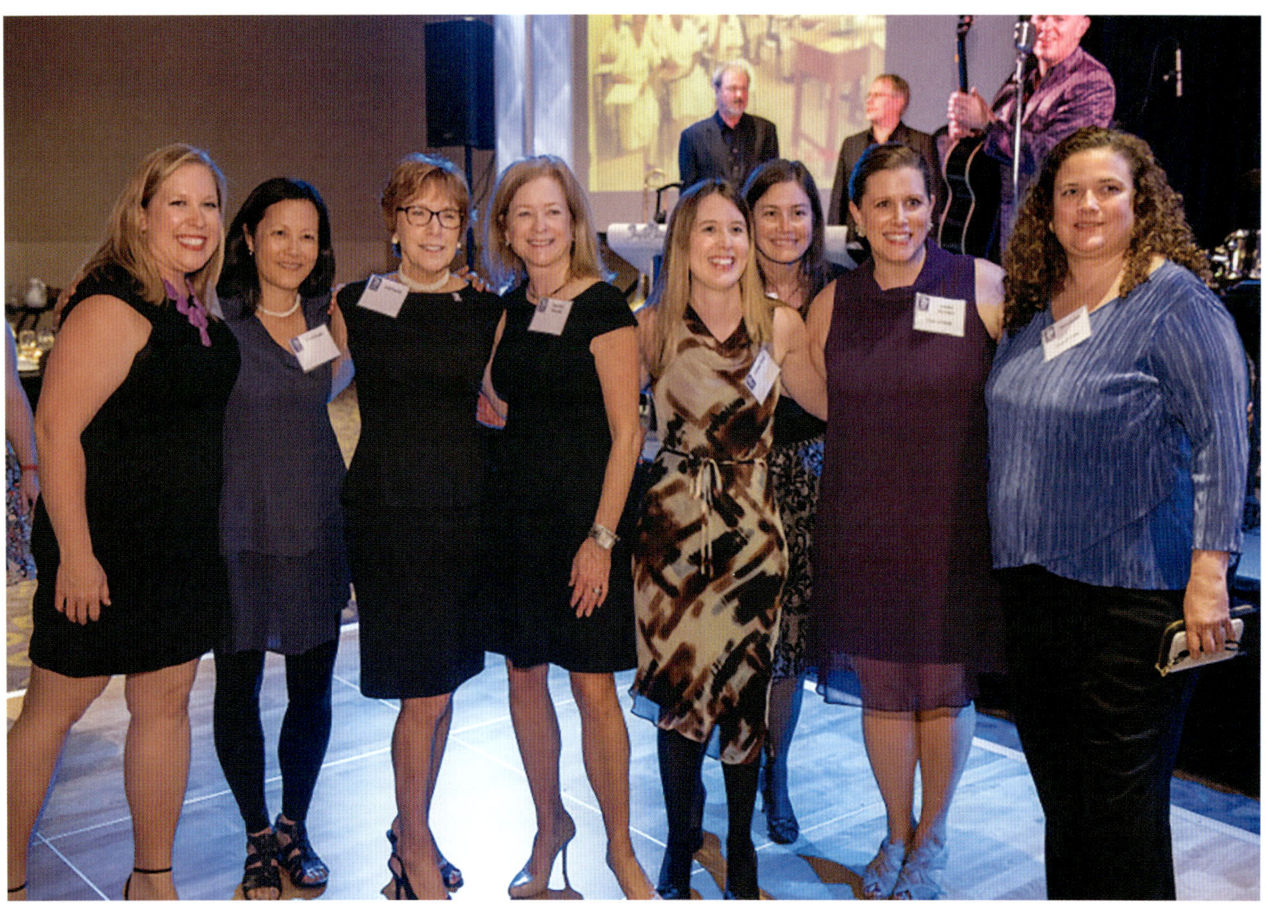

L-R, Leslie Zimpelman, Carol Howe, Andi Smith, Marinda Allender, Caitlin Dodd, Andrea Erwin, Lisette Saleh, and Kara Keeton Griffin at the 70th Anniversary Gala.

recognize and express their emotions in appropriate ways. (*see* https://journals.sagepub.com/doi/abs/10.1177/1059840509339738?journalCode=jsnb for article details).

A third example demonstrated how synergistic relationships between service learning partners and faculty members opened the door for conversations about the integration of immigrants. Pam Frable established a partnership with the Ministries with African Immigrants at the First United Methodist Church in Hurst to address needs of English-language learners. In a short time, immigrants from Africa, Asia, the Middle East, and the Central, South, and Caribbean Americas joined the Church's English language program. Public health nursing students completed community assessments that demonstrated the need for an immigrant welcome center in Northeast Tarrant County and identified the evidence-based features for the center. Subsequent cohorts built on this work, developing evidence in support of family coaching and conversation partner initiatives. These clinical experiences helped nursing students learn about immigration and hone skills for communicating and providing nursing care across languages and cultures. The students' work also helped community members understand the scope of nursing practice.

A service learning conference, Promoting Health and Wellness through Community Campus Partnerships: Combining Our Strengths for a Better Tomorrow, also took place during the 2011–12 academic year. Faculty, students, and professionals from a variety of health care institutions were active participants (Frable 2011).

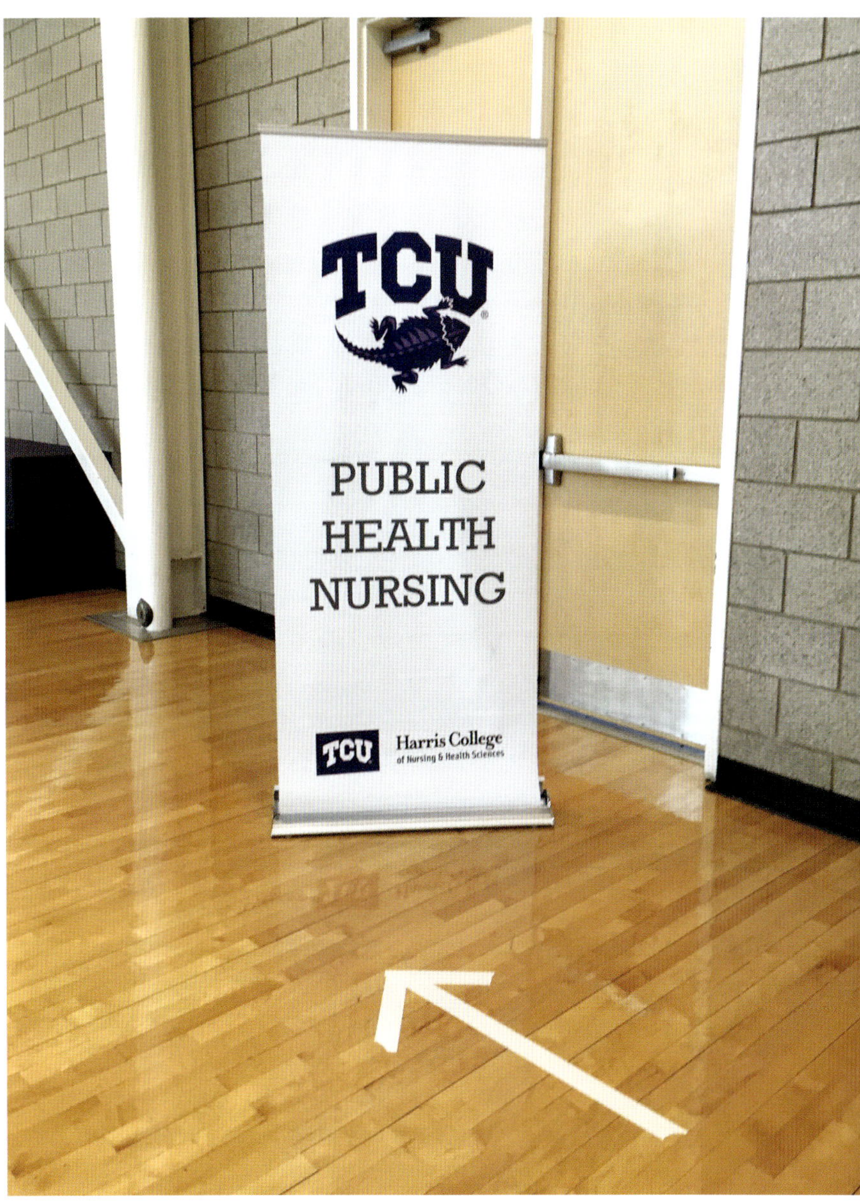

Public health nursing sign at TCU's Flu Vaccine Clinic, 2018.

Under the direction and coordination of Sharon Canclini, who teaches public health nursing, senior students have had the opportunity to provide seasonal influenza vaccinations to TCU students, faculty, and staff since 2009. This was initiated through partnerships between Harris College of Nursing & Health Sciences (HCNHS), the TCU Recreation Center, and the TCU Health Center. The clinic originated through a collaboration between Canclini and the late Steve Kintigh. The notion was to develop a service learning opportunity for nursing students while providing a needed service on the TCU campus. Over time, the clinic has grown from a twelve-member team of nursing students offering five hundred doses of vaccine to a twenty-four-member leadership team with forty volunteers per hour providing doses of vaccine in a one-day clinic. In the fall of 2018, over three thousand recipients were vaccinated.

As a part of a capstone project in the public health nursing course,

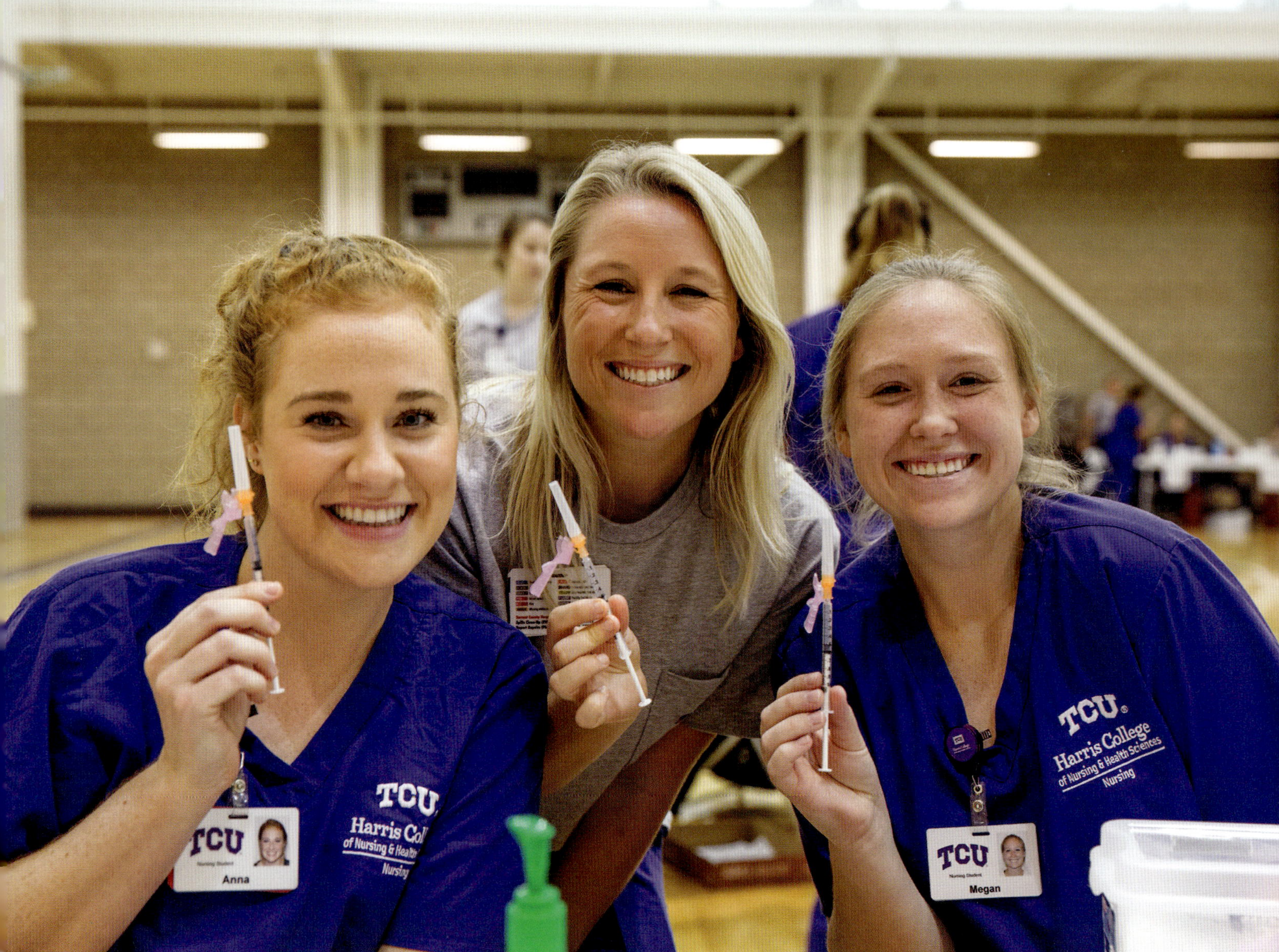

Students with flu vaccines, in current uniforms, 2018.

two teams of Senior II nursing students work together to plan, organize, and implement the seasonal influenza vaccine clinic during the fall semester of each year. Students design the vaccine clinic, which is open to the entire campus community, using best evidence and community assessment data. One team takes the lead for marketing the event throughout the campus. This team develops a marketing strategy and a brand. The marketing strategy includes outreach activities customized for particularly vulnerable members of the TCU population, such as housekeepers, groundskeepers, and freshmen students. The second team takes the lead for all the logistics for the event, including the set-up in the recreation center—the latter a demonstration of how to develop a point of distribution in the event of a disaster.

Students are involved in many activities, including greeting those who come for the vaccinations, obtaining informed consent to receive the vaccine, and administering the vaccination. In addition, student leadership team members are trained in fainting, anaphylaxis, and allergic reaction response protocols. Senior II students assist faculty members with supervision of Senior I students, who prior to joining the Senior II students at the administration tables must attend a Just-in-Time training, which involves giving one another their vaccinations, and then in turn administering the vaccination to a client. Alumnae also participate in the event by pulling the medicine into syringes and supporting the students.

In the fall of 2015, a revised bachelor of science in nursing degree plan was implemented. Changes in the curriculum included the integration of interprofessional education activities (IPE) in collaboration with the University of North Texas medical school, pharmacy, and physician assistant programs. These IPE activities also include HCNHS social work students (Stephanie Evans, pers. comm., 2018). Pathophysiology, health assessment, and three clinical reasoning and simulation courses are now stand-alone courses.

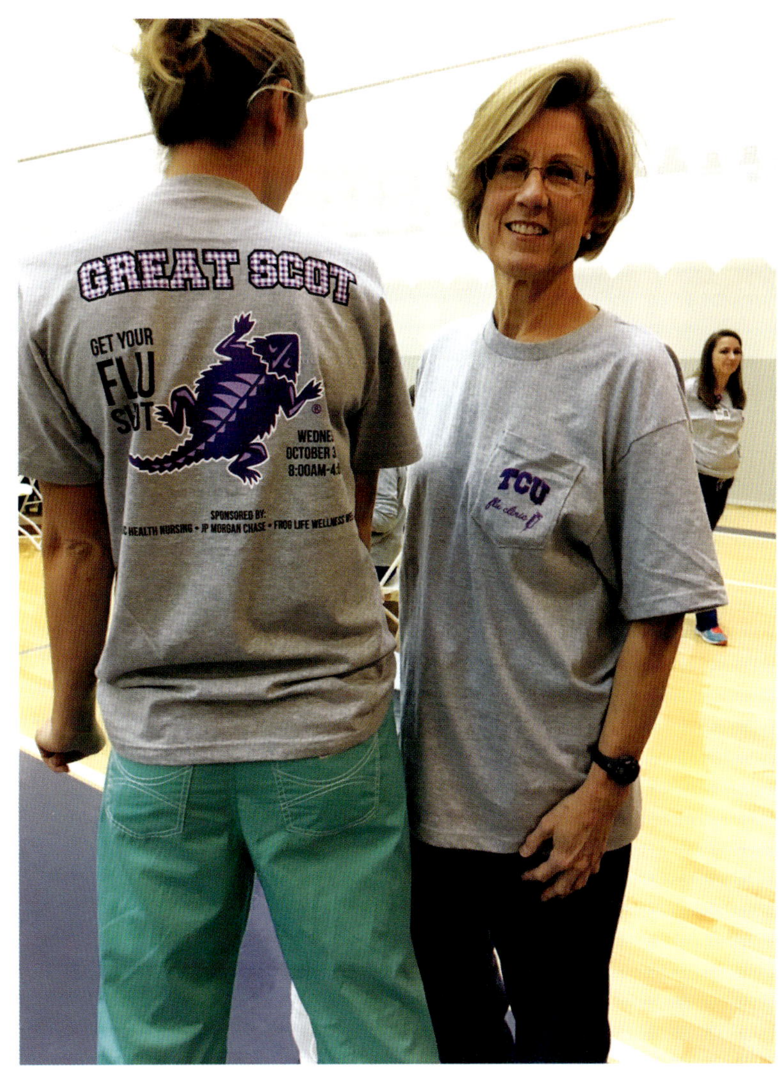

Sharon Canclini and student at TCU's Flu Vaccine Clinic, 2018.

Faculty

Nursing faculty members continue to be honored with a variety of awards. Three individuals received the Deans' Teaching Award: Kathy Baldwin (2010), Diane Hawley (2013), and Sharon Canclini (2014). Suzy Lockwood (2010) and Jo Nell Wells (2016) received the Deans' Research Award.

The Wassenich Award for Mentoring in the TCU community celebrates faculty and staff who serve as role models, advisers, and guides to students. The award, in

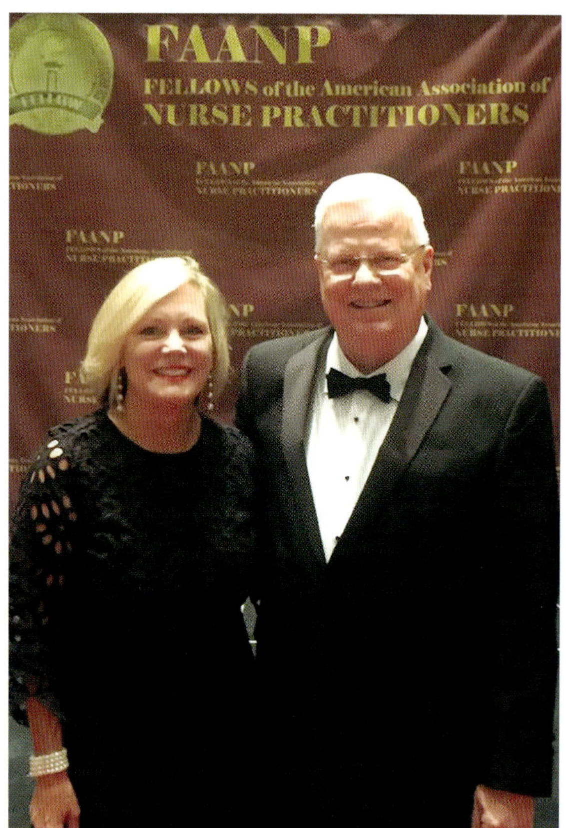

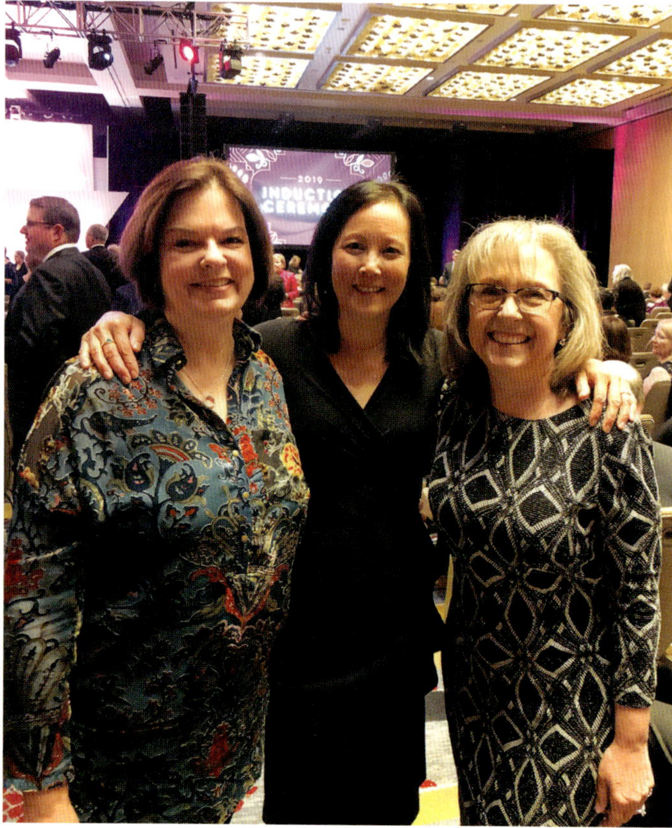

(Left) Kathy Ellis and Kenneth Lowrance at induction, American Association of Nurse Practitioners, 2017. (Right) L-R, Kathy Baker, Carol Howe, and Suzy Lockwood at the American Academy of Nursing.

honor of Linda and Mark Wassenich, TCU alumni, was presented to Diane Hawley at the Fall Convocation in 2013.

Other nursing faculty were nominated for the Chancellor's Award for Distinguished Research or Creative Activity: Linda Curry (2011), Suzy Lockwood (2012), and Charles Walker (2014). Debbie Rhea was the recipient of the Chancellor's Award in fall 2018 and became the first university-level winner from the college. Six adjunct faculty members received the DAISY Award between 2013 and 2018: Phyllis Allen (2013), Cindy Cochrane (2014), Elisa Stehling (2015), Kathy White (2016), Gayle Wilkins (2017), and Joyce Putnam (2018). Jo Nell Wells received the Outstanding Mentor Award from the TCU Evidence-Based Practice Fellowship in 2016. The Woman of the Year Award by the American Association of University Women was given to Glenda Daniels in 2017. Two faculty members, Kathryn Ellis and Kenneth Lowrance, were inducted as Fellows into the American Association of Nurse Practitioners in 2017. In 2018, the Texas Nurses Association posthumously honored

Emeritus Professor Mildred Hogstel at the Legacy Banquet. In 2019, Carol Howe was inducted into the American Academy of Nursing.

Faculty members continue to serve in many leadership roles at the local and national levels. Locally, Marinda Allender serves on the Board of Trustees of Medical City North Hills, while Lisa Bashore is president of the Board of Directors of Shine Therapy. Suzy Lockwood serves on the Baylor All Saints Board and Weeks is the chair of the board for Harris Southwest as well as a system level board member for Texas Health Resources. At the national level, Kathryn Ellis serves on the board of directors for the National Organization of Nurse Practitioner Faculties. Melissa Sherrod, who has been active in the American Association for the History of Nursing, serves as the second vice president. Many other faculty members provide service in a variety of organizations at the local, state, national, and international levels.

At the beginning of the 2018 fall semester, the nursing faculty consisted of fifty-three full-time members and twenty-nine part-time members.

Staff

Zoranna Jones, director of the Academic Resource Center, received the 2017 Wassenich Award in recognization of her extensive support and mentoring of students.

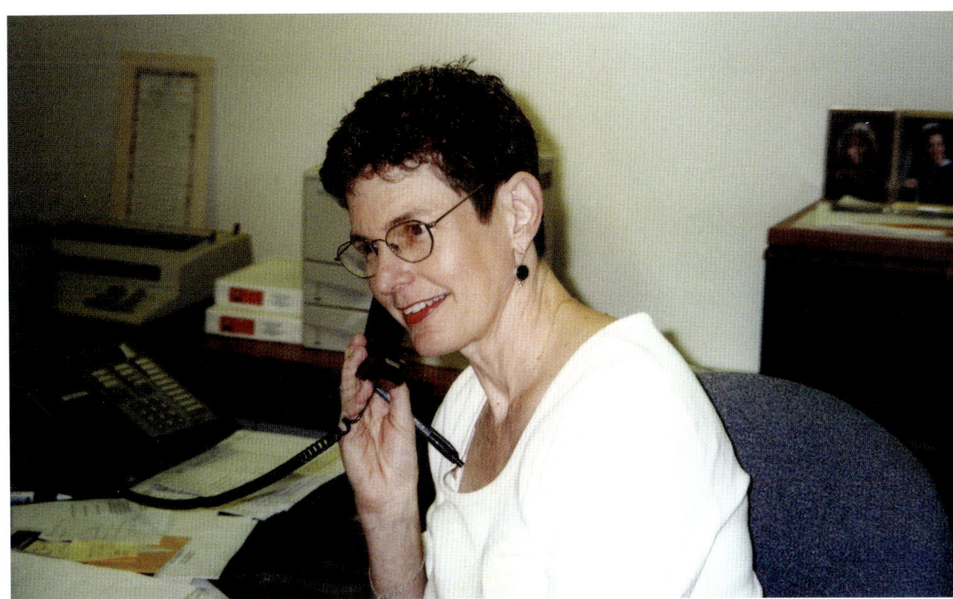

Susan Moore in her office, 2000.

In 2017, Susan Moore was featured in *Harris: Magazine of Harris College of Nursing & Health Sciences* for thirty-five years of service as an administrative assistant in the dean's office. Working under five previous deans and an interim dean in 2018, she has seen many changes—from using a computer instead of an electric IBM typewriter to the addition of many academic programs. June Seely, assistant to the dean, said that Moore serves as the "backbone" of the dean's office and tackles "innumerable and varied responsibilities with due diligence" (Salinas 2017). Former dean Susan Weeks recognized Moore as a "constant source of information and support" and provider of knowledge about the roles and functions of the dean's office (Salinas 2017). She left no stones unturned

Susan Moore's 35 Years

By Meghan Salinas '17

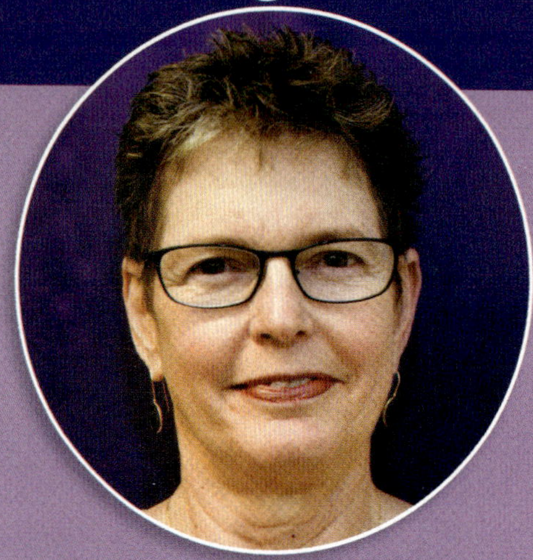

When making a phone call to the Dean's Office at Harris College of Nursing & Health Sciences, you'll probably hear the friendly voice of Susan Moore on the other end of the line. And, if you happen to visit the college to meet with an advisor or professor, Moore will likely be the smiling face greeting you at the door.

In 1982, when the college was still simply known as Harris College of Nursing, Moore arrived on campus to interview for a position under then-Dean Patricia Scearse. After securing the job, Moore came on board and joined the Harris family as an administrative assistant, a position she still holds today.

Five deans and 35 years later, Moore has borne witness to tremendous change in the halls of Harris College, originally beginning her departmental work the old-school way -- on an electric IBM typewriter.

"The technology has certainly changed, and it's been both a benefit and a good challenge," said Moore. She added, "Harris has really grown a lot, especially in the academic areas offered here."

Moore's ability to adapt to change, along with her hands-on professional style, have contributed to her upstanding reputation as both a skilled assistant and a steadfast friend.

"Susan Moore serves as the backbone of the Harris College Dean's Office and tackles her innumerable and varied responsibilities with steady diligence," said June Seely, assistant to the dean. "I am so thankful to work with such a kind and dependable colleague and friend."

Throughout the years, Moore has built strong bonds with her fellow officemates. She says one of her favorite aspects of the job is interacting with her colleagues, all of whom she considers to be more comrade than coworker.

And, certainly, Moore is just as beloved by her friends at Harris as they are to her.

"She was truly my go-to person when I had questions about anything related to the faculty, the staff, nursing, or the college," said Sharon Hudson, former assistant to the dean. "Her knowledge, dependability, work ethic, and loyalty to TCU and [Harris College] is truly amazing"

Today, Moore continues to have a quiet, yet incredibly immense impact upon the success of Harris College. Students and colleagues alike appreciate all she has done to support the mission of the organization.

"Susan Moore has been a constant source of information and support since I arrived at TCU in 1994," said Dr. Susan Weeks, dean of Harris College of Nursing & Health Sciences. "When I was asked to serve as the acting dean in December of 2013, she provided guidance to help me understand the functioning of the Dean's Office. She remains a valued colleague. I can't imagine doing my job without her!"

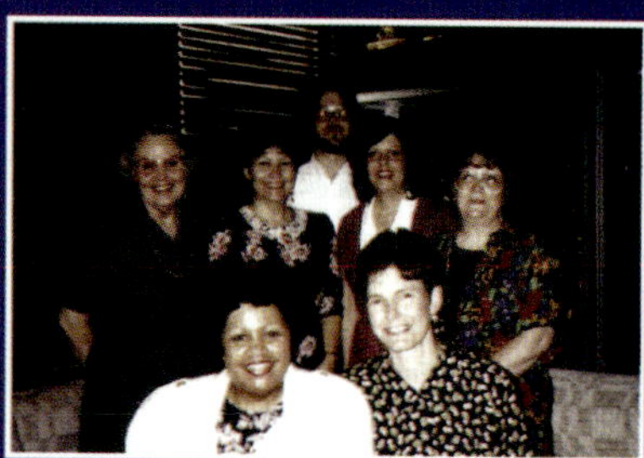

Left: Susan Moore (bottom right) and other Harris College faculty and staff pose for a photo in 1993.
Courtesy photo: Susan Moore

When Moore isn't on campus, she's usually spending time with family — daughters Sara, Lori, and Jaime, all TCU graduates, along with her son-in-law, Nathan; and grandchildren Blake, Holland, Myles, Cayson and Everett. The family enjoys taking road trips together, especially to the Texas Hill Country. Moore's faithful dog, Stormy, is always at her side.

Susan Moore, featured in **Harris Magazine** *for thirty-five years of service as an administrative assistant in the dean's office, 2017.*

to assist in locating and verifying resources for this book and provided unwavering support and assistance to the authors.

Students

Thirty-five students at Harris College were enrolled in the Army Reserve Officers' Training Corps (ROTC) as nurse cadets in 2011. Tierra Boykins followed in her father's and grandfather's steps by enrolling in the program (Smith 2011). Another student, Valerie Grenald, said her Panamanian immigrant parents' "spirit of giving back to their adopted homeland" influenced her to sign up for the program. Nursing cadets, in addition to learning nursing skills, also learned how to lead army units and "master skills such as land navigation, map reading, and patrolling" (4).

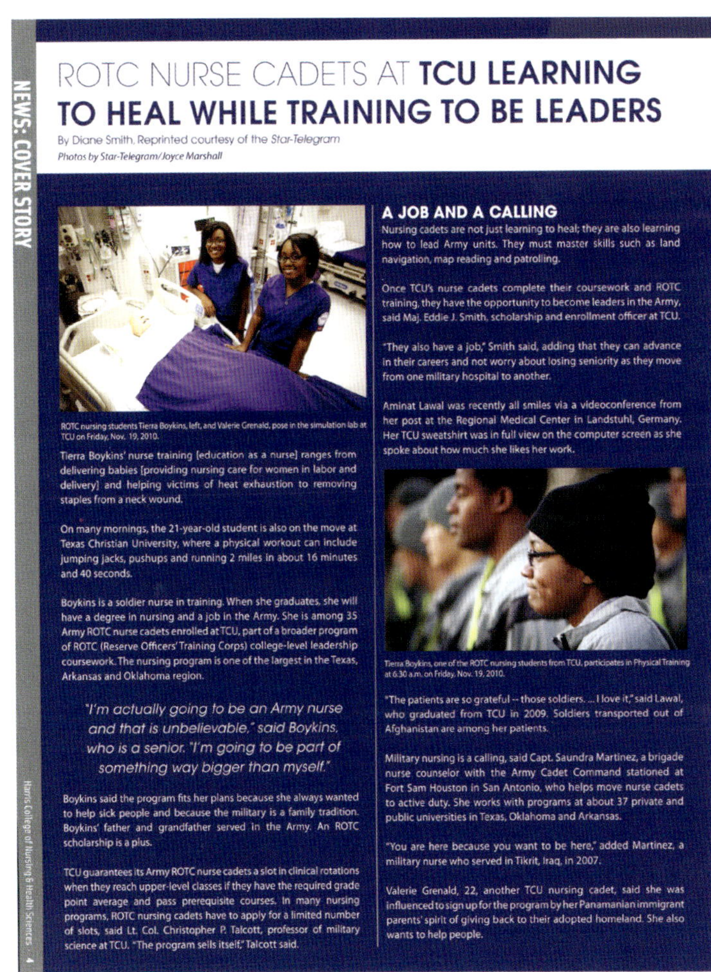

NEWS: COVER STORY

ROTC NURSE CADETS AT **TCU LEARNING TO HEAL WHILE TRAINING TO BE LEADERS**

By Diane Smith, Reprinted courtesy of the *Star-Telegram*

Photos by Star-Telegram/Joyce Marshall

ROTC nursing students Tierra Boykins, left, and Valerie Grenald, pose in the simulation lab at TCU on Friday, Nov. 19, 2010.

Tierra Boykins' nurse training [education as a nurse] ranges from delivering babies [providing nursing care for women in labor and delivery] and helping victims of heat exhaustion to removing staples from a neck wound.

On many mornings, the 21-year-old student is also on the move at Texas Christian University, where a physical workout can include jumping jacks, pushups and running 2 miles in about 16 minutes and 40 seconds.

Boykins is a soldier nurse in training. When she graduates, she will have a degree in nursing and a job in the Army. She is among 35 Army ROTC nurse cadets enrolled at TCU, part of a broader program of ROTC (Reserve Officers' Training Corps) college-level leadership coursework. The nursing program is one of the largest in the Texas, Arkansas and Oklahoma region.

"I'm actually going to be an Army nurse and that is unbelievable," said Boykins, who is a senior. "I'm going to be part of something way bigger than myself."

Boykins said the program fits her plans because she always wanted to help sick people and because the military is a family tradition. Boykins' father and grandfather served in the Army. An ROTC scholarship is a plus.

TCU guarantees its Army ROTC nurse cadets a slot in clinical rotations when they reach upper-level classes if they have the required grade point average and pass prerequisite courses. In many nursing programs, ROTC nursing cadets have to apply for a limited number of slots, said Lt. Col. Christopher P. Talcott, professor of military science at TCU. "The program sells itself," Talcott said.

A JOB AND A CALLING

Nursing cadets are not just learning to heal; they are also learning how to lead Army units. They must master skills such as land navigation, map reading and patrolling.

Once TCU's nurse cadets complete their coursework and ROTC training, they have the opportunity to become leaders in the Army, said Maj. Eddie J. Smith, scholarship and enrollment officer at TCU.

"They also have a job," Smith said, adding that they can advance in their careers and not worry about losing seniority as they move from one military hospital to another.

Aminat Lawal was recently all smiles via a videoconference from her post at the Regional Medical Center in Landstuhl, Germany. Her TCU sweatshirt was in full view on the computer screen as she spoke about how much she likes her work.

Tierra Boykins, one of the ROTC nursing students from TCU, participates in Physical Training at 6:30 a.m. on Friday, Nov. 19, 2010.

"The patients are so grateful -- those soldiers. ... I love it," said Lawal, who graduated from TCU in 2009. Soldiers transported out of Afghanistan are among her patients.

Military nursing is a calling, said Capt. Saundra Martinez, a brigade nurse counselor with the Army Cadet Command stationed at Fort Sam Houston in San Antonio, who helps move nurse cadets to active duty. She works with programs at about 37 private and public universities in Texas, Oklahoma and Arkansas.

"You are here because you want to be here," added Martinez, a military nurse who served in Tikrit, Iraq, in 2007.

Valerie Grenald, 22, another TCU nursing cadet, said she was influenced to sign up for the program by her Panamanian immigrant parents' spirit of giving back to their adopted homeland. She also wants to help people.

Harris College of Nursing & Health Sciences 4

Tierra Boykins and Valerie Grenald in Sim Lab, 2011.

The baccalaureate nursing program became the first DAISY in Training Award partner in Texas in 2015. The DAISY in Training Award recognizes students for "above-and-beyond" care and compassion shown to families. Criteria include a commitment to compassionate care of patients and families, a connection with patients, families, and peers by building trust and respect, advocating for patients, and demonstrating exceptional skill. Nominations may be made by patients and their families, staff members, coworkers, physicians, preceptors, instructors, or fellow students.

The first student to receive the award was Jenny Van Beber in 2015. She was nominated by a faculty member for her empathy with a cancer patient. This initial student award was presented to Van Beber during the TCU Nursing's Pinning Ceremony in May (Marinda Allender, pers. comm., 2018). Subsequently, the award has been presented at the Annual Celebration of Leadership Dinner sponsored by the Leadership Department of TCU. Other DAISY in Training Award recipients have been Grace Cable in 2017 and Bridget Davis in 2018.

In the summer of 2012, Amberle Durano, a bachelor of nursing science student, was selected for a competitive internship with the World Health Organization. As part of the internship, she worked on data related to the provision of antiretroviral therapy and the pediatric population.

In 2013, Reagan Elliott became the first undergraduate student to complete a systematic review as a part of her honors project along with her faculty adviser Diane Hawley, as the principal investigator, and Sharon Gunn, a clinical nurse specialist at Baylor Scott and White in Dallas. The systematic review investigated best evidence as to whether pleural chest tubes should be drained by suction or by gravity in resolving a pneumothorax. The review was later published in 2014 in the *JBI Database of Systematic Reviews & Implementation Reports.* The review was selected as the inaugural winner of the TCU JBI Systematic Review in the 2013–14 academic year.

The 2013–14 academic year provided additional opportunities for students to broaden their experiences. Sharon Gunn, a doctor of nursing practice student, participated in an internship with the International Council of Nurses in Geneva, Switzerland.

In 2017, two undergraduate nursing students engaged in internships focused on their special interests. Before her final semester at TCU, Rachel Kellogg, described as an "advocate of preventive care," spent a summer in Washington, DC, where she interned with the US Senate Committee on Health, Education, Labor, and Pensions. During the summer, along with four other interns, she worked with the Health Policy Office, which "focuses on public health, immunizations, emergency preparedness, and global health." In this role she had the responsibility to "track changes to health care bills" and summarize them for the health team. Based on her experiences as an intern, she is considering potential career opportunities as a research assistant in global health policy in either the Office of Global Affairs or the Office of Disease Prevention and Health Promotion (Farason 2018).

A second student, Crysta Coomer, completed an internship with the World Health Organization in Switzerland. During her six weeks in this role, she participated as a data collector in selected research projects related to HIV and AIDS among young girls and women within southern and eastern Africa. She also had the opportunity to attend seminars related to current projects and their findings. For example, one researcher discussed his research related to "the lack of sexual education for adolescents in public schools in Texas." Coomer, who was on her first trip abroad, also noted that the internship helped her develop people skills and gave her the opportunity to interact with people who were different from her (Farason 2018).

A reunion between Israel "Izzy" Sanchez, a Navy veteran and nursing student at TCU, and Rear Admiral Rebecca McCormick-Boyle occurred in November 2017 when Boyle spoke to his class during TCU's Navy Week. Sanchez joined the Navy in 2003, served in the Naval Hospital Great Lakes in 2005, and served under McCormick-Boyle when she was the executive officer in the clinic where he worked. He noted her focus on education, leadership, and health promotion, and considered her a mentor. Entering the BSN to doctor of nursing practice (DNP) program at TCU will be his next step in becoming a nurse practitioner (Harris College/TCU Nursing 2017).

Student Nurses Association (SNA)

In the spring of 2018, an invitation was sent to the current officers in the TCU Student Nurses Association (SNA) asking them to participate in interviews about their motivation for becoming nurses, their involvement in the SNA, and the major challenges and rewards of their roles in the organization. Three students (the vice president, the secretary, and the president-elect for 2018–19) responded.

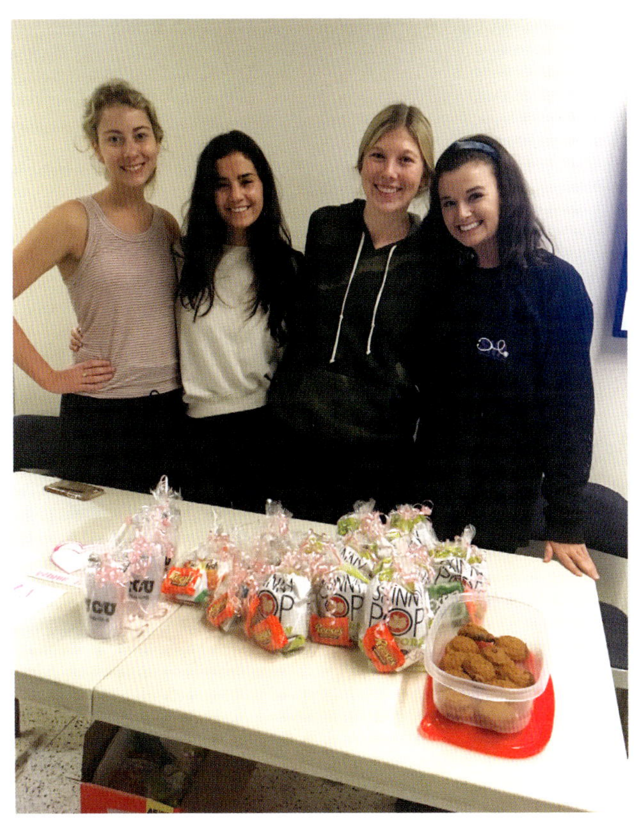

SNA students fundraising. L-R, Georgia Ginn, president; Marissa Ulibarri, treasurer; Caroline Scully, secretary; and Rachel Federer, membership director, February 11, 2020.

Caja Norman, the secretary of SNA, who was Junior II in the spring of 2018, chose to become a nurse after her sister died in 2000. She wanted to be able to care for babies like her and considers her to be the "motivation and reasoning behind all she does" (Caja Norman, pers. comm., 2018). Participation in SNA provided the opportunity to interact with people who had similar goals. Norman hoped to lead her peers toward experiences during college that would prepare them to become better nurses in the future.

Claire Bordeaux, who graduated in spring 2018 and served as vice president of SNA, was also motivated by a desire to be in a helping profession, to be involved in something that would allow her to give to and serve others (Claire Bordeaux, pers. comm., 2018). Claire saw her involvement in SNA as an opportunity to learn about the nursing world outside of TCU, as it allowed her to hear and learn from speakers in a wide range of health care fields. It was also an opportunity to connect with other nursing majors at TCU.

Savannah Hale, who became the president of SNA in fall 2018, participated in SNA committees when she was a freshman (2016–17) and was the treasurer and parliamentarian during the 2017–18 academic year. Savannah cannot cite a "single reason" she chose nursing, although her mother was a licensed vocational nurse (LVN). She had originally thought of majoring in business, but when she arrived at TCU, her "heart was pulling her towards nursing." She joined SNA to become more involved in the nursing department and "to get as much out of it as possible . . . and to be able to give back to a department that I know has so much to give me" (Savannah Hale, pers. comm., 2018).

Savannah chose to run for office as she was both motivated and encouraged by older students who were already on the executive committee. She has "always had a passion for leadership" and wanted the opportunity to put her ideas into action. Challenges included the difficulties in balancing class, clinical, and "regular life." Hale noted that there is "something very special about Harris College . . . the relationship between students and professors." She added that she never feels like she is alone in her journey and that she has people behind her who support and believe in her (Savannah Hale, pers. comm., 2018).

Norman, Bordeaux, and Hale all described one or more activities in which they had participated as SNA members and officers. They include blood drives, organizing study events, and organizing care packages that students receive from their parents during finals. The latter involved contacting parents, ordering supplies, assembling boxes, and distributing personal letters from parents to students' mail boxes.

Sponsors for SNA during the 2017–18 academic year were faculty members Barbara Patten and Susan Fife, with Jodie Weatherly joined joining Fife as a second sponsor in 2018 upon the departure of Patten.

Harris Fellows, Harris Ambassadors, and Harris Peer Partners

Harris Fellows, junior-level students who are nominated by faculty based on a minimum 3.5 GPA, are selected for participation in a one-year academic enrichment program that was initiated in 2012 for nursing majors, but included all Harris majors in 2013. Activities include leadership development, invitations to research events, hospital tours, and service events such as volunteering to provide Halloween and Valentine parties for residents of the Presbyterian Night Shelter. Approximately twelve to fifteen students participate each year.

Harris Ambassadors, students also nominated by faculty based on a minimum 3.0 GPA, serve as representatives of Harris College. These individuals provide assistance with activities such as Green Chair events, the Nursing Pinning Ceremony, and college and career fair events.

Harris Peer Partners, junior and senior students, serve as mentors to freshmen. To participate, they complete an application, receive training related to their responsibilities, and are oriented to the university resources for students. They also attend university events together to help incoming students integrate in the university. Thirty-four pairs participated in the academic year 2017–18.

In 2014, the Arnold P. Gold Foundation (APGF) and the American Association of Colleges of Nursing collaborated to fund one hundred schools of nursing to pilot the White Coat Ceremonies. The first White Coat Ceremony for BSN students at TCU was held in January 2016. Originally a rite of passage in medical schools, it was designed to "promote humanistic patient-centered care" (Arnold P. Gold Foundation 2018).

The January 2018 ceremony was held at University Christian Church in Fort Worth, where seventy-three BSN students recited an oath to provide the highest quality care and services. This ceremony included a processional, a welcome by Marinda Allender, division director of the Undergraduate Program, and a presentation by Lynnette Howington, director of administrative and clinical affairs for TCU Nursing. This was followed by the donning of white coats and a recitation of the White Coat Ceremony Oath. The most recent ceremony was held in August 2018, with Interim Dean Suzy Lockwood bringing the welcome to 116 students. The speaker for the ceremony was a 2017 BSN graduate.

White Coat Ceremony Oath

As a nurse dedicated to providing the highest quality care and services, I solemnly pledge that I will

- Consider the welfare of humanity and relief of suffering my primary concerns;
- Act in a compassionate and trustworthy manner in all aspects of my care;
- Apply my knowledge, experience, and skills to the best of my ability to assure optimal outcomes for my patients;
- Exercise sound professional judgment while abiding by legal and ethical requirements;
- Accept the lifelong obligation to improve my professional knowledge and competence;
- Promote, advocate for, and strive to protect the health, safety, and rights of the patient.

With this pledge, I accept the duties and responsibilities that embody the nursing profession. I take this oath voluntarily with the full realization of the responsibility with which I am entrusted by the public.

Discover TCU Nursing

In the summer of 2018, students entering their junior or senior year of high school had the opportunity to "discover what nursing is really like" (2018). The first nursing camp at TCU was held in July 2018 and offered students a firsthand look at the nursing profession, the opportunities for nurses, and the challenges and rewards of the profession. Lockwood presented the idea to faculty and asked for interested persons to participate. With the ongoing support of Rose Davis, administrative program specialist, the program was marketed to prospective participants who were supported by her throughout the initial process. Stephanie Evans was appointed the program coordinator (Stephanie Evans, pers. comm., 2018). Thirty-two campers from throughout the state of Texas and one from California participated in the activities in 2018.

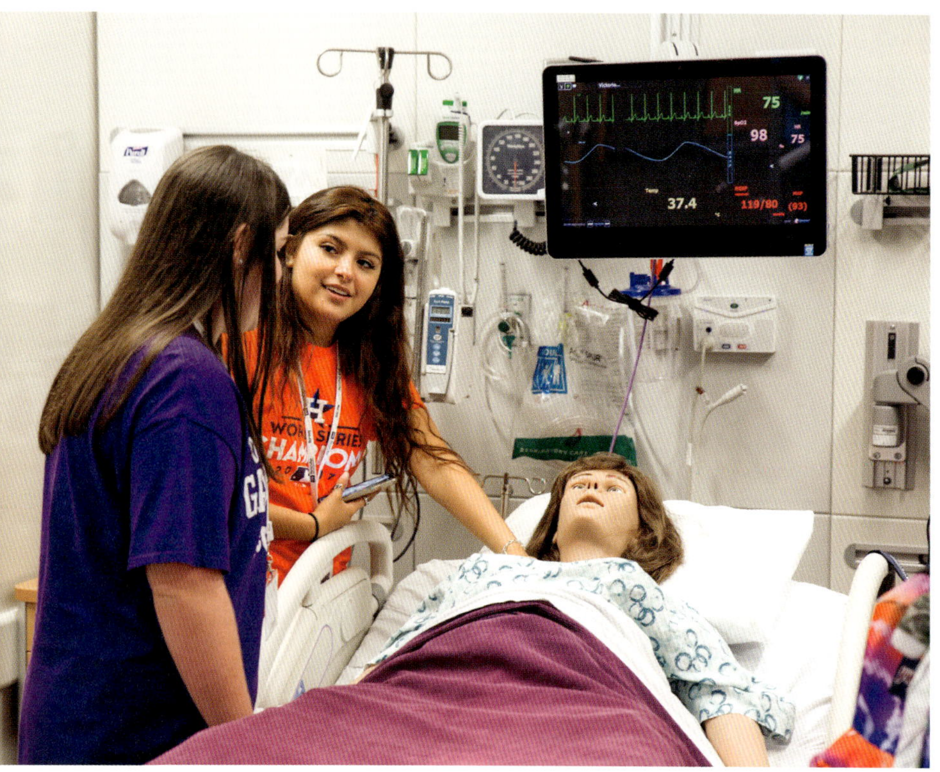

Students at the Discover the TCU Nursing camp.

Prospective campers submitted an application form, a current high school transcript, and a letter of recommendation from a science teacher or school counselor. They also answered an essay prompt: "Why I am interested in exploring a career in nursing and how the Discover TCU Nursing camp will impact my plans for the future." Twelve current nursing faculty members, one microbiology faculty, and nine current nursing students participated in the camp. Nursing students guided the campers through program activities on campus such as lunches in the Brown-Lupton University Union and in the Annie Richardson Bass Building, where they completed an American Heart Association CPR course, interacted with human patient simulators, and practiced effective communication skills.

The camp, which was held from 8:30 a.m. to 5:00 p.m. for five consecutive days, offered participants the opportunity to practice effective communication skills, explore nursing skills such as taking vital signs and caring for wounds, and learn how knowledge from the sciences is used by nurses.

Three students, Joshua Clift, Cile Baker, and Karina Gonzales, and faculty member Libby Slone volunteered at the Carnival de Salud sponsored by the Hispanic Wellness Coalition in the summer of 2018. Services provided by the students included keeping track of attendees by issuing wristbands to children and adults, greeting members from the community and showing them the various services that were available, and translating for Spanish-speaking individuals. Gonzales commented that it was an honor to represent TCU at the Hispanic Wellness Coalition, and she hoped that future nursing students would continue to volunteer (Karina Gonzales, pers. comm., 2018).

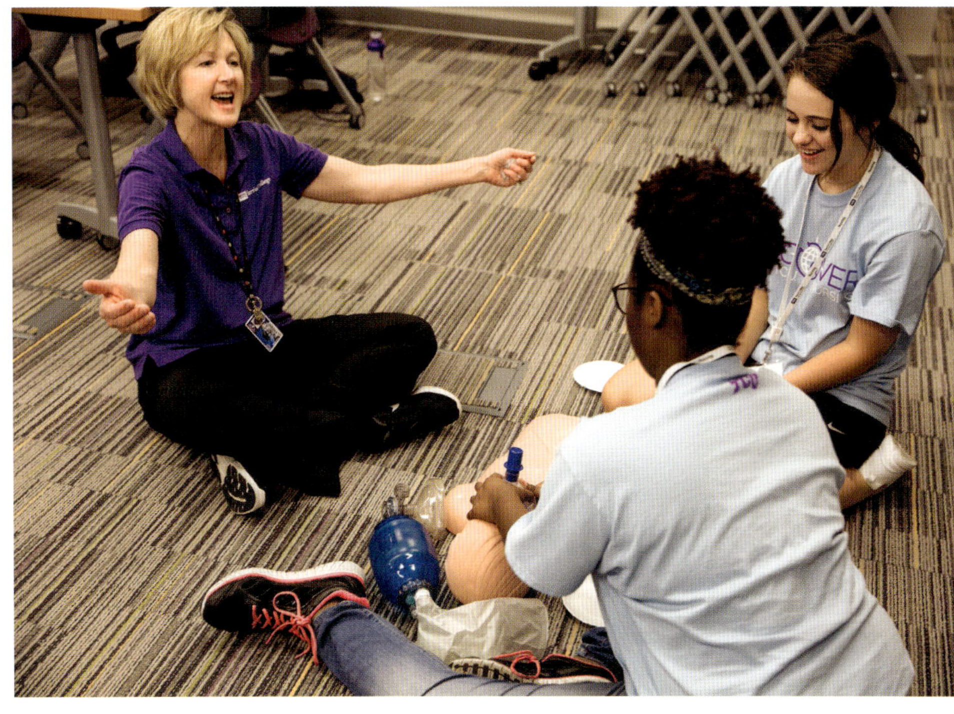

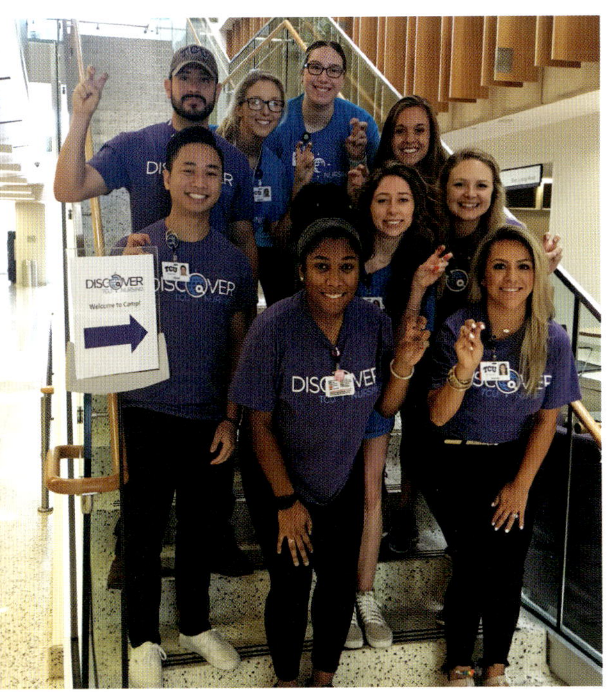

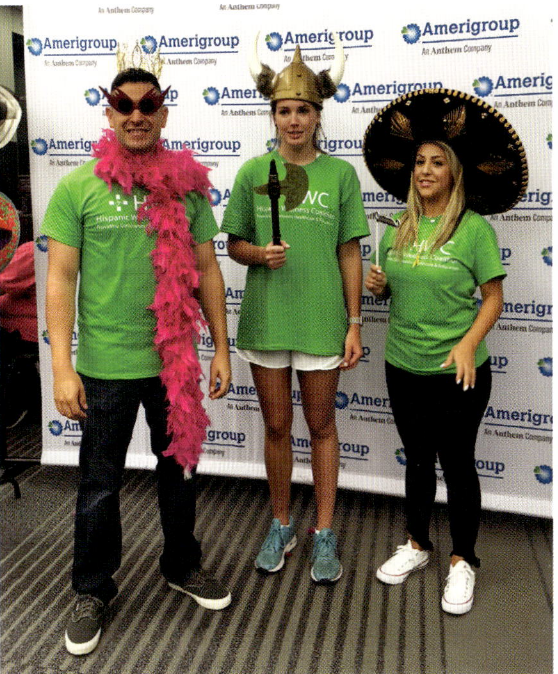

(Above) Laura Thielke and students at the Discover TCU Nursing camp, 2018.

(Far left) TCU Nursing camp participants, summer 2018.

(Near left) Having some fun at the Carnival de Salud, 2018.

Graduate Programs

In 2015, all graduate programs were reaccredited for another ten years, through 2025. In 2016, TCU's first nurse practitioner program, a post baccalaureate to DNP Family Nurse Practitioner (FNP), was launched. This program prepares graduates entering with a BSN to obtain a terminal practice degree as advanced practice nurse in the role of FNP. FNPs provide direct clinical care at the individual patient level with a focus on the care of the family across the lifespan. The Adult-Gerontology Acute Nurse Practitioner Program was approved in April 2018 and will begin admitting students in summer 2019.

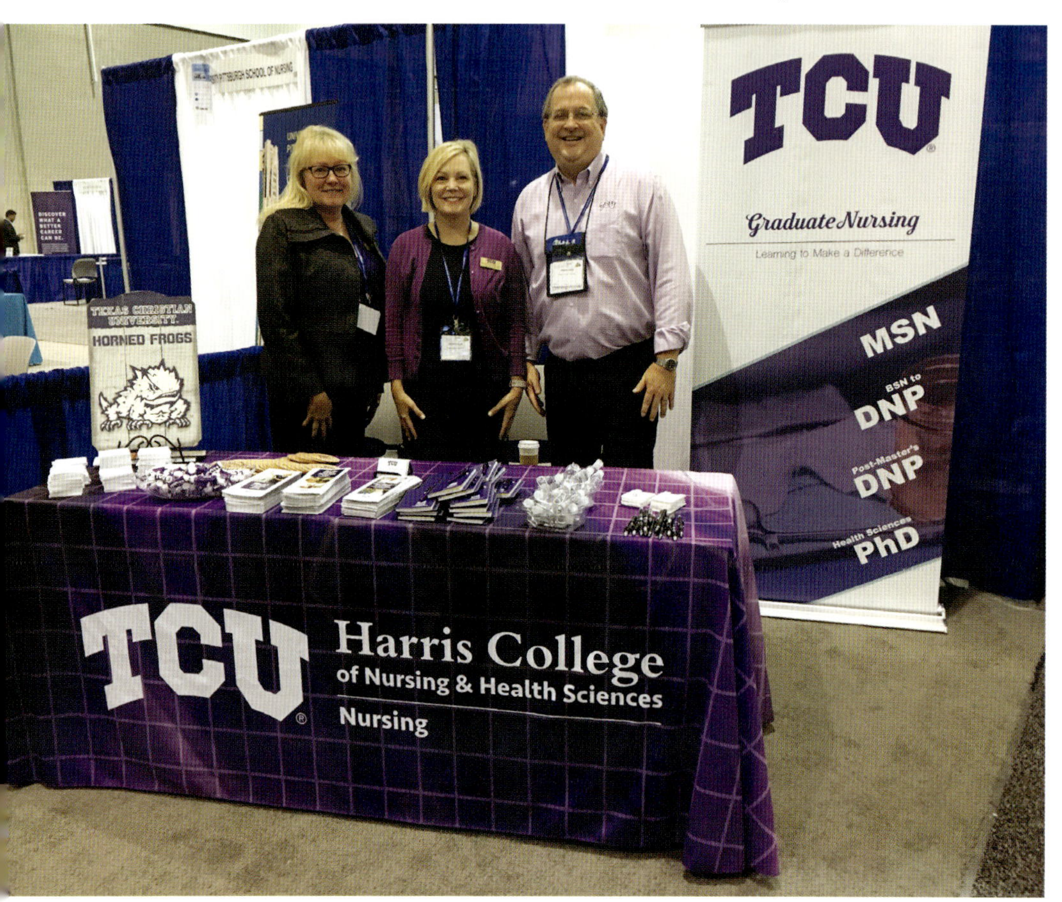

L-R, Roseann Diehl, Kathy Ellis, and Dennis Cheek recruiting for nursing graduate programs.

In addition, the existing MSN Clinical Nurse Specialist (adult-gerontology and pediatric) program was transitioned to BSN to DNP in 2016 to be consistent with the AACN recommendation that all APRNs be prepared at the doctoral level.

The Doctor of Philosophy (PhD) in Health Sciences, which began in fall 2018, prepares individuals for research and teaching careers in academia and industry by offering two tracks: physical health sciences and social health sciences. The physical health sciences track focuses on physiological and epidemiological issues related to the human body from one of four different graduate departments in Harris College: Communication Sciences and Disorders, Kinesiology, Nurse Anesthesia, and Nursing. The social health science track focuses on psychosocial issues of human beings from one of the five different graduate departments in Harris College: Communication Sciences and Disorders, Kinesiology, Nurse Anesthesia, Nursing, and Social Work (Harris College of Nursing & Health Sciences 2018).

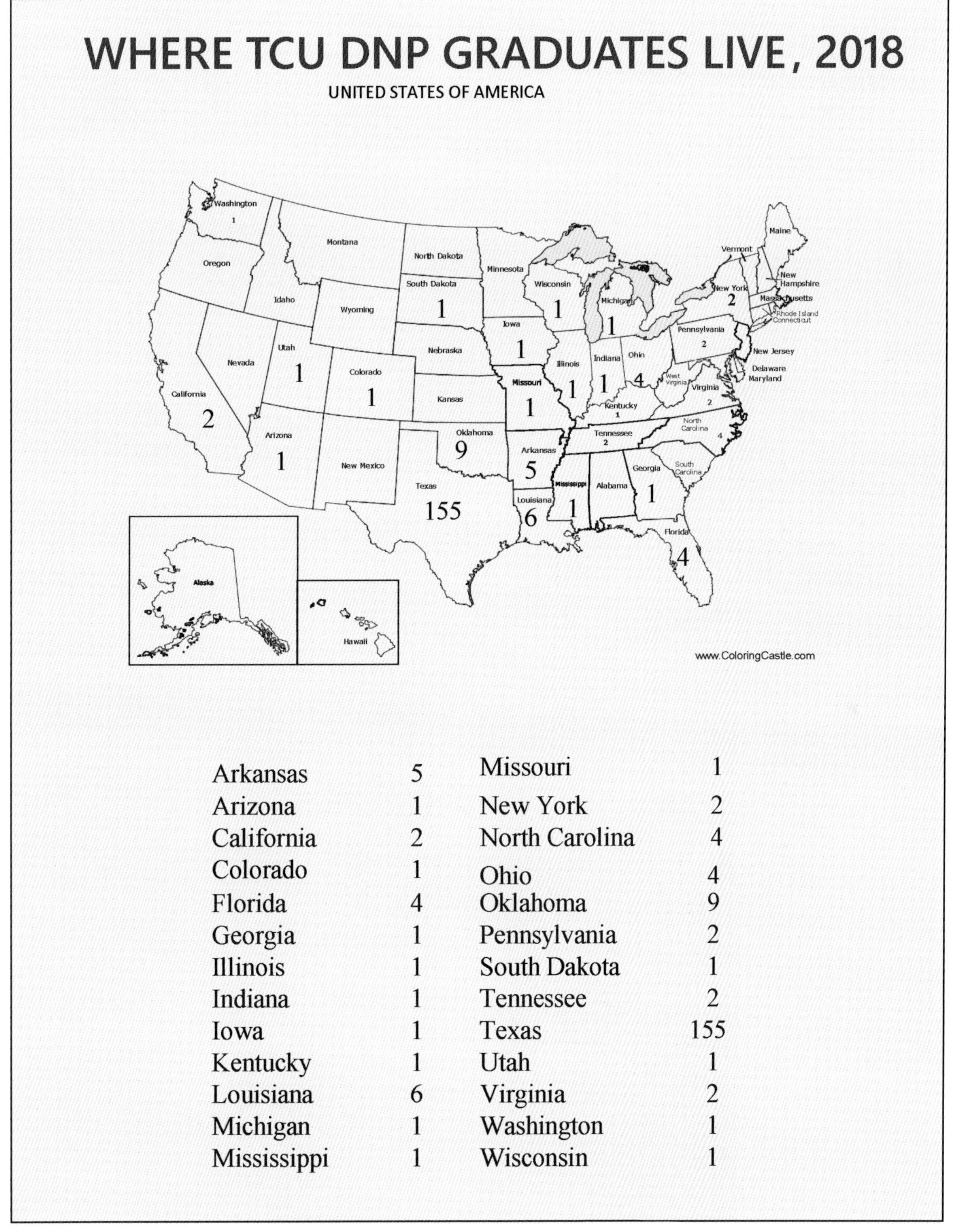

Arkansas	5	Missouri	1
Arizona	1	New York	2
California	2	North Carolina	4
Colorado	1	Ohio	4
Florida	4	Oklahoma	9
Georgia	1	Pennsylvania	2
Illinois	1	South Dakota	1
Indiana	1	Tennessee	2
Iowa	1	Texas	155
Kentucky	1	Utah	1
Louisiana	6	Virginia	2
Michigan	1	Washington	1
Mississippi	1	Wisconsin	1

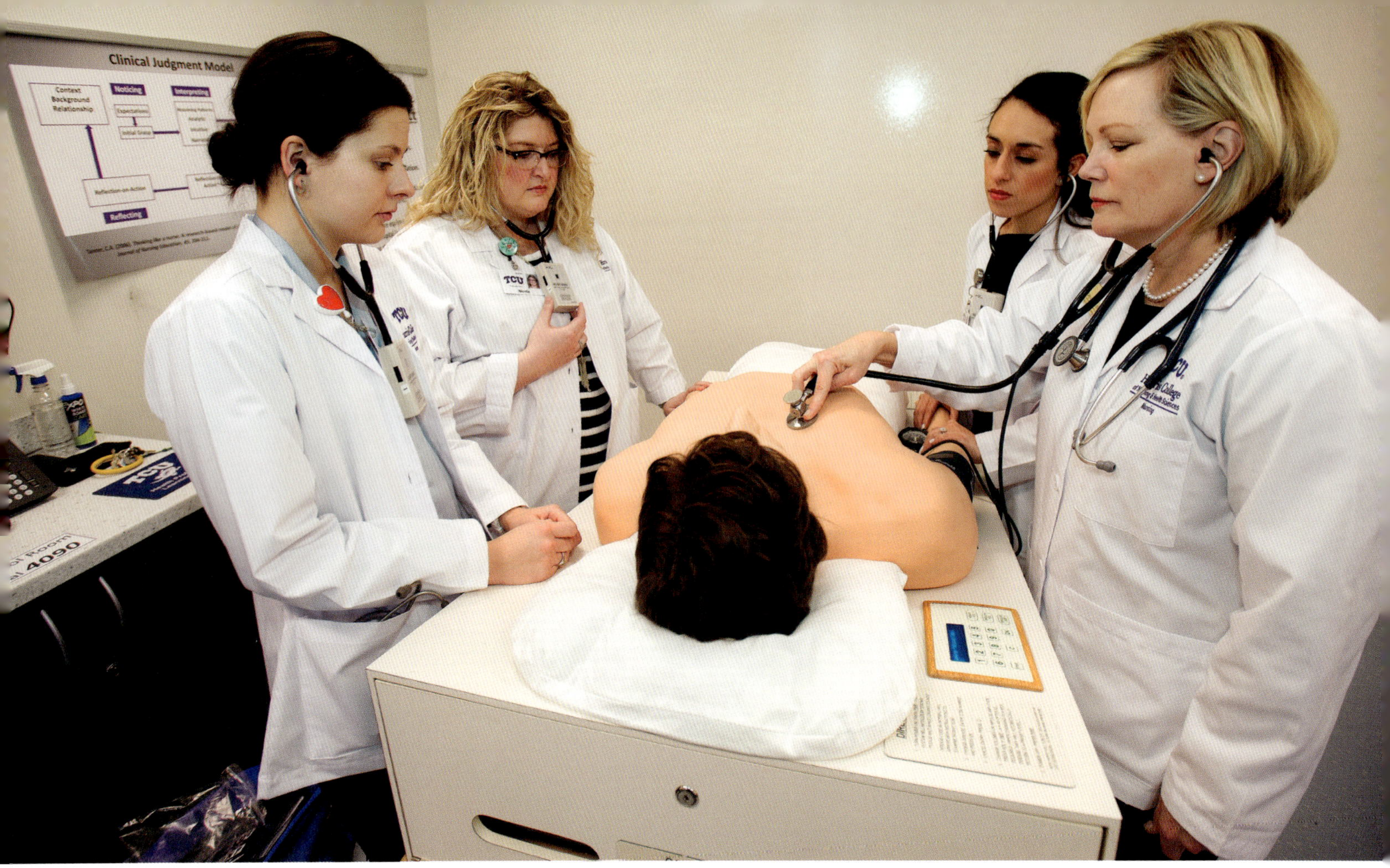

(Above) Kathy Ellis and students in the Simulation Lab.

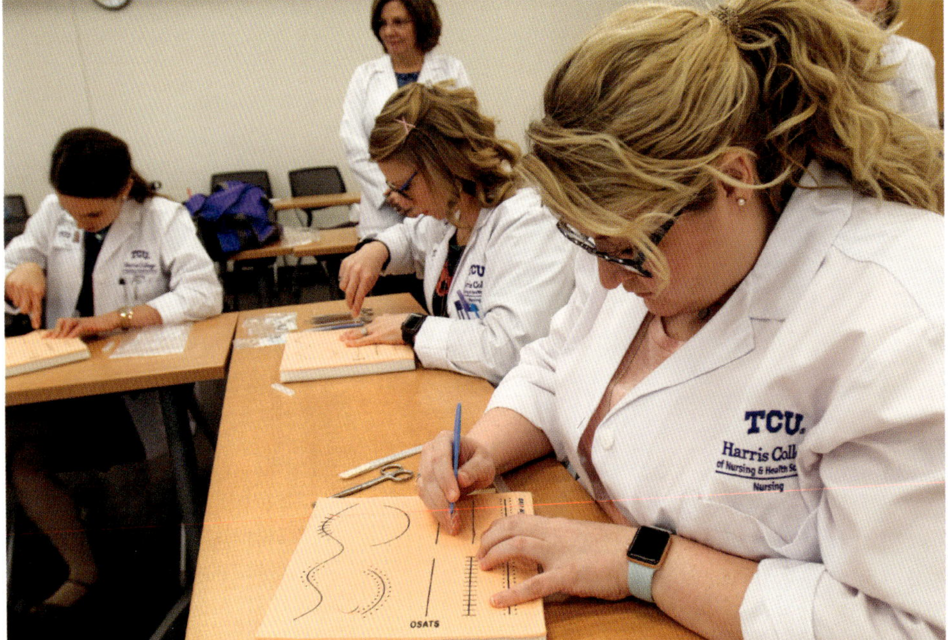

(Right) Students in wound class.

Study Abroad

Global Perspectives in Health continued to be offered in London in 2010, though in 2012, 2014, 2016, and 2018 the course was modified to include one week in Geneva and two weeks in London. Participating in these trips were faculty members Susan Weeks, Diane Hawley, Sharon Canclini, Marinda Allender, and Amy Anderson.

Weeks indicated that the addition of time in Geneva allowed the expansion of course content to focus on global health and health care. The decision was made to start the course in Geneva to ease the students into a new culture. The intense pace of London was often perceived as overwhelming to the average student, even though all spoke English. Geneva has a small but international community feel, which was the perfect setting to begin the study abroad experience for students. The World Health Organization helped students understand the broad and varied nature of

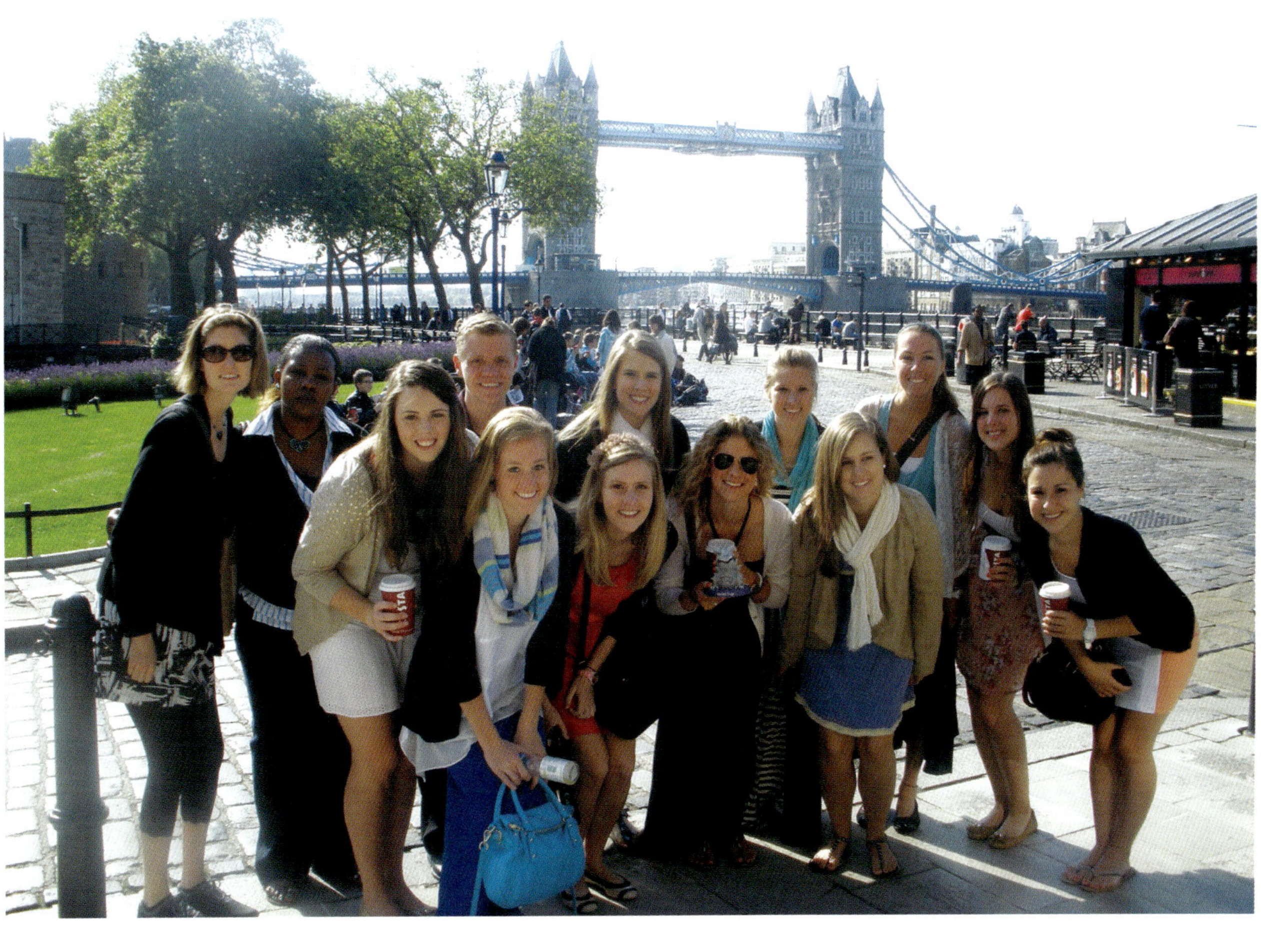

Students at London Bridge, summer 2012.

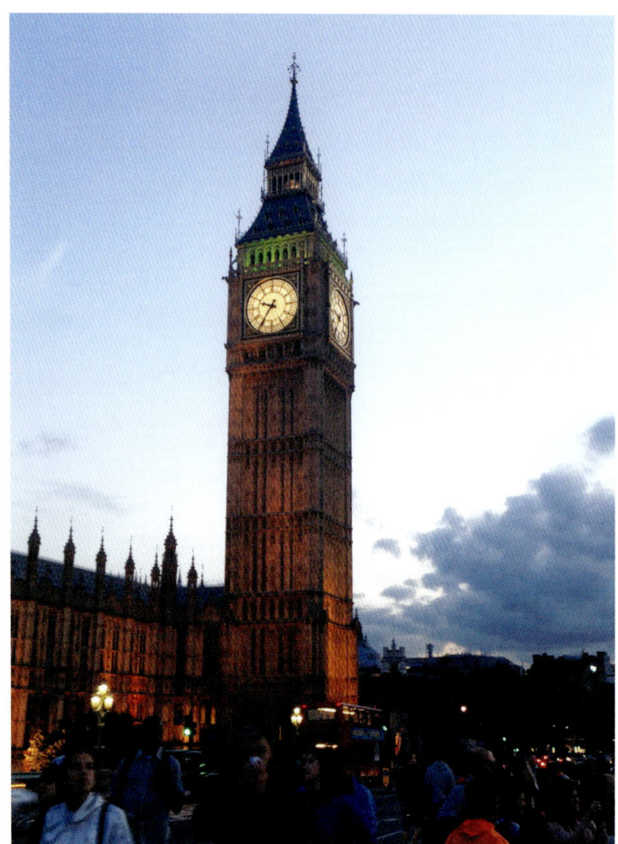

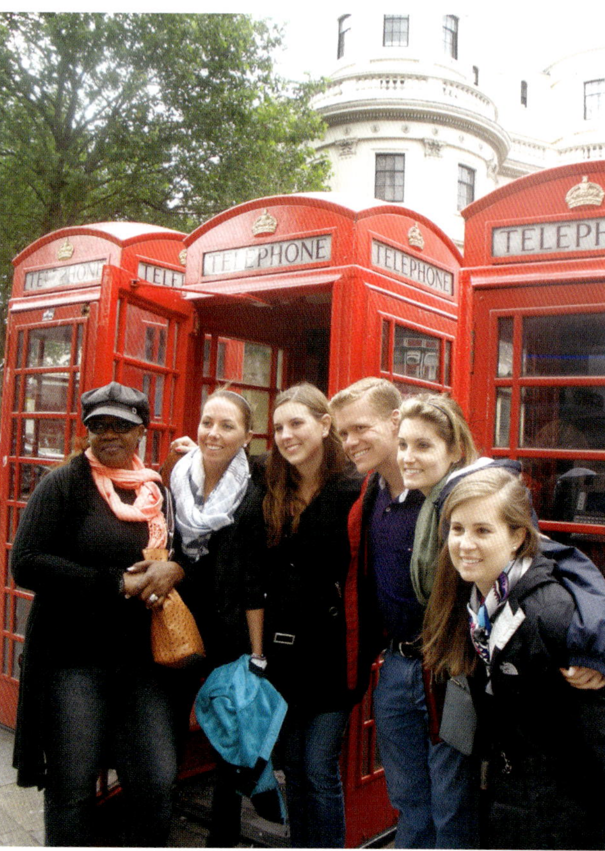

(Left) Big Ben. (Right) The iconic phone booths of London, summer 2012.

health concepts within the global community. The United Nations (UN) European Headquarters provided glimpses into the way health has become a political issue. Students learned about the Millennium Development Goals and subsequent Sustainable Development Goals offered by the UN and how each relates to the social determinants of health. The headquarters of the International Red Cross and the International Council of Nurses provided the opportunity for students to learn about the scope and role of large international organizations. Also included in the Geneva portion of the course was a day trip to a rural community outside of Geneva, where the students completed an assignment comparing urban and rural aspects of health.

During each course, health care delivery sites such as hospitals and clinics were visited to assist students in their comparison of the US, British, and Swiss health care systems. The ability to compare and contrast each system of care, as well as the care settings, helped students understand the vast resources that are dedicated to health care. The Swiss health care system happens to be a nice blend of the US health care system, at one end of the spectrum, and the British National Health Service

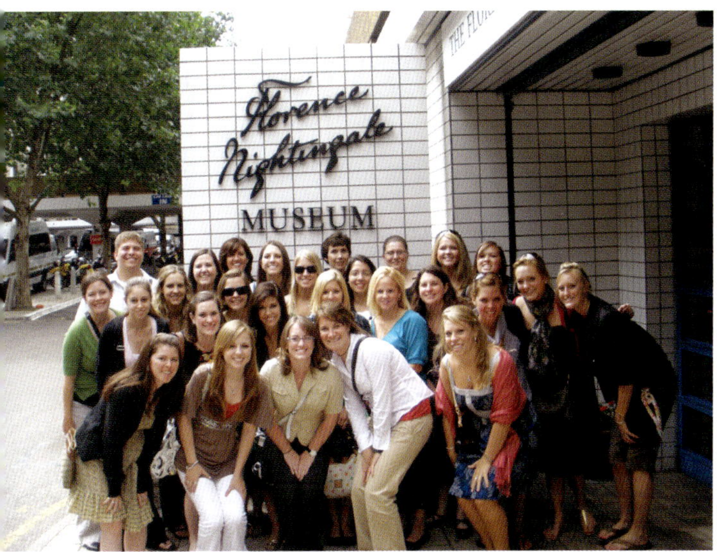

Students at the Florence Nightingale Museum.

at the other.

Students were also able to study in Reggio Emilia and Florence, Italy, in 2013, 2015, and 2017 to explore the country's historical development as it relates to modern health, illness, and the health care system. The inaugural trip to Reggio Emilia, a Sister City of Fort Worth, occurred in 2013 and was led by faculty members Sharon Canclini and Lea Montgomery, accompanied by Dean Paulette Burns.

Students explored the historical development, the social-political and bio-physical factors related to health beliefs, and the health care delivery system in Italy. Field trips, visits to historical and health-related sites, lectures, and hands-on experiences provided them an opportunity to observe the role of the nurse and other health care workers in a variety of settings. In addition, students learned about health and wellness as part of the Mediterranean diet and lifestyle.

Students reported that during their many tours, the concept of "cultural humility and awareness" was ever present. This was exemplified by many of the brochures about the country being written in multiple languages to accommodate all visitors. A special event was the opportunity to observe the Sala (Room) del Tricolore, the birthplace of the Italian flag. Representative of the bond between many cultures, the flag is flown constantly. Upon returning from Italy, students delivered a presentation about their experiences living and learning in Reggio Emilia to the Fort Worth Chapter of Sister Cities International. These citizens support the intercultural relationship between the two cities.

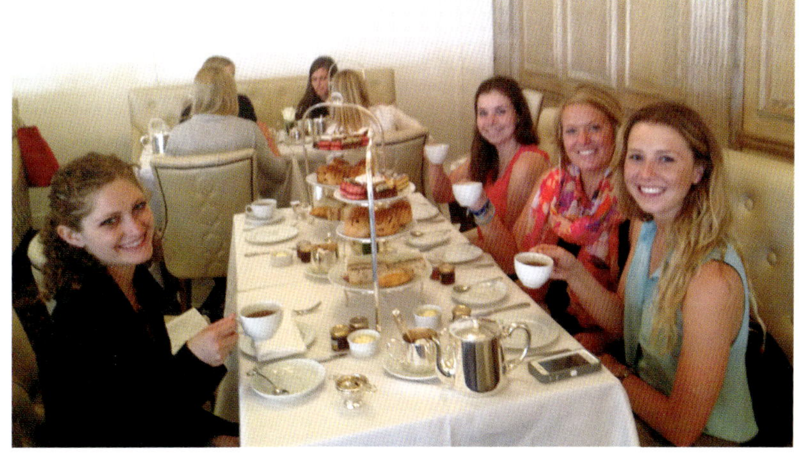

Students at High Tea, summer 2014.

In the summer of 2017 another twenty students traveled to Reggio Emilia and Florence with Sharon Canclini and Diane Hawley. Four months after the completion of the course, students vividly recalled some of their experiences (Students who participated in study abroad, pers. comm., 2017). One student commented that she "learned a lot about the bigger picture of everything and how there are so many different things that impact and influence health." She had gained a new appreciation for other health care systems "and how daily lifestyle and nutrition play a big role in health" (pers. comm., 2017). Still another student noted that the elderly were "so fit and agile . . . because of years of good health practices," which were credited as a means of prevention (pers. comm., 2017).

One student experienced the health care system firsthand with a dental emergency (fractured tooth) midway through the trip. While on a field trip to a cancer hospital, the student could no longer tolerate the pain and an attending doctor provided enough medication to manage the pain until help could be secured. This was followed by a call to a Fort Worth-Reggio Emilia Sister City contact who identified

Students at the World Health Organization, 2014.

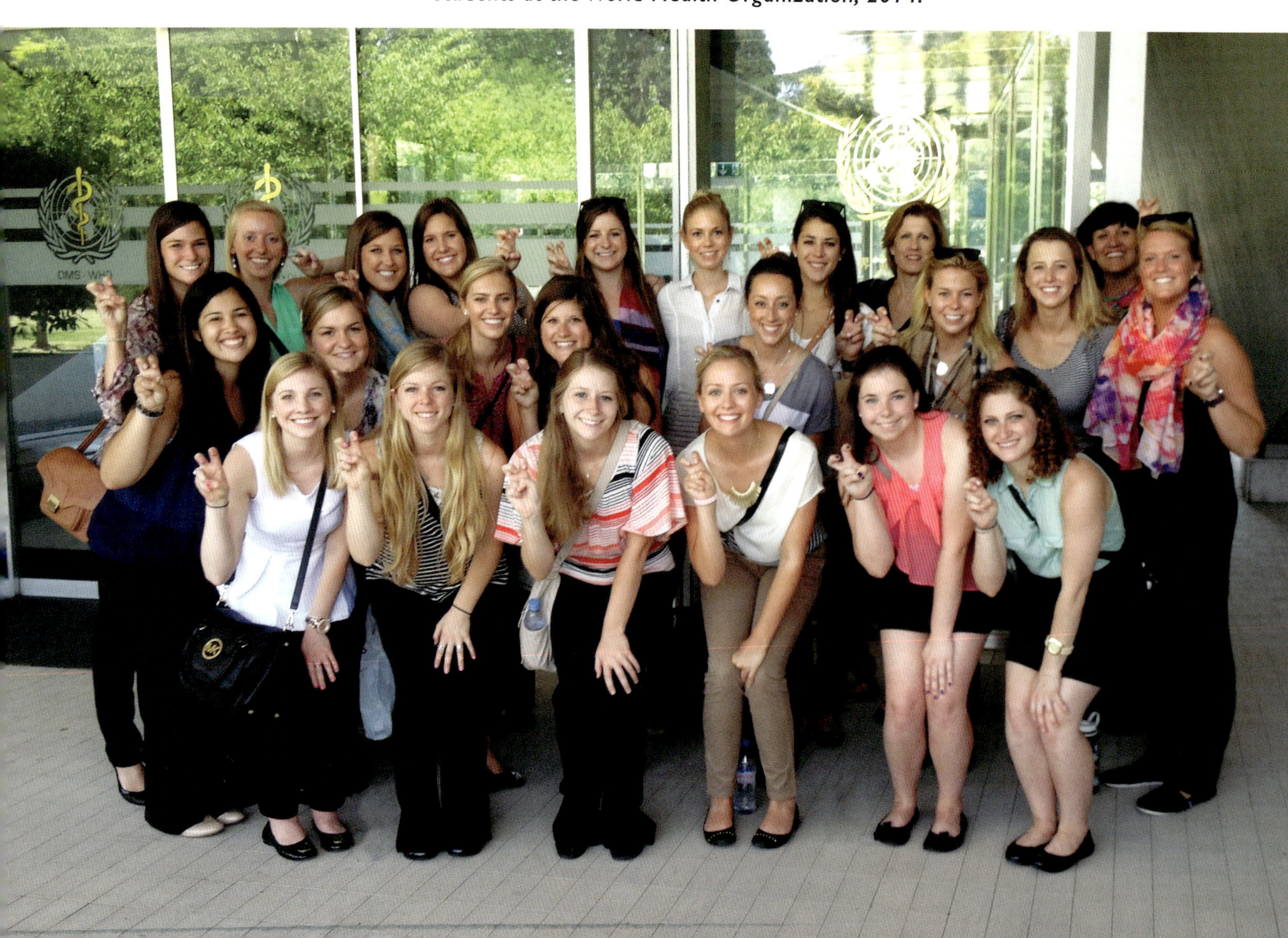

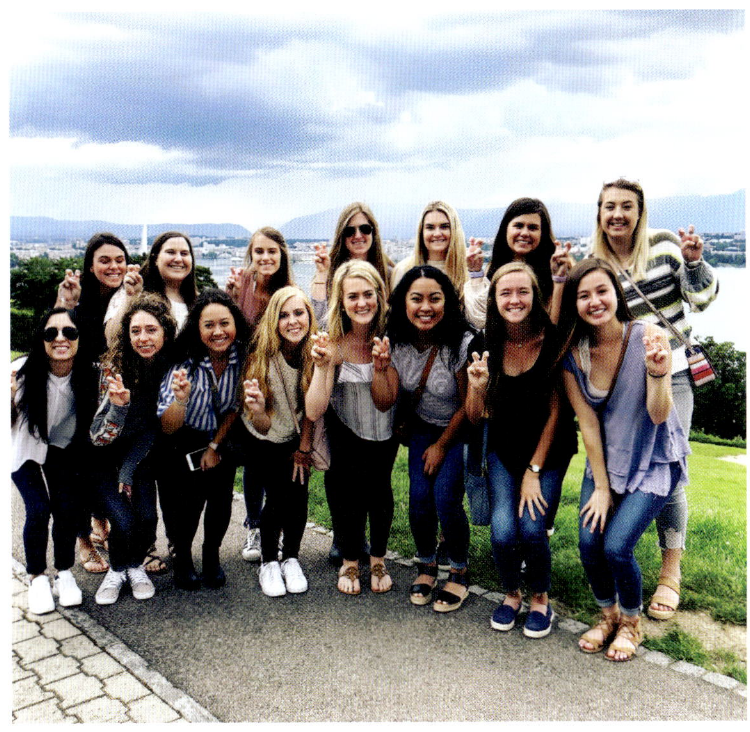

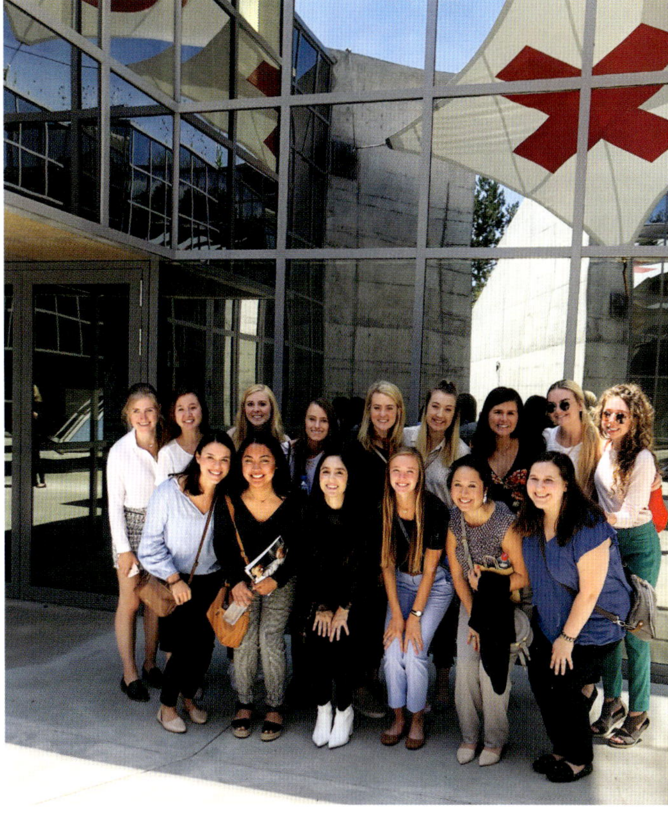

(Above) Students exploring Geneva, 2018.
(Right) Students visit the International Red Cross, 2018.

a dentist for immediate treatment. Reflecting on her experience, the student commented that the "care was very personable, with short wait times, clean and brightly lit rooms, and a friendly atmosphere." And, no charges!

The consistent "friendliness" of the Italian individuals with whom the students interacted was a highlight of the trip (pers. comm., 2017). Students commented that their perspectives on a different culture and health care within a different system would impact the way they thought about their health system and ways in which care is delivered in different countries.

Chile and Argentina

In 2017, study abroad options were expanded to include the first trip to Chile and Argentina, where students examined the health beliefs and practices of two South American countries and the role of health professionals with whom they interacted. Directed by Suzy Lockwood and Irmgard Payne from Communication Sciences and Disorders, ten students traveled to Santiago, Chile, where they interacted with individuals from Universidad Mayor. While in Santiago, participants engaged in lectures and discussions that focused on historical aspects of health, illness, and delivery

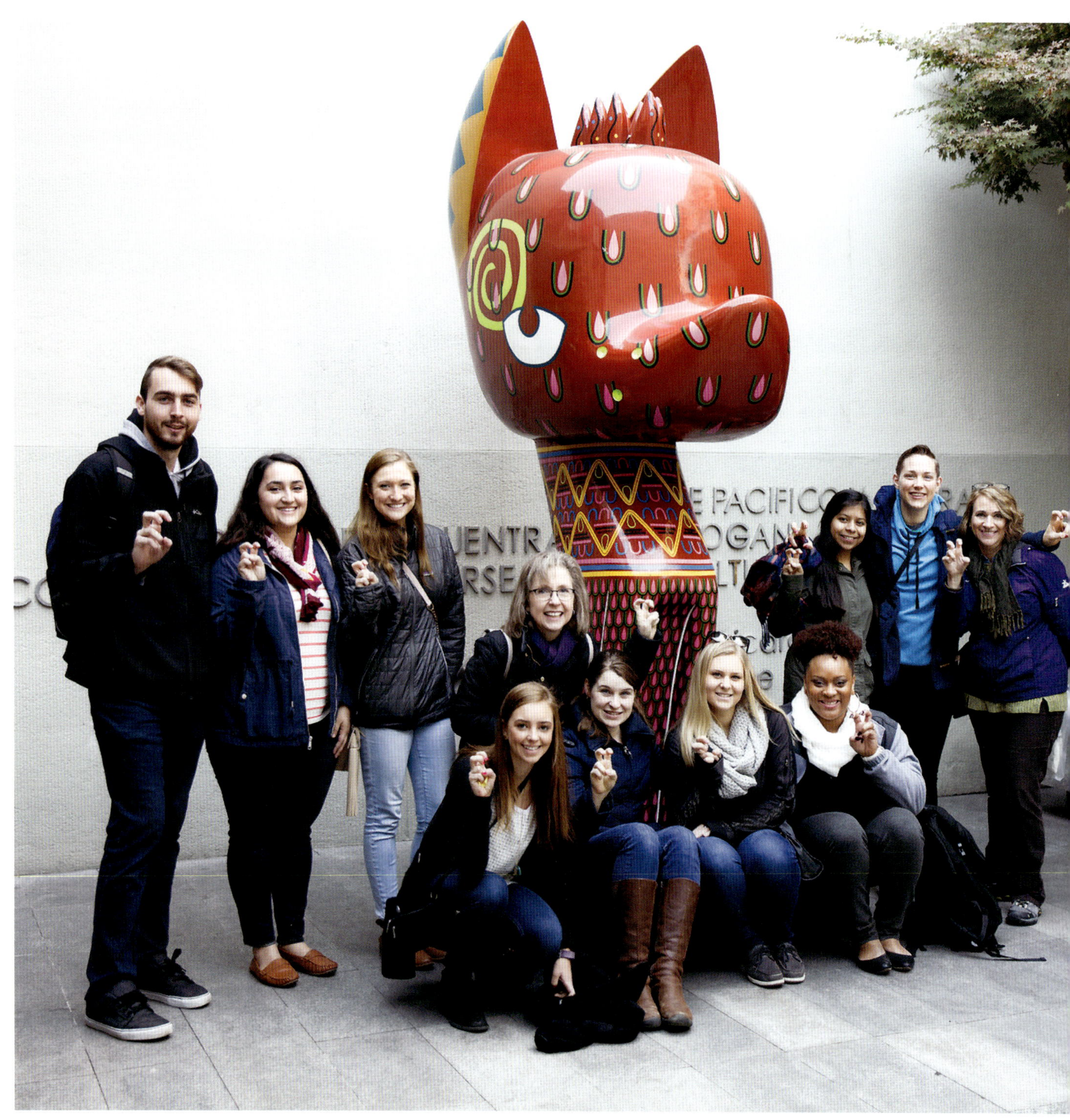

Students with Dr. Suzy Lockwood and Irmgard Payne at Statue Santiago.

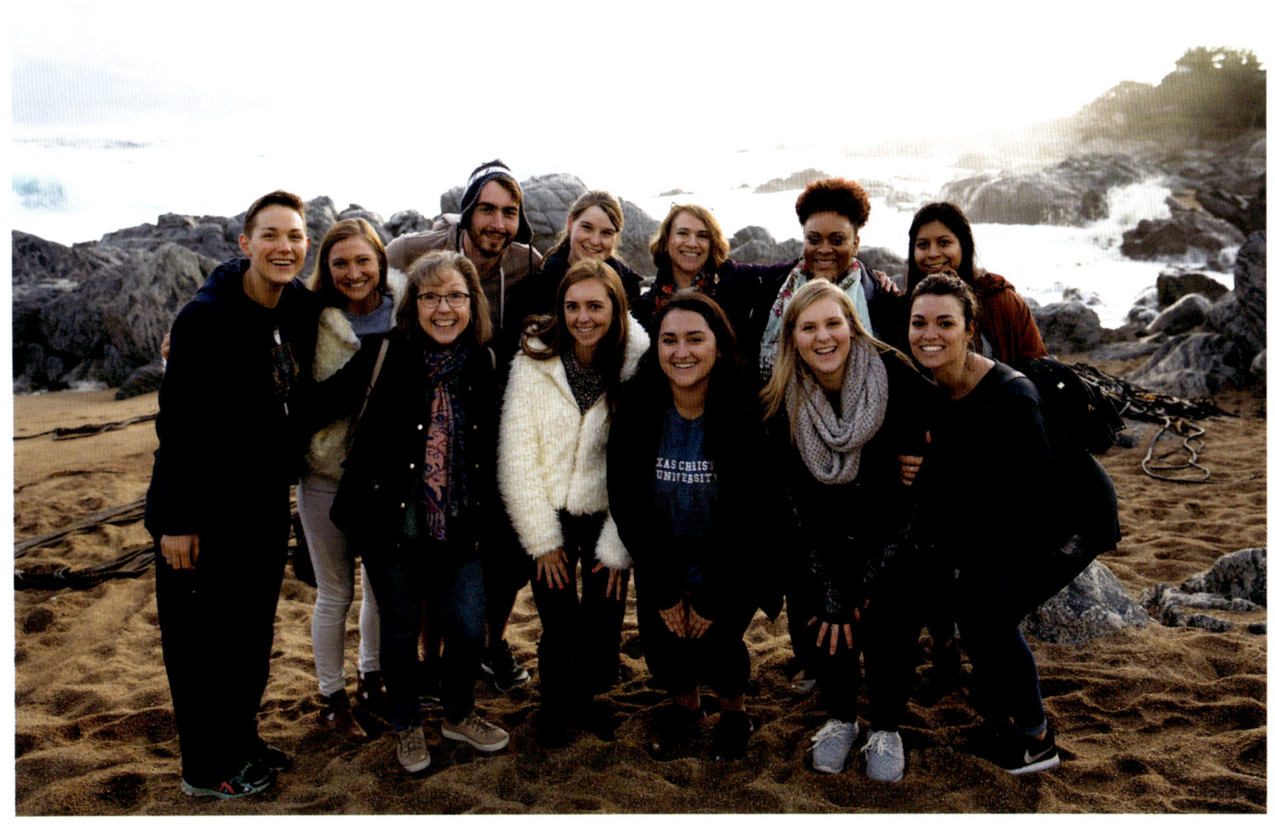

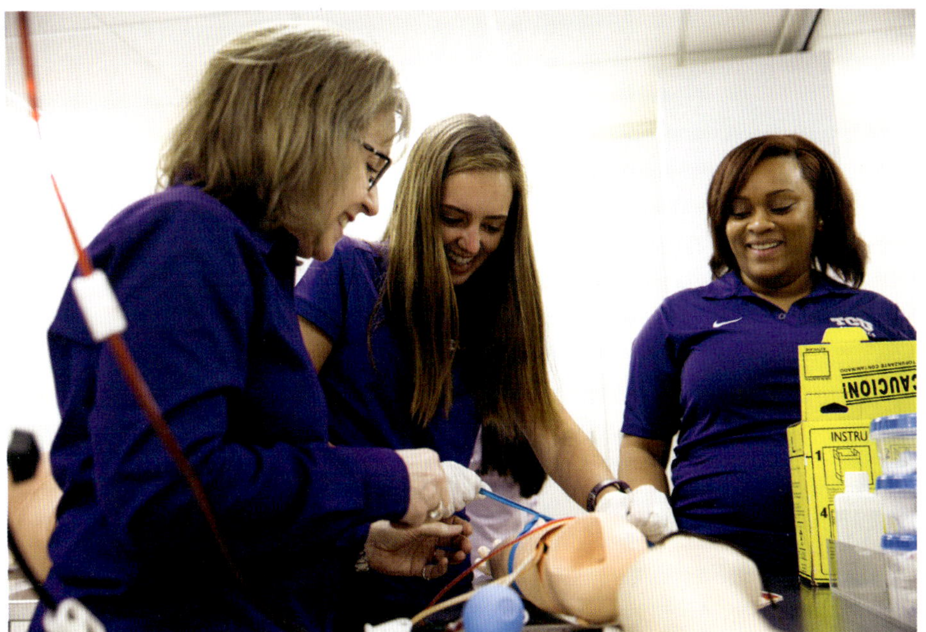

(Above) Students with Dr. Lockwood and Irmgard Payne at Isla Negra, 2017.

(Left) Dr. Lockwood and students in simulation lab in Santiago, 2017.

systems, along with cultural beliefs and practices. Field trips to selected clinical sites such as a family health clinic, speech and hearing clinic, and a nursing simulation lab provided a glimpse into the health care system and roles of the health care providers.

The time spent with host families was a highlight for students and faculty, who were able to continue discussions of health care beyond academic settings. Students said that the families made them feel very welcome in their homes.

In Argentina, students and faculty were guided by an on-site program coordinator from abroad who welcomed them with a tango dinner and gave them tango lessons. They visited health care sites such as Foundation for the Fight against Neurological Illnesses of Infants, Hospital Italiano de Buenos Aires, Hospital de Niños Dr. Ricardo Gutiérrez, and attended lectures from faculty of the Universidad del Museo Social Argentino.

In addition to field trips to cultural and health care sites students engaged in a debate as a final evaluative exercise. Faculty members assigned students to groups which would argue either for or against the proposition that health care systems should refuse to pay for lifestyle-influenced health conditions such as cardiac disease among the obese, respiratory disease among smokers, and liver disease among alcohol abusers. They also debated whether the government had the responsibility to mandate or provide health care for all. This exercise further allowed students to compare and contrast the experiences they had while in two different countries and

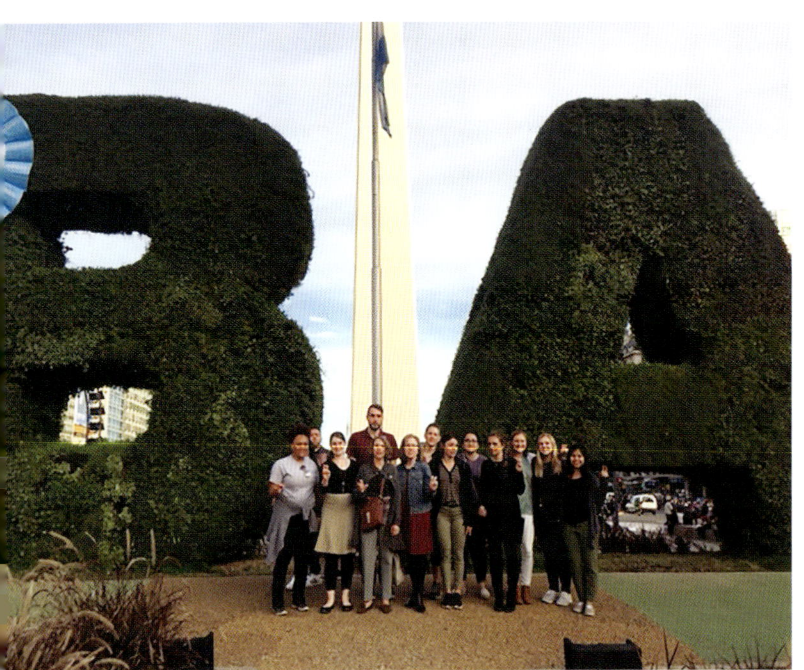

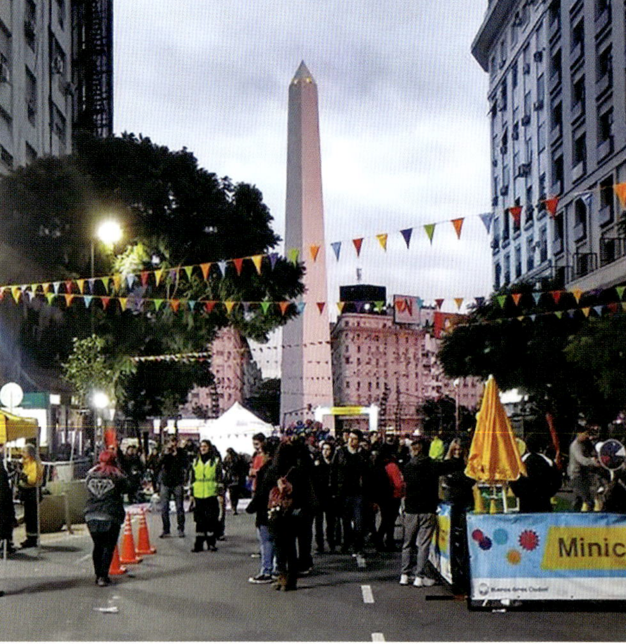

(Left) Students in Buenos Aires, 2017. (Right) The Buenos Aires Market, 2017.

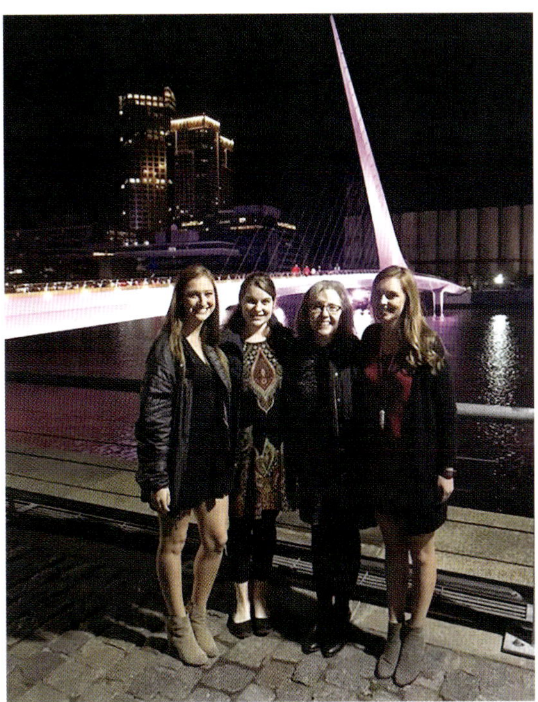

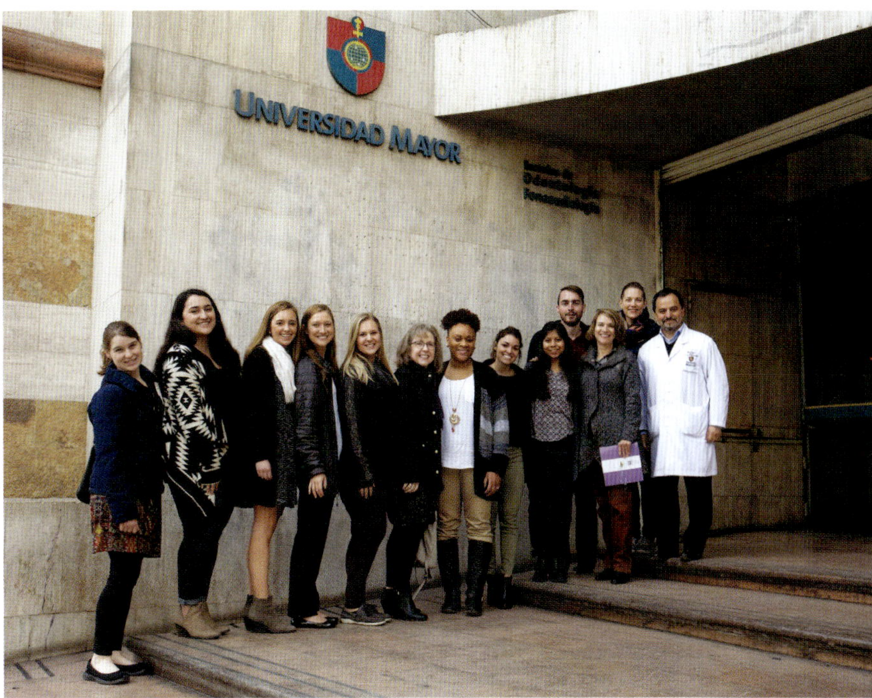

(Left) Dr. Lockwood and nursing students at Womens' Memorial Bridge in Buenos Aires, 2017. (Right) Students and faculty from TCU at Universidad Mayor in Buenos Aires, 2017.

provided additional opportunities for reflection on cultural and global awareness.

Upon completion of the course, students were asked to identify five major things they had experienced or observed in Chile or Argentina that would change their personal values, their professional practice, or their view on life. One student commented that even though the health care systems were very different, many therapies were the same. . . . "it feels [like] home even though thousands of miles away." Another commented that it was "important to go with the flow . . . leave the Type A time schedule and enjoy 'Chile-Argentina time.'" Host families were credited with providing a unique cultural perspective. Reflecting on the differences in culture and language, another student commented, "It doesn't take more than a few minutes to find common ground."

Selected Organizations

Beta Alpha Chapter of Sigma Theta Tau International won its first Chapter Key Award in 2011. Melissa Sherrod, chapter president, accepted the award at the biennial conference in October.

In December 2012, Lambda Eta Alpha Beta Chapter of Chi Eta Phi Sorority was chartered at TCU. Marisol Sigala, a junior nursing student at TCU, received a scholarship from the Lambada Eta (graduate) Chapter in 2011, and felt motivated to help Traci Murray, a former TCU nursing student; Glenda Daniels; Janie Robinson; and Thelma Love, president of the graduate chapter, establish an undergraduate chapter of the sorority. Chi Eta Phi Sorority, Inc. is a national sorority of registered professional nurses and nursing students founded in 1932. Chi Eta Phi's mission is to serve humanity, elevate nursing, and promote interest in the nursing profession. Activities include the pursuit of continuing education, recruitment programs for health careers, the stimulation of a close and friendly relationship among its members, the development of working relationships with other professional groups, and the identification of a core of nursing leaders who affect social changes at the national, regional, and local levels (Lambda Eta Alpha Beta, 2012). Programs include disease prevention and health promotion; programs for seniors, youth, and young adults; community outreach; leadership development; research; scholarships; and recruitment and retention.

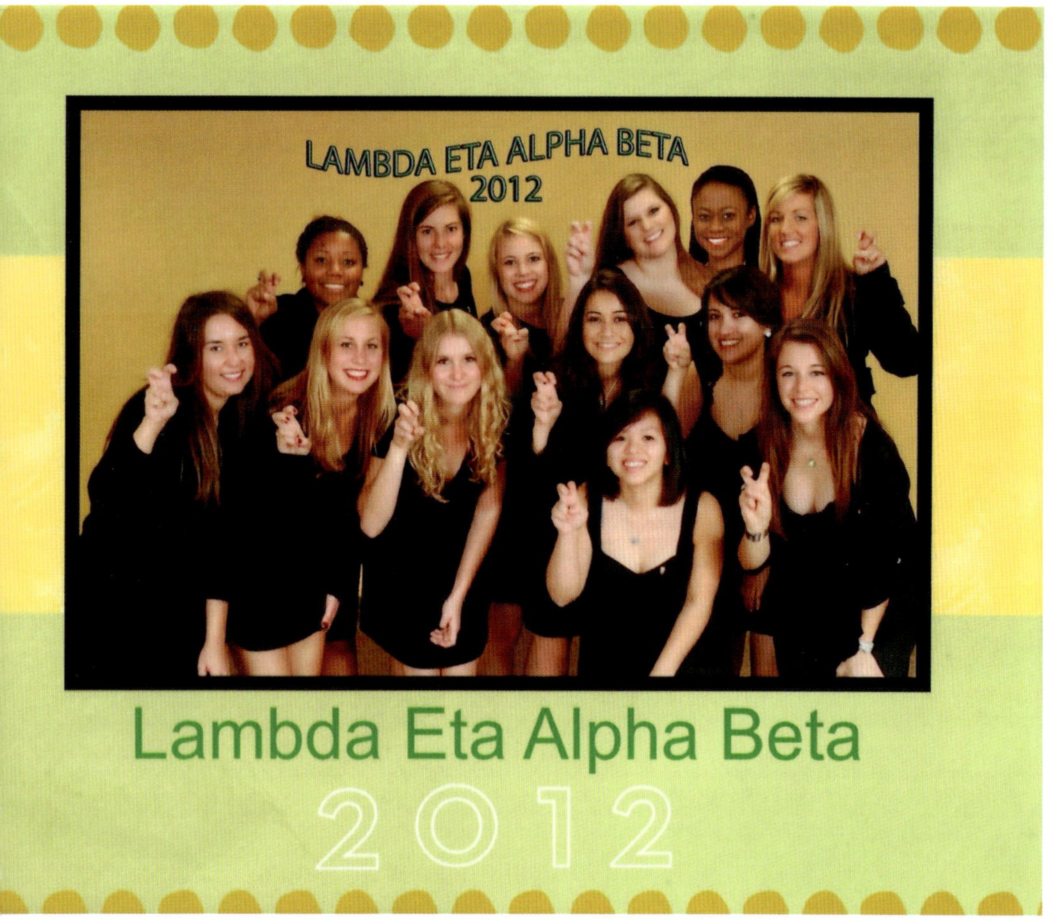

Lambda Eta Alpha Beta, 2012.

Daniels serves as the sorority's Beta Sponsor and Robinson serves as the sorority's faculty adviser. Currently, the TCU chapter is composed of twenty-one members who meet approximately three times a semester. Local events have included educational activities on the TCU campus (programs about sexually transmitted infections [STIs], flu vaccine, melanoma, mental health awareness, the March of Dimes, graduate school, and dress to impress); community educational activities (speaking with young adults about the profession of nursing, STIs, and heart disease awareness); and community events (participation in health and wellness expos, including

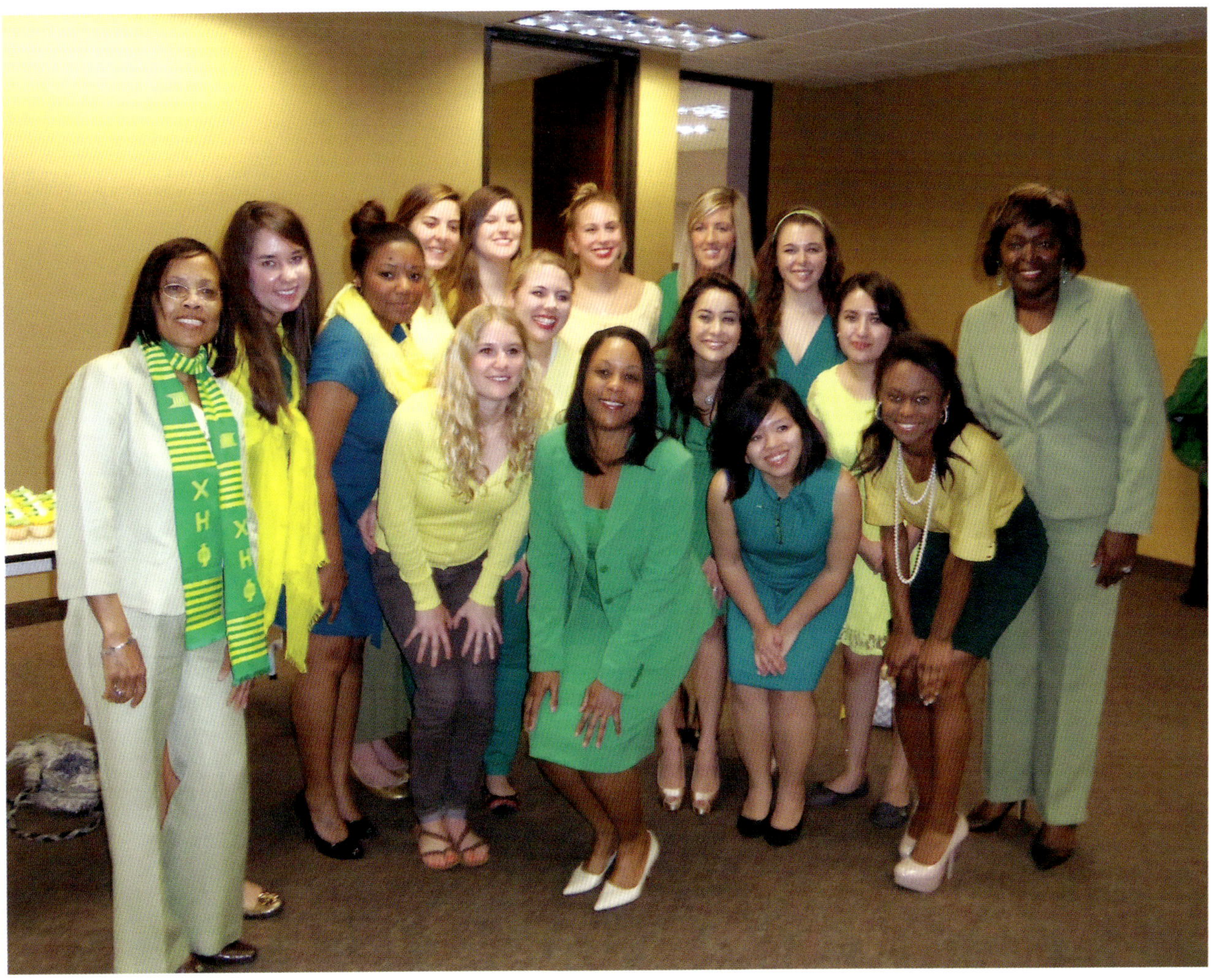

Lambda Eta Alpha Beta, 2012.

Go Red for Women, winter clothing drives for homeless people, and collecting items for the Women's Shelter).

Selected Activities of MSN Graduates

Ashley Neal, a 2012 graduate, was recognized with the Mosaic Award from Texas Health Denton Hospital in 2013. The Mosaic Award recognizes a staff member who embodies cultural diversity and awareness in their daily practice and advocates for culturally sensitive care with patients and families. Mary Spears, also a 2012 graduate, was elected to the Texas Nurses Association District Three Secretary and

Membership Committee along with Danell Stengem, a 2012 alumna, who was elected to the District Three Nominating Committee.

TCU Nursing was well represented at the Clinical Nurse Leader (CNL) Summit in California in 2014 with alums presenting papers. Michael Culver (2009) presented "Too Hip to be Square and Too Hip for Surgical Site Infections." Cory Franks (2011) spoke on "How a Microsystem Assessment Helped Improve the Discharge Process on a Medical SurgicalUnit." Danell Stengem (2012) presented "The Role of the CNL in Creating a Culture of Certification and Professional Development." Dianne Thomas (2012) spoke on the "Evolution of the CNL Workgroup for a 14 Hospital System," and Flame Uytico (2012) presented "Clinical Nurse Leader's Role in Advancing Quality Stroke Care at a Micro, Meso, and Macro Systems Level." Joe Hafley (2012) presented "Building and Leading a Team to Decrease t-PA Usage for PICC Line Clots." Esther Gosdin (2013) spoke on "Interventions to improve Staff Responsiveness and Patient Satisfaction through Call Light Management and Purposeful Hourly Rounding." Ginu Philip (2013) presented "Discharge Planning to Prevent Re-Admissions and Improve Patient Satisfaction."

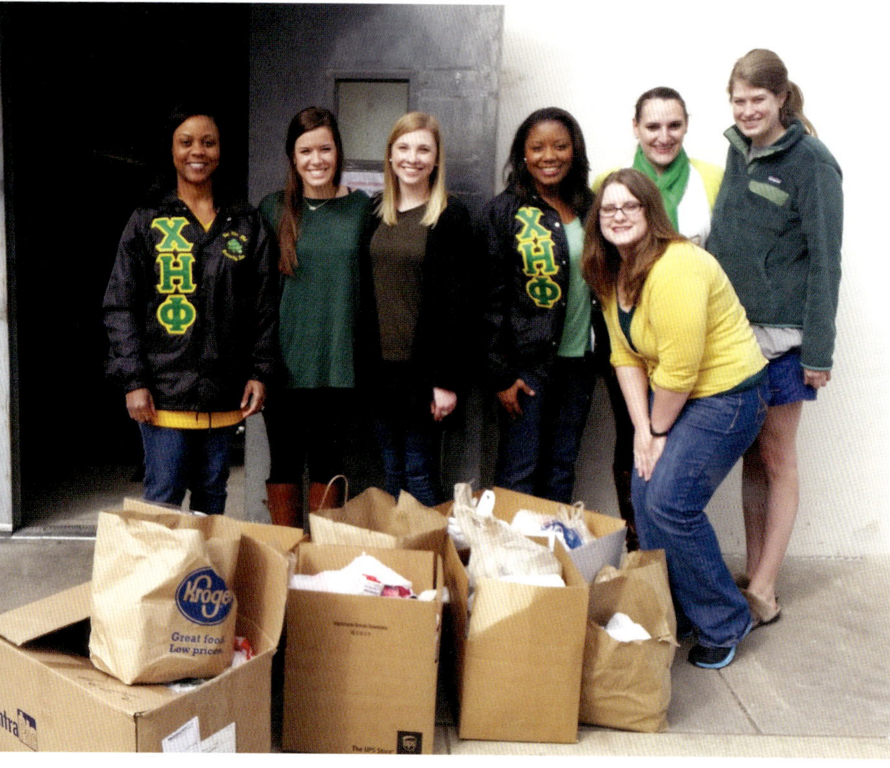

Saturday of Love.

In 2014, Les Rodriguez, a 2008 graduate of the MSN Clinical Nurse Specialist Program, was inaugurated as the president of the National Association of Clinical Nurse Specialists. This "New President's Message" was later published in *Clinical Nurse Specialist Journal.*

Selected Activities of DNP Students

Cole Edmonson (2011), former vice president of Patient Care Services and chief nursing officer at Texas Health Presbyterian Dallas, served as president of the

Texas Organization of Nurse Executives and received their Excellence in Leadership Award. He was also a coauthor, with June Marshall (2011), of "Balancing Interests of Hospitals and Nurse Researchers: Lessons Learned," published in *Applied Nursing Research* in 2012. Wendy Fletcher (2012) was appointed to the Kentucky Board of Regents for a five-year term beginning in April 2018. Laura Garza-Gongora (2013) received the Joanna Briggs Institute "Best Convention Concurrent Session Award" in Adelaide, South Australia, in 2013. Erin Kiser (2015) traveled to Togo, West Africa, in 2016, where she taught microbiology at a nursing school sponsored by a US mission hospital. She subsequently published "Fighting Ebola in Sierra Leone," in *Nursing 2018*. Teresa Whited (2015) was promoted to director of the master's program at the University of Arkansas for Medical Sciences, Little Rock, in 2016. Claire Zangerle (2017) was appointed chief nurse executive for the Allegheny Health Network in Pennsylvania in 2016. Collectively, DNP graduates published a total of twenty-three manuscripts between 2014 and 2017 as part of a writing course developed and taught by Kathy Baker and Suzy Lockwood. Several of these focused on the clarification of the role of the nurse; one example is "The Clinical Effectiveness of a Nurse Practitioner versus a Non-Nurse Practitioner on Hospital Admissions of Older Adults Residing in Skilled or Long-Term Care Facilities: A Systematic Review Protocol" (Hamby and Christian 2015).

ALUMNI EXAMPLES OF CHANGING ROLES

Defining the Role of the Nurse as a Global Nurse Leader

An Interview with Ayla Landry, BSN 2010

Ayla Landry recalled that at eighteen years of age, she found thinking about "college and career as daunting and overwhelming responsibilities," but she desired to make the world a better place; she chose nursing as it seemed to directly align with her goals (Landry, pers. comm., 2018). She loved asking questions and felt comfortable with math and science. She said that the influence of her mentors led her to "jump into leadership roles" at an early point in her college career. She was selected to work as a teaching assistant to Wayne Barcelona, faculty member in Anatomy and Physiology (A&P). This became one of her "most beloved experiences," where she simultaneously was being mentored by "Dr. B" and, in turn, mentored younger nursing students who were taking A&P. Ayla's joy in nurse education was born then and persists today.

While at TCU, she also solidified her Spanish language skills and gained a passion for serving in Latin America. She spent the summer of her sophomore year in the Dominican Republic, where she took courses at a local university and worked

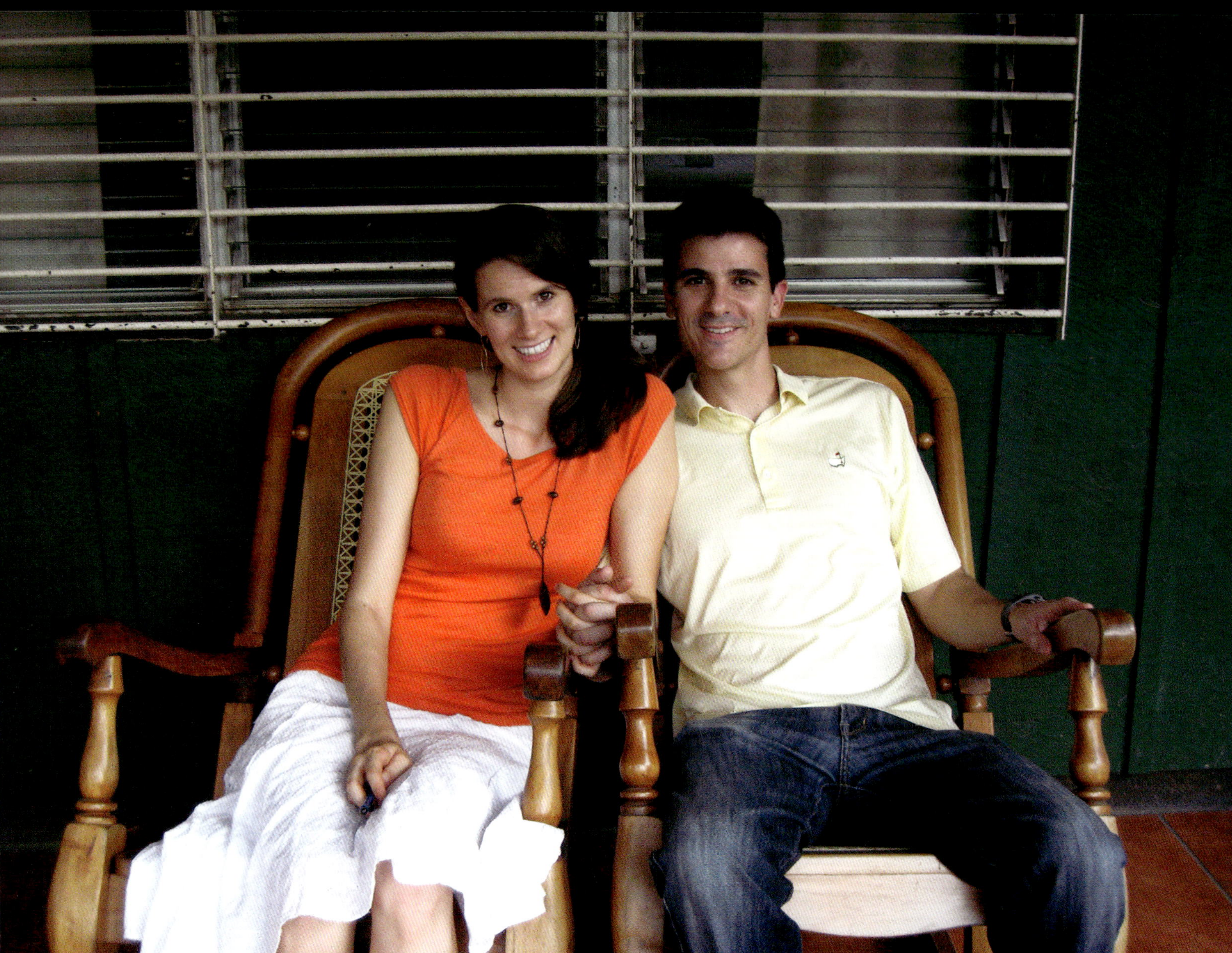

Ayla Landry and husband in Nicaragua, 2018.

with an organization (Caritas), where she served alongside Catholic nuns to deliver "much needed" medications and basic health care to rural communities. During subsequent spring breaks, Landry traveled to Nicaragua to volunteer with a multifaceted national campaign to address cervical and breast cancer.

She credits Sharon Canclini for cultivating her interest and shaping her trajectory in community health nursing and introducing her to the Sight's Global Health and Innovation conference at Yale University. This and other experiences "helped solidify" her desire to be a global health nurse.

Landry moved to Nicaragua in 2011 and served as a school nurse with a Christian nonprofit organization, the Nicaraguan Resource Network, where she developed a sustainable program, alongside a local Nicaraguan pediatrician, to provide primary care for nearly two thousand students. After involvement in several organizations, including the Nurses for Nurses International, she realized she needed to expand her knowledge to effectively promote global health and serve the developing world. She returned to the US, where she received a master's in nursing and a master's in public health from Johns Hopkins University, with a certificate in global health, a certificate in maternal child health, and a Nurse Educator Certificate.

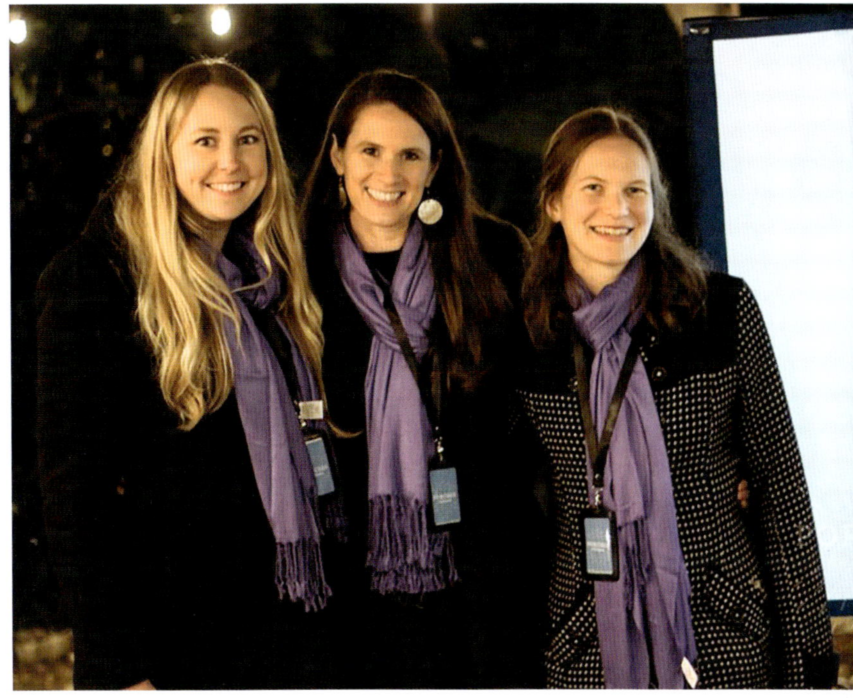

Ayla Landry (center) with coworkers, Porches Board Roadshow, December 2017.

Following graduate school, Landry worked at a Federally Qualified Healthcare Center in Texas as a program design manager, where she led a federal grant-funded care improvement model for patients with chronic diseases, behavioral health issues, and socio-economic barriers. She and her husband Ryan (a TCU alum) moved to the remote agricultural town of Nueva Guinea in Nicaragua and adopted a Nicaraguan teenager. After completing an assessment of priority community health needs and subsequent analysis, which often took place on the porch of her Nicaraguan home, Landry, her sister Elyse, and fellow 2010 Harris College of Nursing graduate Whitney Winters established the 501(c)3 nonprofit organization, Porches for Progress. The organization's mission is "to propel ideas for progress within resource-poor communities through collaboration, micro-grants, and the power of opportunity." Grant applications are accepted for community improvement projects related to seven target categories based on the United Nations Sustainable Development Goals. The next step is to identify competent local leaders to manage the grants and test them in various resource-poor countries.

Landry sees global health nursing as an emerging specialty, with its roots in the work of nurses like Florence Nightingale and Lillian Wald. She credits the Harris College of Nursing for "teaching her to love the lifelong journey of nursing and the quest for knowledge and skills needed to make a difference" (Ayla Landry, pers. comm., 2018).

Defining the Role of the Nurse as a Program Adviser at World Relief

An Interview with Amberle Durano Brown, BSN 2013

Amberle Durano Brown felt "an internal motivation to serve vulnerable communities and individuals in low-resource settings" since she was very young. She was further motivated by the privilege she believed nurses have to be present and care holistically for people during "some of life's most fragile moments" (Amberle Brown, pers. comm., 2018).

Upon entering nursing school, her goal was to become a missionary nurse and provide care for those who would not otherwise have access to it. Between her sophomore and junior years at TCU, she interned with a missionary nurse in Port-au-Prince, Haiti, where she provided primary care to urban and rural populations. The following summer she interned at the World Health Organization (WHO) in Geneva, Switzerland, where she designed and conducted a systematic review on the role of community health workers in HIV care and treatment. This, plus her first hospital job in an intensive care unit, helped form her view of health systems and public health. She acknowledged the assistance of Dean Paulette Burns, Diane Hawley, and Susan Weeks in making it possible for her to intern at the WHO, an experience that she credits with "altering the trajectory of her life." The WHO internship gave her an opportunity to work with "brilliant minds . . . learn about collaboration, research, and synthesis . . . and gain a unique insight into global health" (Amberle Brown, pers. comm., 2018).

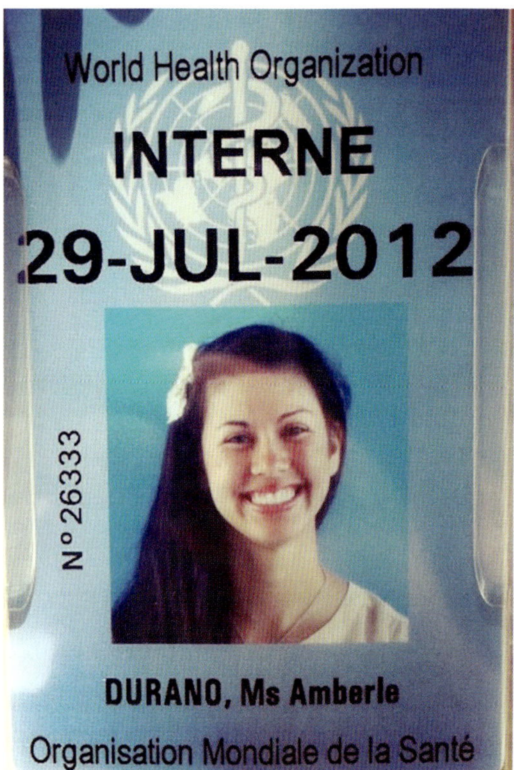

Amberle as an intern at the World Health Organization.

Brown's experiences in the Honors College Community Service (HCCS), the Chancellor's Leadership Program, and Study Abroad also provided "service and leadership experience that expanded my horizons and allowed me to dream beyond my prior categories." Other extracurricular activities, such as volunteer work with Refugee Services of Texas and World Relief, offered her real-world experience that helped shape her professional goals. She also credits the public health nursing class at Harris College with "providing me language to define my career hopes" (Amberle Brown, pers. comm., 2018).

Following completion of a master's in public health and master's in nursing, Brown assumed the role of program adviser for Health and Nutrition in the International Programs department of World Relief, a Christian global health and development non-governmental organization (NGO). In this role, she oversees maternal and child health and HIV programs in Cambodia, Burundi, Malawi, and Haiti, where she works with local staff to "ensure excellence of implementation, positioning for influential opportunities, and thorough monitoring systems to build the evidence base for our interventions" (Amberle Brown, pers. comm., 2018).

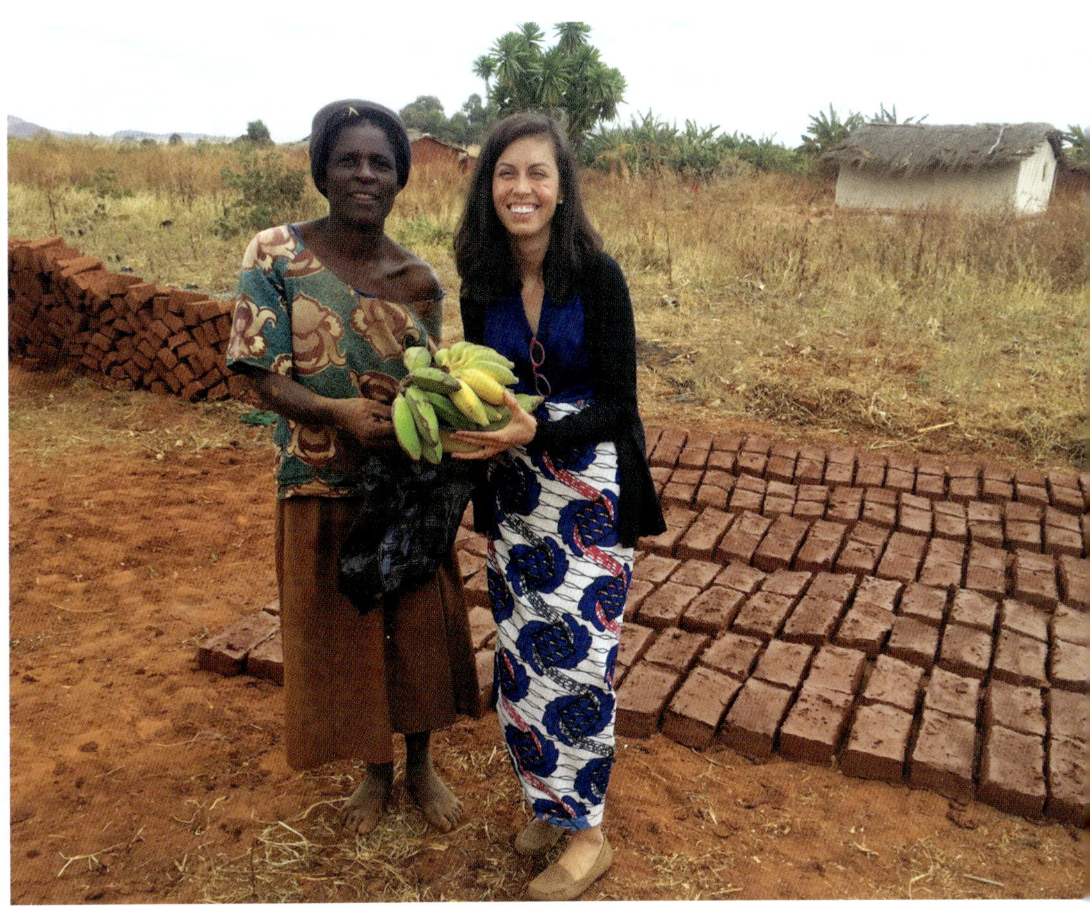

Amberle Durano Brown (right) and villager in Africa.

Brown is "deeply grateful" to work in a role "where the daily goal is to improve the lives of some of the most vulnerable on the planet." She stated that she continues to learn from people all over the world—from mothers in rural Cambodia to professors at top-tier universities. Discouragement comes when she sees children who are "stunted and wasted" and people who don't have transportation to get to their treatment. She closed the interview by saying that the "problems are too big for me to solve . . . and can be discouraging." She believes, however, that through collaboration we can "together make this world a healthier place" (Amberle Brown, pers. comm., 2018).

Chapter Six

Defining the Role of the Nurse as a Consultant to the Surgeon General

An Interview with Jo Ellen Schimmels, DNP 2011 (TCU)

Lieutenant Colonel (LTC) Jo Ellen Schimmels's distinguished career may be characterized by continuous learning, and in turn, by service in multiple roles. Her desire to help people motivated her to enter nursing school as a cadet at Viterbo University; she graduated in 1998. Subsequently, she was commissioned into the US Army. Although her initial practice was in medical-surgical and pediatric nursing, she had a long-term interest in psychiatric nursing and became credentialed as a psychiatric nurse practitioner in 2007. She holds a postgraduate certificate as a behavioral health nurse practitioner. For LTC Schimmels, education never ends. She is also a family nurse practitioner, a graduate of TCU's Doctor of Nursing Practice Program, and a current student in the PhD program in Health Professional Education at the United States Uniformed Health Services University (USUHS) in Bethesda, Maryland. When asked what motivated her to seek her PhD, she responded that she wanted to become a better instructor (at USUHS)—one of her multiple current roles, in which she teaches classes and supervises clinical practica in behavioral health (Schimmels, pers. comm., 2017).

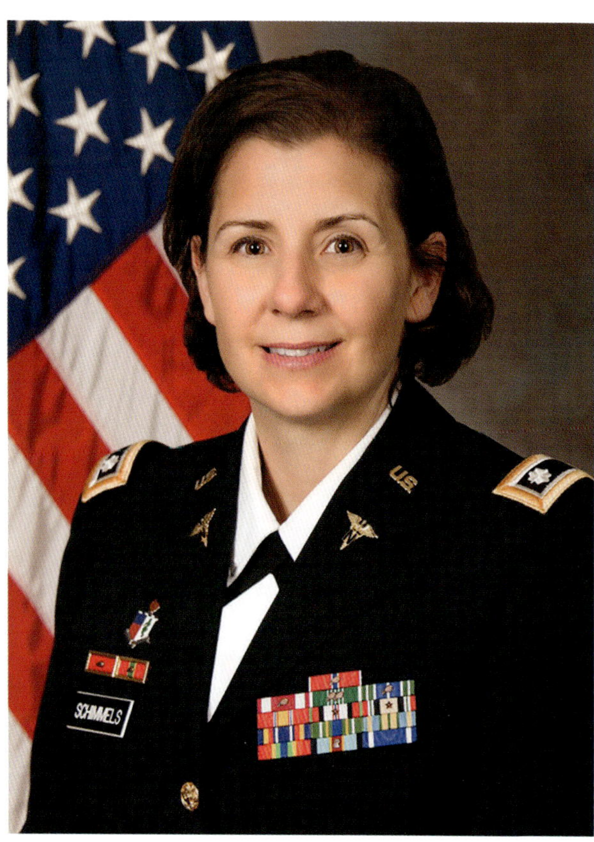

Jo Ellen Schimmels.

Currently, LTC Schimmels serves as a consultant to the Surgeon General for behavioral health nursing. Selected for this voluntary role through a competitive process, she will complete a four-year term that includes membership on multiple committees and the opportunity to review policies related to behavioral health nursing and provide feedback to the Surgeon General. When asked about the challenges in this role, she acknowledged time pressures, lack of authority, and the realization that her recommendations may not be accepted. Time in getting recommended policies approved was also noted as a challenge.

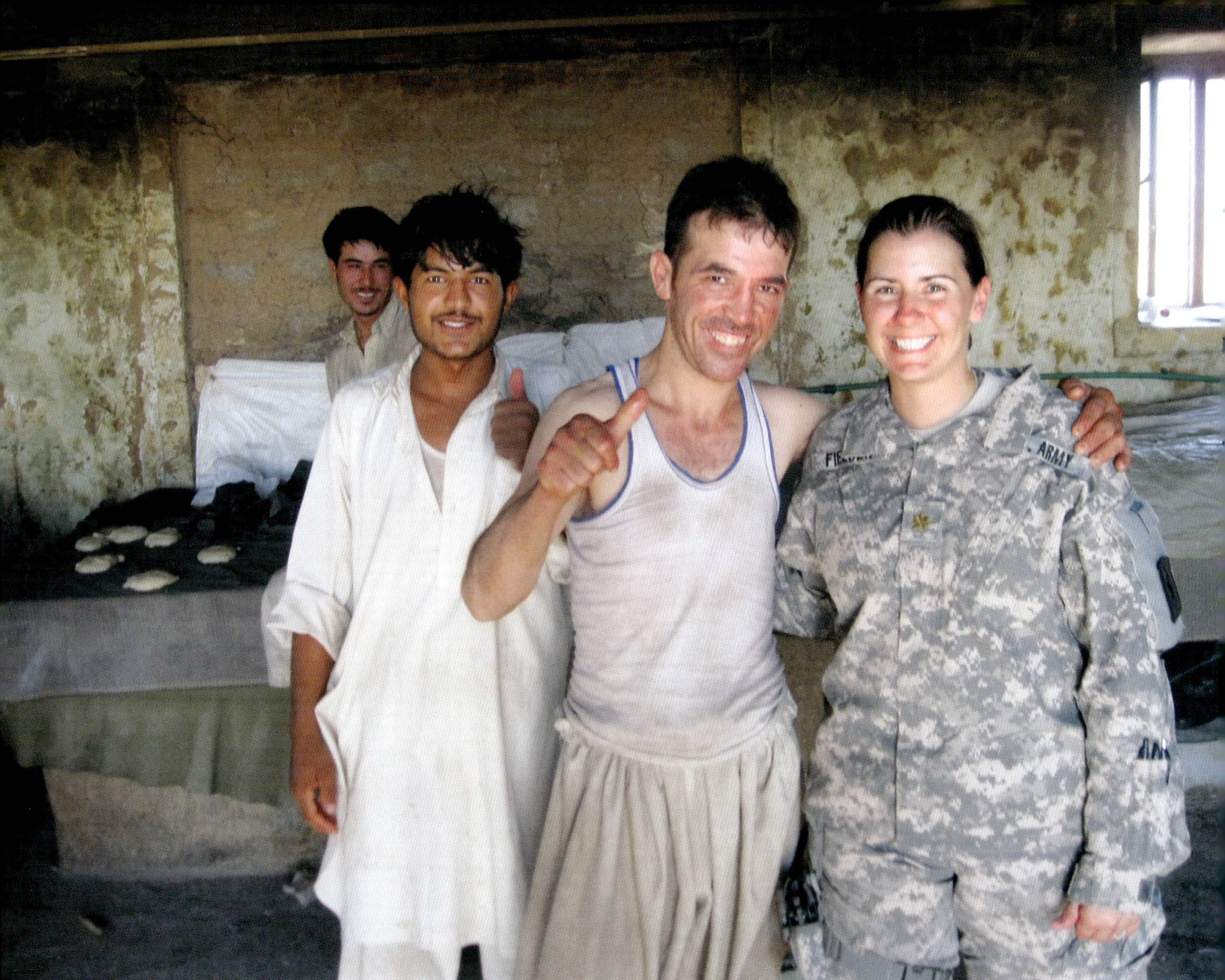

Jo Ellen in work clothes with students.

A major reward in her current role is having the opportunity to mentor soldiers and nurses. She traces her desire and ability to do this to the mentors she had while she was a student in the DNP program at TCU. They were cited as faculty members who not only mentored her personally but who gave her a "taste" of education and policy that "made her a better practitioner" and motivated her to make and use policies. When deployed, her focus was on prevention through frequent screening of soldiers for potential post-traumatic stress syndrome (PTSS) (Jo Ellen Schimmels, pers. comm., 2017).

Defining the Role of a System Chief Nursing Officer

An Interview with Dian Adams, DNP 2013

Dian Adams shared that she "wished she could say that nursing was a calling," but her decision was "purely circumstantial." Having switched majors several times in college, she switched to nursing after learning that all the biological science classes she took when she was enrolled in premed applied to nursing. Today, however, she said "I wouldn't change a single part of this great adventure of being a nurse. . . . I cannot think of another profession that is as rewarding or has as much versatility." Although she did not know what nursing role she wanted upon graduation, she accepted her first position in a neonatal intensive care unit, where her brother was an intern. She later became involved with HCA Healthcare, the largest for-profit health care system in the US, where she worked for twenty-four years and was afforded the opportunity to "build her skill set and grow as a leader practicing nursing leadership across the United States" (Dian Adams, pers. comm., 2018).

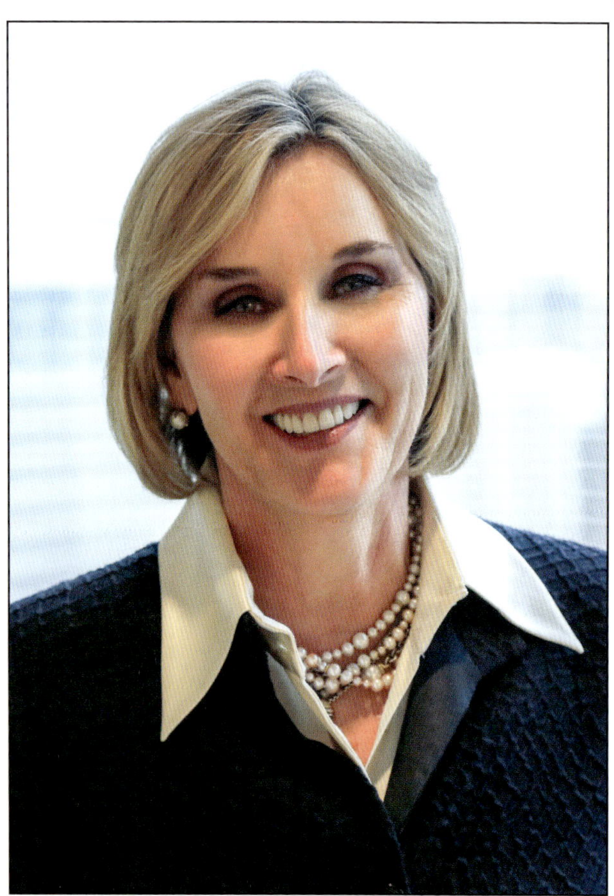

Dian Adams.

As the chief nursing officer in Tenet Health, Dian has the opportunity to apply all she has learned "while driving the practice of nursing forward" (Dian Adams, pers. comm., 2018). She represents more than 40,000 nurses at the corporate level in a partnership with the Chief Medical Officer as they drive clinical practice and advance care. She believes that it is very important for nurses and nurse leaders to have a seat at the table when it comes to decision-making for clinical, operational, and strategic initiatives. She also has operational responsibility for patient safety, performance excellence, emergency preparedness, and clinical research.

Adams said that the biggest challenge in her role is "staying strategic and executing in an environment of change and uncertainty" (Dian Adams, pers. comm., 2018). She sees the biggest rewards as being able to connect with the nurses and patients and staying focused on making a difference in the lives of others. She commented that "going to TCU was the single best educational investment I made," as it complemented her practical experience and "helped make me confident that I could assume an expanded role" (Dian Adams, pers. comm., 2018).

Defining the Role of President of a National Organization, Author, Clinician

An Interview with Vicki Good, BSN 1989; DNP 2016

A "two-time" graduate of nursing from TCU, Vicki Good began her studies in business and mathematics. After her initial classes, she decided that the major was not a good fit and began her nursing studies at Tarrant County College before entering Harris College of Nursing. Motivated by her observations of the "caring and compassion" of nurses with whom she came into contact during her initial studies, she also became aware of the vast number of opportunities for nurses providing direct patient care, support services, and leadership, and she realized that she wanted to be in a leadership role (Vicki Good, pers. comm., 2018).

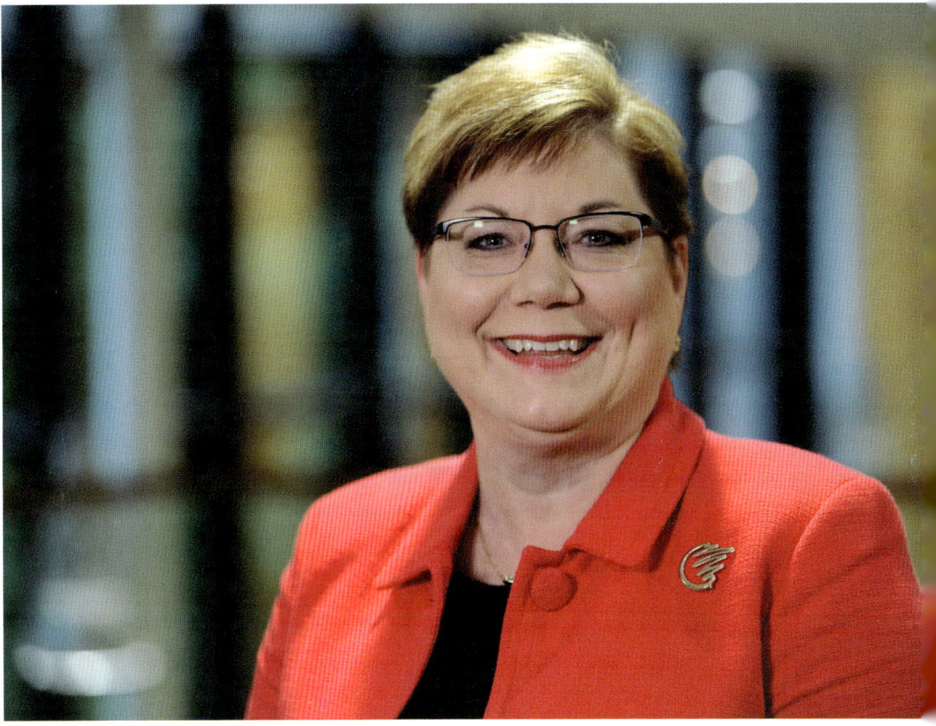

Vicki Good.

Influenced by her mother's and another nurse colleague's role in critical care, she enrolled in the Parkland Trauma Nurse Internship program, an eight-month postgraduate training program for critical care nurses. She became an assistant nurse manager early in her career. With the TCU faculty's encouragement to become involved in professional associations, she also became involved in the American Association of Critical-Care Nurses (AACN) during her senior year (Vicki Good, pers. comm., 2018).

Good remembers that early in her career she sat at the national conference of the AACN and watched the board members and president "guiding and leading crucial conversations related to the value of the registered nurse and thought to myself, one day that will be me!" (Vicki Good, pers. comm., 2018). During her master's degree program at Seattle Pacific University, she was invited by Karen Carlson, her mentor, to be a section editor for the AACN Advanced Critical Care Textbook. While working on the book, she made numerous professional contacts across the country and within AACN, where she was nominated and served on the board of directors.

Currently, Good works with multidisciplinary teams in the area of Quality and Patient Safety. She was named by *Becker's Hospital Review* as one of the fifty leaders in Patient Safety in 2014. She has also served on several expert panels and advisory boards for the National Patient Safety Foundation and currently works with the American Association of Critical Care Nurses and the Critical Care Societies Collaborative on Burnout in the Critical Care Health Professions (Vicki Good, pers. comm., 2018).

Good says that finding time to get all the important work done is her biggest challenge. The reward she cherishes most is the impact she can make on others' careers. She credits Billie Hightower, TCU faculty member from 1972 to 1993, and Rhonda Keen-Payne, current faculty member, for encouragement, support, and instilling in her the belief that "I can do it" and that "I can do anything I set my mind to do: I do not need others' permission, but I need my desire and hard work" (Vicki Good, pers. comm., 2018).

CHALLENGE TWO

Research to Determine What Effects Variables in Nursing Care Have on the Health of People

Context and Trends

The National Institute of Nursing Research (NINR) celebrated its twenty-fifth anniversary of nursing science at the National Institute of Health (NIH) in 2010-2011. A series of workshops and a dialogue with stakeholders from 2013-2014 was undertaken via a public website to identify future research directions within its focus areas. The purpose was to explore unanswered questions, promote "results-oriented research, and guide the science over the next five to ten years" (National Institute of Nursing Research 2016).

Sigma Theta Tau International (STTI) added three grants to their repertoire of research awards in 2013 and 2014. The Global Nursing Research Grant was established in 2013 in honor of STTI's former chief nurse executive, Patricia Thompson. In 2014, the American Nurses Credentialing Center Evidence-Based Practice Implementation Grant and the Chamberlain College of Nursing Education Research Grant were awarded for the first time (Patricia Thompson, pers. comm., 2018).

The National League for Nursing continued to fund research in nursing education by its members. The research priorities for the years 2016–19 are:

1. Build the science of nursing education through the discovery and translation of innovative evidence-based strategies;
2. Link student learning to sentinel health indicators to promote health, prevent disease, and manage the symptomatology of illness;
3. Examine the science of learning in the academic context related to health transitions.

(National League for Nursing 2016)

Harris College, TCU Nursing

Research in this decade continues to increase in a variety of areas. Studies cover both clinical topics and aspects of nursing education research and are conducted by individuals and teams composed of faculty, students, and other professional colleagues. Two Beta Alpha Chapter members of STTI presented their research at the biennial convention in 2017 in Indianapolis. Between 2010 and 2018, five Hogstel Research Awards and six Beta Alpha research grants were awarded to support selected studies.

Hogstel Awards went to such studies as "The Effect of Reminiscence on the Older Adult" (Elizabeth Long) and "Mediating Factors of Technology Adoption by Senior Adults" (Kathy Daniel of the University of Texas at Arlington). Studies receiving Beta Alpha Awards included "Stressors in the Older Adult with End Stage Renal Disease" (Janie Wells), "An Exploratory Study of Head and Neck Cancer and the Quality of Life in Survivorship" (Suzy Lockwood and Kathy Baker), "The Quality of Prenatal Care and Pregnancy Outcomes Comparing Centering Pregnancy Versus Traditional Prenatal Care" (Lisette Allender), "Personal Disaster and Preparedness and the Ability and Willingness of Nurses to Report to Work in Time of Disaster" (Lavonne Adams), and "Nazdrovya: A Qualitative Inquiry of the Russian-American Immigrant Population and the Effects of Cultural Change" (Melissa Sherrod).

FACULTY/STUDENT RESEARCH: SELECTED EXAMPLES

Nursing Education Research—Laura Posluszny and Diane Hawley

Laura Posluszny, a BSN graduate, and Diane Hawley conducted a study that compared professional values of sophomore and senior baccalaureate nursing students.

The study was conducted using the Nurses Professional Values Scale-Revised (NPVS-R). Two study questions were posed to participants: "What is the relative importance of professional values for beginning and graduating baccalaureate nursing students" and "Are there differences in professional values between these students?"

Trust, caring, and justice were found to be more important than activism to sophomore-level students. Senior-level students perceived trust as more important than activism and professionalism. NPVS-R scores were not significantly different between the two groups, but senior students scored significantly higher on activism than the sophomore students.

The researchers concluded that the study suggests an opportunity for faculty to reevaluate the curriculum with reference to ethics. Findings suggest that values of activism and professionalism should be reinforced.

Nursing Education Research—Ashley Franklin and Caitlin Dodd

Ashley Franklin's program of research stems from teaching experiences at TCU in the simulation lab. Franklin investigated how simulation helps novice nurses improve their competence for managing multiple patients in medical-surgical settings. Franklin conducted a pilot that was a randomized control trial to evaluate the effect of three simulation preparation methods (reading assignments, voice-over PowerPoint lectures, and expert modeling videos) on twenty-one novice nurses' competence and self-efficacy. Bandura's Social Cognitive Theory guided implementation of the expert modeling intervention, and a modified National League for Nursing (NLN) Self-Confidence Learning Survey was used to evaluate self-efficacy. Two blinded raters scored novice nurses' performances in pre- and post-test simulations using the Creighton Simulation Evaluation instrument. Results from the pilot study indicated that the expert modeling intervention was twice as effective as using voice-over PowerPoint to help novice nurses prepare to provide care for multiple patients simultaneously. This study was funded with $5,000 by the Joan K. Stout Research Grant from STTI.

Franklin and TCU Nursing colleague Caitlin Dodd extended this line of inquiry with a multi-site, randomized control trial in 2016, in a study where the same interventions were implemented with TCU Nursing students and on the campus of Oregon Health and Science University. Findings from the full-scale, multisite trial with seventy-three novice nurses revealed no difference in the competence score among three study groups, although there was a statistically significant difference in the pre-test and post-test scores. Change in self-efficacy did not correlate with change in competence. These findings were interpreted to be meaningful to shape how nurse educators use multiple patient simulation experiences in capstone clinical courses. They also provide a better understanding of how novice nurses benefit from repeated multiple patient simulation activities. The study was funded with $20,000 by the Joyce Griffin-Sobel Educational Research Grant from the National League for Nursing following receipt of the $5,000 Joan K. Stout Research Grant from STTI and

$3,000 from Beta Psi Chapter of STTI to pilot the study.

Clinical Research

Carol Howe, Danielle Walker, and Jordan Watts (2017) conducted a cross-sectional study with 522 diabetes educators to determine their use of and perceived effectiveness of recommended communication techniques as they taught patients diabetes self-management, and to determine differences in communication by educator characteristics. The American Medical Association (AMA) Communication Techniques Survey was used to assess the results.

Findings indicated that simple language, written patient education materials, and using teach-back were the most frequently reported techniques. The least reported were follow-up phone calls and drawing pictures. Educators who used significantly more communication techniques included Hispanics, those with more than sixteen years of practice, and those who provided sixteen hours or more of education per week. Nurses also used more communication techniques than dieticians. No significant differences in routine communication techniques were found by education level or certification status. The authors noted that the findings provide a baseline assessment of diabetes educator communication practices and suggested that opportunities exist for "interprofessional health literacy communication and research."

Glenda Daniels has been involved in a number of studies related to gastrointestinal conditions. A recent study about bowel management strategies used by veterans with long-standing spinal cord injuries is her most recent publication (Schmelzer, Daniels, and Baird 2017). In this qualitative study, the researchers described strategies that eighteen veterans used to achieve control over bowel function. Recordings of participant interviews were analyzed to identify major themes.

Data revealed that fourteen of the eighteen participants had gained control of their bowel function. The importance of positive attitudes was emphasized along with "listening to their bodies" (2017), remaining physically active, and using trial and error in order to find the best bowel control strategies. The value of peer support was emphasized. Participants also provided "practical advice for adapting strategies" (2017) they had learned during rehabilitation for long-term control following dismissal and return to their homes.

Lisa Bashore, in collaboration with Joyce Bender, a clinical social worker at Cook Children's Health Care System in Fort Worth, conducted a descriptive, qualitative study to explore long-term benefits experienced by families of childhood cancer survivors derived from attending a weekend family retreat, which was held at least twelve months prior to the time of the study (Lisa Bashore, pers. comm., 2017).

Semistructured questions were used as the interview guide for three separate audiotaped focus groups composed of seven families. Through qualitative analysis, three themes emerged. Findings included major benefits in reconnecting with families or others in a therapeutic environment, changing their outlook on life, and putting life into perspective.

Kathy Baker's ongoing program of research has focused on quality of life (QOL). Her initial study was a pilot of QOL in liver transplant recipients and focused on their perceptions of QOL following transplantation. The study reveals the importance of physiological, psychological, social, spiritual, family, and socioeconomic aspects of QOL for liver transplant recipients. Building on her pilot work, Baker continued her study with larger mixed methods, multi-site study of QOL, self-transcendence, illness distress, and fatigue in liver recipients. The findings emphasize the need to minimize post-transplant co-morbidities like fatigue and illness distress, while enhancing self-transcendence in order to enrich the transplant recipient's QOL experience. An unexpected finding was that participants demonstrated a very distinct trend toward optimism or pessimism related to their transplant experience. Baker has presented her work at the New Zealand Gastro Conference, Southern Nursing Research Society, International Transplant Nurses Society in Rotterdam, Netherlands, and at the Society of Gastroenterology Nurses conferences.

As a followup to initial studies, Baker is currently collaborating with Suzy Lockwood in an investigation of survivorship experiences for individuals with complex diagnoses, including pancreatic, head, neck, and gynecologic cancers. The experiences and perspectives of cancer survivors' families and friends are also being documented. Initial findings suggest the QOL needs of survivors demonstrate both similar needs and needs that are unique, based on the cancer diagnosis. Survivors and their families are very interested in sharing their experiences and have specific recommendations about how to enhance QOL. Additionally, health care providers are often not aware or are not addressing these QOL issues.

A large portion of Baker's scholarly efforts have been with the collaboration, consultation, and mentorship of other nurses in both practice and academic settings. Her expertise in evidence-based practice, qualitative methods, and systematic review methods, as well as her consultation with the Health Innovations Institute at TCU, have resulted in publications with students and colleagues in a variety of journals, including the *American Journal for Nurse Practitioners, Journal of Advanced Nursing Studies, Gastrointestinal Endoscopy, Perioperative Nursing Clinics, American Journal of Nursing, Applied Nursing Research, American Association of Nurse Anesthetists (AANA) Journal Pharmacogenomics,* and *Nursing Management.*

Baker has made presentations in South Australia, Belgium, Canada, Ireland, Czech Republic, New Zealand, Uruguay, South Africa, and Thailand. The dissemination of her work has made a significant contribution to the body of knowledge that informs how nurses determine actions potentially affecting the health outcomes of their patients, one of the challenges identified by founding dean Harris in 1973.

The Evidence-Based Practice and Research Collaborative has continued and expanded from twenty to forty participating institutions. The Evidence-Based Practice Fellowship has graduated 457 Fellows and produced 441 Evidence-Based Projects. An exemplary project incorporated a "nurse-driven neonatal neck-neutral positioning and low movement protocol for < 1500 gram birth weight premature infants that resulted in a reduction of serious grade 3-4 brain bleeds from 28.6% to 0%"(Smith, pers. comm., 2018). Fellows and partners have made a significant contribution to practice changes and improved patient outcomes. The work of the DBP Fellowship was instrumental in Dean Susan Weeks and TCU Nursing being asked to participate in the US-Sino Nursing Forum, a collaborative of leading universities in the US and China. The participating universities from the US include Duke University, Johns Hopkins University, New York University, University of Pittsburgh, Yale University, and TCU.

In summary, TCU Nursing had many reasons to celebrate in the decade beginning in 2010. The addition and renovation of the Annie Richardson Bass Building provided faculty and students a state-of-the-art facility in which to conduct educational initiatives. The success of the Joanna Briggs Institute Collaboration Center facilitated collaboration with other international centers to promote effective health practices and improve patient outcomes. Four centers joined together to become the Health Innovation Institute (HIATT) to increase advancement of each of the center's missions.

The undergraduate curriculum continued to offer two tracks: the traditional track and the accelerated track. Curricular changes incorporated multiple opportunities for interprofessional education. A Post-Baccalaureate Doctor of Nursing Practice (DNP) was added with a focus on the family (Family Nurse Practitioner). In fall 2018, a PhD in Health Sciences began with collaboration across disciplines. Faculty and students in all programs remained active in local, national, and international professional undertakings. Between the fall 2010 and spring 2018, there were 1,516 BSN graduates, 146 MSN graduates, and 188 DNP graduates.

Chapter Seven

TCU Nursing

Creating the Future

After reflecting on the vision, mission, and core values of TCU Nursing and the current and future status of nursing and nursing education, the faculty revised and approved the departmental strategic initiatives for 2018–23. The mission, "to equip individuals to deliver evidence-based care, advance nursing scholarship, and lead practice innovation" flows from the vision of being a "leader in nursing education, practice, and scholarship" (TCU Nursing Faculty 2018).

Core Values

Eight core values guide the work of the school's administrators, faculty, and staff. These are altruism, autonomy, civility, human dignity, innovation, integrity, social justice, and teamwork.

Altruism refers to the "concern for the welfare and well-being of others, a commitment to caring and compassion." Faculty members believe that "in professional practice, altruism is reflected by the nurse's concern for the welfare of patients, faculty members, other nurses, members of the healthcare team, and populations" (TCU Nursing Faculty 2018).

Autonomy is defined as "professionalism, lifelong learning, personal wellness, and responsibility, while upholding the right to self-determination." According to TCU nursing faculty, "Autonomy is demonstrated when the nurse respects patients' rights to make decisions about their health." They further stated that "autonomy is demonstrated when the nurse exercises independent and interdependent decision-making in accordance with the scope and standards of nursing practice" (TCU Nursing Faculty 2018).

Civility is defined as "an authentic respect for others that requires time, presence, willingness to engage in genuine discourse, and intention to seek common ground that governs both speech and behavior towards others" (Clark 2016). TCU nursing faculty have provided an example of civility and promoted it "through a culture where others feel validated and valued." This includes peers, patients, and caregivers. They also have emphasized that "civility must be present for professionalism to occur" (TCU Nursing Faculty 2018).

Human dignity is the "respect for the inherent worth and uniqueness of individuals and populations, exercising civility in all circumstances, promoting wellness and holism, confidentiality and privacy." Faculty members have further reinforced the belief that in professional nursing, practicing human dignity "is reflected when the nurse values and respects all patients, family members, colleagues, and populations" (TCU Nursing Faculty 2018).

Innovation refers to the "commitment to creativity, ingenuity, and curiosity in practice and scholarship, teaching/learning, and improved performance and outcomes." In professional practice, innovation has been interpreted by TCU nursing faculty as the nurse's use of "updated knowledge to develop a new or novel approach which enhances health and education" (TCU Nursing Faculty 2018).

Integrity is the "commitment to accountability, transparency, stewardship, citizenship, honesty, and veracity, in accordance with an appropriate code of ethics and accepted standards of practice." Integrity is demonstrated in practice "when the nurse is honest and provides care based on an ethical framework that is accepted within the profession" (TCU Nursing Faculty 2018).

Social justice is the "dedication to upholding moral, legal, and humanistic principles." TCU nursing faculty members believe that social justice is evidenced "when the nurse advocates assuring equal treatment under the law and equal access to quality health care for all" (TCU Nursing 2018).

Teamwork, as defined by the faculty, is a "respect for the value of interprofessional collaboration, effective communication, academic-practice partnerships, and community engagement." When "change agency and transformation among patients, community members and members of the healthcare team" is evidenced, teamwork has been accomplished (TCU Nursing 2018).

Strategic initiatives for 2018–23 not only serve as venues for fulfilling the vision and mission of Harris College, but they also respond to the challenges posed by Dean Harris in 1973 and the imperative for creating a positive future in nursing. Initiatives were identified as excellence in teaching and scholarship, high-quality students, faculty, and staff, transformational community engagement, and a world-class learning environment.

Excellence in Teaching and Scholarship

Initiatives in teaching and scholarship demand "faculty excellence within each domain of the teacher-scholar-practitioner model." TCU Nursing defines the teacher-scholar-practitioner model as one in which nursing practice is the foundation for scholarship and teaching, and through which nursing knowledge is generated, shared, and applied in a variety of settings. TCU Nursing faculty integrate ways of knowing as teachers and scholars to facilitate the holistic education of students (Harris College of Nursing & Health Sciences 2018).

The TCU Nursing action plan calls for the development of a variety of activities. For example, the action plan calls for a commitment to support student engagement in scholarship. Potential activities include the development of an interprofessional education (IPE) seminar for students which focuses on research, the establishment of funding for student engagement in scholarship at both the undergraduate and graduate level, and an increased support for honors advising (Harris College of Nursing & Health Sciences 2018).

High-Quality Student, Faculty, and Staff

To recruit and retain diverse, high-quality applicants to both undergraduate and graduate programs is a high priority for the coming years. Following the recruitment of students, the plan calls for collaboration with the Harris College of Nursing & Health Sciences Academic Resource Center and the TCU Counseling and Mental Health Center to develop programs for supporting students. Scholarships for students in all nursing programs was identified as another high priority.

A commitment was made to the recruitment and retention of a diverse faculty and staff with exceptional knowledge, skills, and abilities related to their position. This commitment also includes support for faculty, staff, and faculty associates to obtain leadership in national organizations.

Transformational Community Engagement

Future activities within Harris College include maintaining and building mutually beneficial academic-practice partnerships within the community. The maintenance and expansion of IPE partners will be ongoing. Another goal is to establish a dedicated education unit with practice partners. These partners also may provide the opportunity for IPE research.

To connect young community partners with the campus and the TCU Nursing faculty and staff, a yearly TCU Nursing camp will be held each summer for high school juniors and seniors who wish to explore nursing as a career.

A World-Class Learning Environment

To have a world-class learning environment, the TCU Nursing action plan aims to increase service learning opportunities to increase faculty and students' appreciation of their variety. A marketing plan will also be designed to increase student applications from diverse populations. This goal will focus on expanding scholarship monies for recruitment and retention of diverse populations of students, faculty, and staff.

State-of-the-art instructional and research technologies will support student learning. In order to seek accreditation as a Center of Excellence for Simulation Instruction and Education, Harris College will implement innovative teaching strategies and innovation in simulation at all levels of nursing education.

Global experiences and learning are final goals for students, faculty, and staff. Harris College seeks to develop global experiences at the graduate level and provide experiences that include IPE courses in rural areas of the United States, and will seek funding for student participation in study abroad programs.

REFLECTIONS

From Congresswoman Eddie Bernice Johnson

US Representative from the Thirtieth Congressional District of Texas

When asked about her motivation to become a nurse, Congresswoman Eddie Bernice Johnson indicated that her initial desire was to be a physician, but her high school counselor recommended that girls should be nurses (Johnson, pers. comm., 2018). She quickly commented that a counselor of the current decade wouldn't make the same recommendation. When Johnson arrived at TCU's Harris College of Nursing, she was already a registered nurse (RN) who had passed the state board examination in Indiana after graduating with a diploma from Saint Mary's College in Notre Dame. She returned to her home state of Texas and started working at the United States Department of Veterans Affairs (VA) in Dallas. Her initial interest was in pediatric nursing, and she had done a rotation in a pediatric unit in Indianapolis. The emotional aspects of working on surgical units for infants, however, convinced her that psychiatric nursing would be a good way for her to learn about emotions, and she subsequently changed her focus. Johnson, who was a wife and mother with a full-time job when she was an RN-BSN student, was inducted into Beta Alpha Chapter of Sigma Theta Tau International for her academic accomplishments and commitment to her studies.

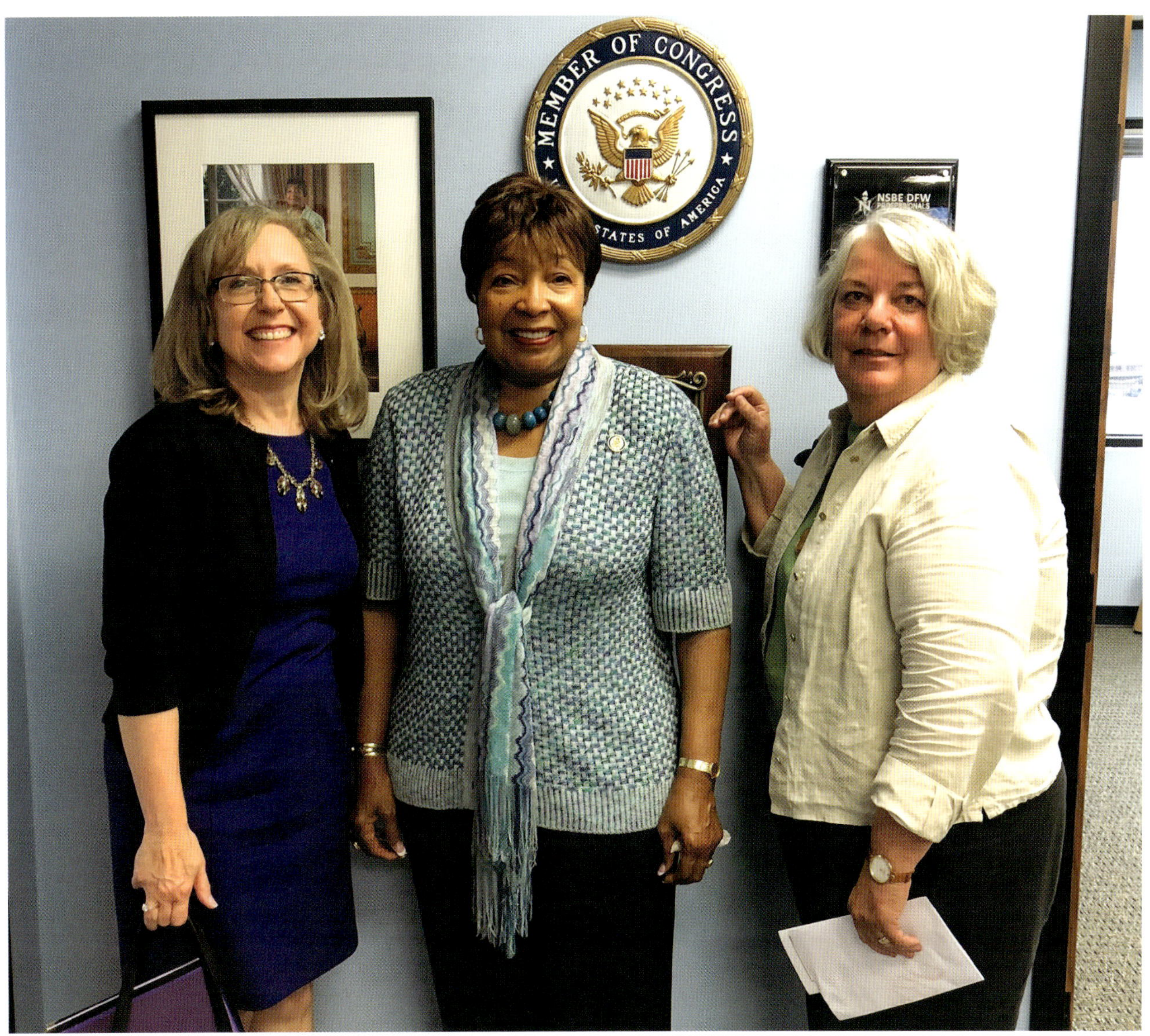

L-R, Suzy Lockwood, Eddie Bernice Johnson, and Rhonda Keen-Payne.

Congresswoman Johnson believes that a particularly good aspect of nursing is its general approach and attention to details, which permit the nurse to make decisions in stressful times while remaining calm. These skills, along with allowing people to be themselves without "judging yourself by that, nor judge them in conjunction with what you are" (Johnson 2018) were cited as being very helpful to the Congresswoman in whatever job she has chosen. She emphasized the importance of not making strong judgments before you know a person. The ability of nurses to develop a strategy and not jump into things without a plan is another important result of their training. Johnson indicated that her nursing experience has provided a very useful framework for many of the roles and responsibilities she has held over the years.

When asked about involvement in organizations at Texas Christian University and Harris College of Nursing, Congresswoman Johnson indicated that she was unable to participate in student organizations as she was married, with a son, and worked full time.

Developing a plan, executing it with a strategy, and organizing one's time, all of which she learned as a nurse, have been critical to her role as an elected official (Johnson, pers. comm., 2018). These same skills can be transferred to one's personal life. She still depends upon this strategy as she makes time for her son and grandsons while she functions in her congressional role.

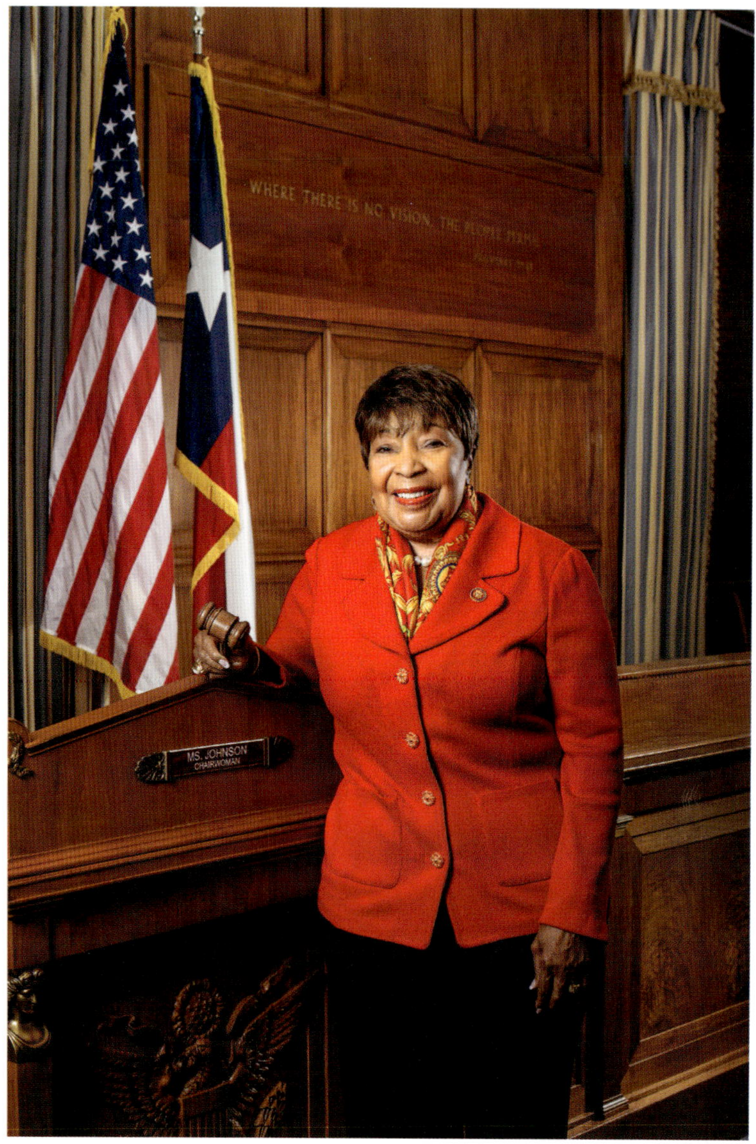

Congresswoman Eddie Bernice Johnson.

Congresswoman Johnson works from two offices: the Washington office, which has responsibility for policy and legislation, and the local district office, a "people office," which assumes responsibility for casework, outreach, and problem-solving. She is typically in her district office on weekends. While the House of Representatives does not hold votes in August, she travels widely to countries where United States personnel conduct research related to science and technology. She has visited colleagues in Switzerland, Australia, France, Finland, Bosnia, Croatia, Germany, and Italy. As she has carried out responsibilities in these countries, she has developed job descriptions for travel and a manual that "comes from the nursing mentality." She is frequently cited as a consultant for others new to public service who travel for the government (Johnson, pers. comm., 2018).

Congresswoman Johnson believes that nurses are prepared for many roles—they can "do most anything— nurses can teach, they can work in a physician's office, they can work in industry—it's boundless" (Johnson, pers. comm., 2018).

During her time in Congress, Johnson sometimes felt that the nursing profession was going to disappear because nurses had not kept watch over what was happening to them. There was a time when she thought that distinctions could not be made between the "occasional nurse, the degreed nurses, and others." She noted that there was a time when there was not a nurse you could call on to get a sense of where the nation was on the issues. She believes that the American Nurses Association has "stepped up" and credits the National League for Nursing that has a collaboration for professions (Johnson, pers. comm., 2018).

In a discussion about the Affordable Care Act, Congresswoman Johnson commented that she found it interesting that there were no health professionals who served on the committees. She did serve on a task force to assist with the wording of the legislation, based on her previous experience with direct patient care. What did she think would happen with health care in the future? "I wish I knew!" she exclaimed. She said they knew from the beginning that the Affordable Health Care Bill was not perfect, and as with Social Security, Medicare, and other major pieces of legislation, Congress could revisit the law to make corrections and improvements. Currently, however, there has been little opportunity to improve it, since "most of the efforts have been directed at dismantling it. . . . There is so much work to be done until before you know it . . . you're staying longer than you ever thought you would" (Johnson, pers. comm., 2018).

Commenting on her experience in Congress, Johnson said, "There's never a dull moment! You meet everybody from every walk of life" (2018). She has worked with governors, mayors, and all types of other professions, believes that nurses can provide invaluable input to Congress, and hopes that more will become involved. She also confirmed the value of the intern experience for students in providing opportunities to become involved in the issues facing the nation.

REFLECTIONS

From Alison Moreland: Board of Visitors Member

Alison Moreland, who arrived at Texas Christian University as a student in 1958 and graduated from Harris College of Nursing in 1961, has assumed a variety of roles throughout her professional career. Having worked in public health nursing, school nursing, and staff development, she joined the College of Health and Human Sciences and became a tenured instructor in 2001. Following her retirement, she returned as an adjunct faculty and served throughout the 2012–13 academic year. Currently, Alison serves as a member of the Board of Visitors of Harris College of Nursing & Health Sciences. As she reflected on the many changes which have taken place over the past sixty years, several themes emerged.

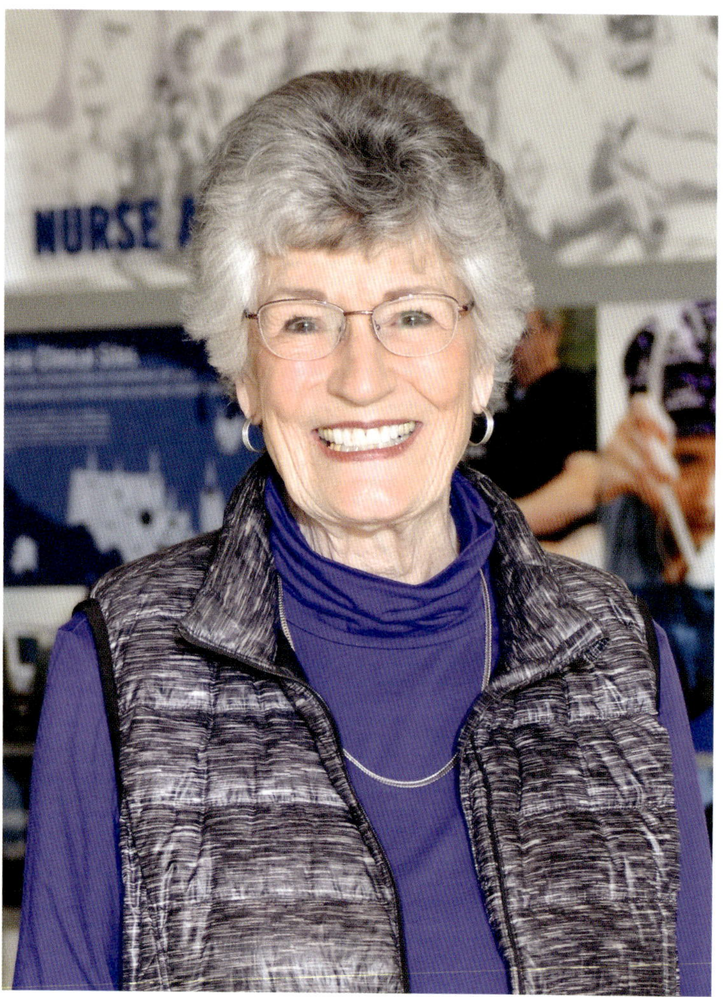

Alison Moreland, 2020.

She first noted the increase in size, along with a significant increase in professionalism within nursing. The nature of collaboration between physicians and nurses has changed dramatically. She noted the value of interdisciplinary activities and the outcomes it can yield for both the caregiver and the recipient of care. The nursing profession's awareness of interdisciplinary collaboration is combined with the inclusion of geriatric content in the nursing curriculum.

One meaningful program that includes both interdisciplinary collaboration and a focus on geriatric care is the Senior Assisting in Geriatric Education (SAGE) program, of which Alison is a participant. SAGE is a collaborative University of North Texas Health Science Center (UNTHSC) and TCU project that pairs seniors with an interdisciplinary team of students in the health professions (nursing, dietetics, social work students attending TCU, and Medicine and Pharmacy students attending UNTHSC). The educational, interdisciplinary program provides students the opportunity to learn together and interact with seniors in their homes.

Moreland believes that research is a strong component of the college's student and faculty work, and was very impressed with the variety of research programs in place. She predicted that a future challenge would be the recruitment of qualified faculty members, especially in the area of geriatric nursing, as growth continues.

REFLECTIONS

From Dr. Kay Bruce: Board of Visitors Member

Kay Bruce, a 1966 graduate of TCU and a current member of the board of visitors of Harris College of Nursing & Health Sciences, knew from the time she was nineteen years old that she wanted to obtain a PhD. As a graduate of the Diploma Nursing Program at Shannon Memorial Hospital in San Angelo, Texas, she came to Fort Worth to continue her education and received a bachelor's degree in nursing at Harris College of Nursing. She taught pediatrics and obstetrics at HCN for five years until she moved to California, where she continued her education and received a master of science degree in nursing from Loma Linda University in 1975, a second master of arts degree in education in 1982, and a PhD in higher education from Claremont Graduate School in 1983.

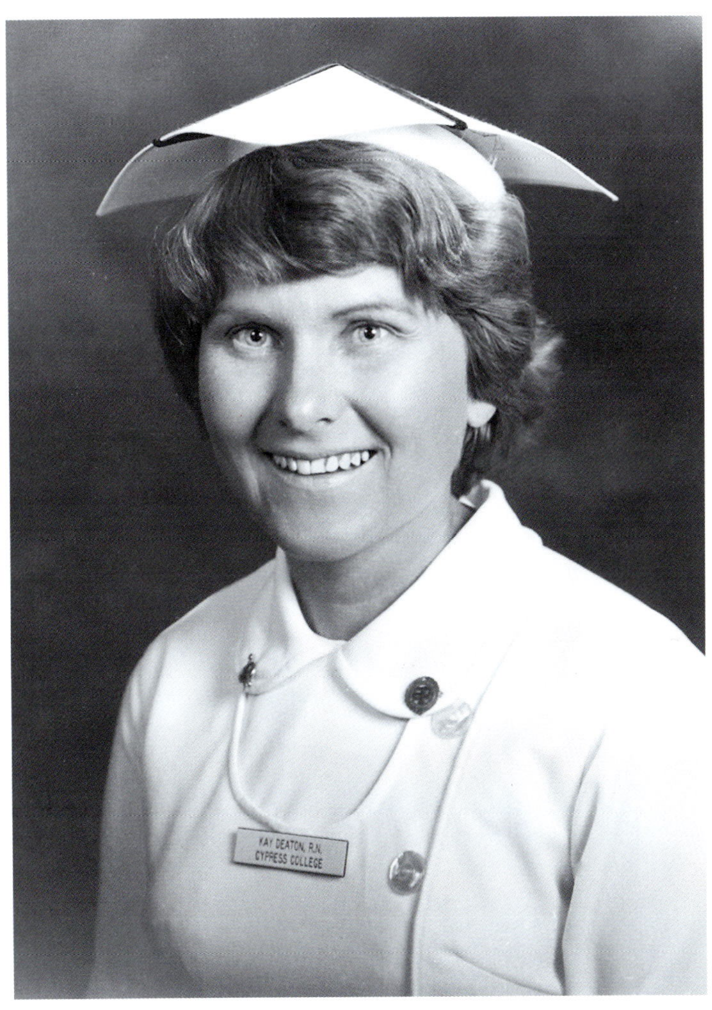

Kay Bruce at graduation.

Dr. Bruce believes that the "wellness model holds the key to the future" (Bruce, pers. comm., 2018). She added that she believed HCN had focused on a wellness model for many years. For example, faculty members prepared professional nurses who focused on the whole person. Self-care was identified as the first part of the equation, so faculty encouraged students to care for themselves by "eating appropriately, exercising, and engaging in spirituality and relationships" (Bruce, pers. comm., 2018).

Bruce believes that the role of the nurse in providing adequate health care depends on the ability to think critically. The nursing process and the use of critical thinking assist the nurse in identifying and solving problems in any area of practice and at all educational levels.

According to Dr. Bruce, health care that includes a focus on the culture of the community is key to the health of citizens. For nurses, this requires an emphasis on general education and liberal arts as well as nursing courses. Travel in a nurse's life is critical in understanding humanity. Study abroad helps nursing students gain perspectives on health from the views of people throughout the world and allows them to become leaders in their communities upon their return home.

Bruce believes the professional nurse has an important role as a leader. This might include serving as a community activist by membership on boards of hospitals, colleges, chambers of commerce, and the United Way. Opportunities for activism can occur at the local, state, national, or international level. She also sees being politically informed as a responsibility of a professional nurse today so that nurses can tell their stories.

Bruce believes that Harris College will continue to be a leader in preparing nurses to establish and maintain wellness in neighborhood settings. As health care delivery changes, the neighborhood nurse is going to be responsible for the level of health in an area. This is not just in our nation but around the world. Wellness will be the goal from conception to death, with issues of illness being of secondary importance. If people accept responsibility for their own health to help prevent illness, then the level of wellness will increase. This is part of the role of the board of visitors: bring forth ideas, recommendations, and money to help change and implement a wellness model.

Bruce would like to see the entrance to practice require a baccalaureate degree, as proposed in the position paper put forth by the American Nurses Association (ANA) in 1965. She asked, "Why is it pharmacy and physical therapy programs have moved to a doctorate level when nursing is still admitting licensure at the Associate Level?" (Bruce 2018).

REFLECTIONS

From Jeanette Lancaster, PhD, RN FAAN

HCN Faculty 1970–77
(Dean Emerita, University of Virginia)

The years that I taught at the Harris College of Nursing were the most formative years for my career. The experienced faculty were supportive and

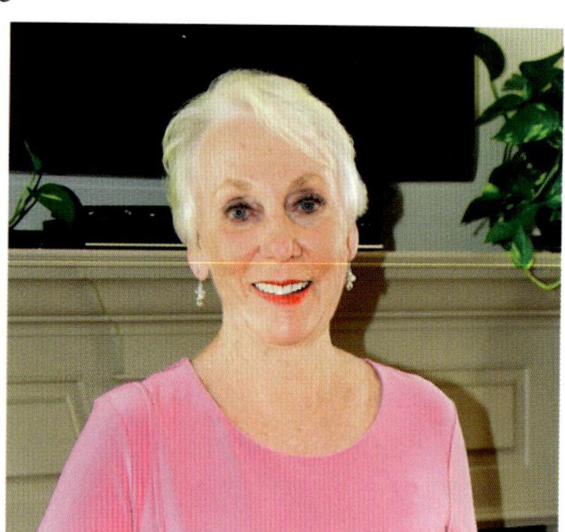

Jeanette Lancaster.

> encouraging; the students were interested in learning; the junior faculty worked well together as we each learned our roles as faculty members; the clinical facilities supported student learning.
>
> Perhaps most of all, Dean Virginia Jarratt was a world-class mentor to me. She continually opened doors to new career opportunities and supported me as I learned my role. It was difficult to say no to her! It has been a pleasure to see the many contributions made to nursing by the TCU nursing faculty, students, and graduates.

In summary, the vision of the future for TCU Nursing is robust. As the role of the nurse has evolved and expanded over the years, TCU Nursing has kept pace with the many changes and multiple opportunities in the health care system and within nursing education. Faculty and staff responded to Dean Paulette Burns's challenge to "be bold." Under the leadership of former deans, interim deans, and the associate dean of nursing, Suzy Lockwood, faculty, and staff created a path to meet the two challenges posed by founding dean Lucy Harris (Appendix 14).

Graduates have clearly demonstrated the fulfillment of traditional and new roles in nursing, including working with colleagues from other disciplines (interprofessional collaboration). Similarly, along with faculty, they have conducted research that shows the potential impact of nursing care on patient outcomes.

Moving forward, TCU Nursing, in collaboration with anesthesia, communication sciences and disorders, kinesiology, and social work, has the visionary mission of transforming global health through education, scholarship, and innovation (Lockwood 2018). Pillars of the college include preparing global citizens, community growth, and excellence with integrity through exceptional teaching, service, high-quality students, faculty, and staff, transformational community engagement, and a world-class learning environment (Appendix 15).

Chapter Eight

The School of Nurse Anesthesia

A Thriving Addition to Harris College

The Doctor of Nursing Practice-Anesthesia (DNP-A) is a practice doctorate designed to prepare experts in specialized advanced nursing practice. There is a sharp focus on practice that is innovative and evidence-based, reflecting the application of credible research findings and theories to improve health care outcomes (TCU graduate catalog 2019).

The Beginning

TCU's Harris School of Nursing was founded by Charles Harris in 1915. Harris Hospital, the original site of nurse anesthesia education in Fort Worth, was also established by Harris. Harris Hospital provided a certificate program in nurse anesthesia from 1946 until the early 1980s, when they partnered with Texas Wesleyan College to offer a master of health science degree in anesthesia.

The TCU School of Nurse Anesthesia (SOA) was founded in 2003. Planning began in the late 1990s, before Jake B. Schrum left Texas Wesleyan University in 2000 to become president of Southwestern University. Wesleyan president Schrum introduced Kay K. Sanders, CRNA, MHS, and director of the Texas Wesleyan graduate program in nurse anesthesia, to Rhonda Keen-Payne, PhD, RN, and dean of the TCU College of Health and Human Sciences. Schrum encouraged collaboration between Texas Wesleyan and TCU. Keen-Payne and Sanders planned an innovative, cooperative program with shared resources; however, the next president of Texas Wesleyan, Harold Jeffcoat, was not in favor of this endeavor. In the fall of 2002, he terminated this collaboration at a meeting of Texas Wesleyan senior administrators.

By that time, community support was evident for a TCU nurse anesthesia program, and an application for a new program had been submitted to the Council on Accreditation of Nurse Anesthesia Educational Programs (COA). Below is an excerpt from the *2002 Capability Review/Self-Study* submitted to the COA in preparation for the initial COA site visit to TCU September 26–27, 2002.

> Following an assessment of the University plant by the Board of Trustees, the campus received $30 million for essential renovation. During the summer and fall of 2001, nearly every space in ARB was improved—new lighting and ceilings, carpet, classroom and office furniture, laboratory equipment replacements and additions, and several small construction projects to reconfigure space. Additionally, every classroom was fitted with new, permanent audiovisual (television, projector) and computer equipment, including network access for instruction.

Some renovations were completed specifically for the program. One large classroom (seating approximately ninety-five) was dedicated to the program and was intended to be the primary location for any video broadcast activity. A second seminar room was prepared for the human patient simulator purchased in early 2002.

As we began development of the program, several key beliefs emerged: first, in order to meet the rigorous demands of a curriculum in nurse anesthesia in a reasonable length of time, we believed that a school separate from the existing nursing school was necessary. Second, we realized that Wesleyan and TCU shared many fundamental beliefs and characteristics and were encouraged that some cooperation might be possible in the future. Third, we remained convinced that regardless of the degree of cooperation, the need for more CRNAs can be partially met by directing TCU's resources toward a new program. Finally, because of these beliefs, we designed a curriculum for faculty similar to Wesleyan's in characteristics, values, and experiences because this not only met our mission and goals, but it also prepared us for possible cooperative ventures in the future. The TCU community had recently voiced an interest in expanding selected graduate professional programs, and the nurse anesthesia program fit well with this goal.

Because the leadership of Texas Wesleyan and TCU programs shared a commitment to high-quality practice, we believed the program's chief outcome, the preparation of nurse anesthetists, would be greatly facilitated.

Initial Personnel

Following the site visit and a national search for a program director, Kay K. Sanders, who served as a consultant to Keen-Payne during the planning and accreditation process, was hired on September 25, 2002, to serve as Clinical Professor, which is

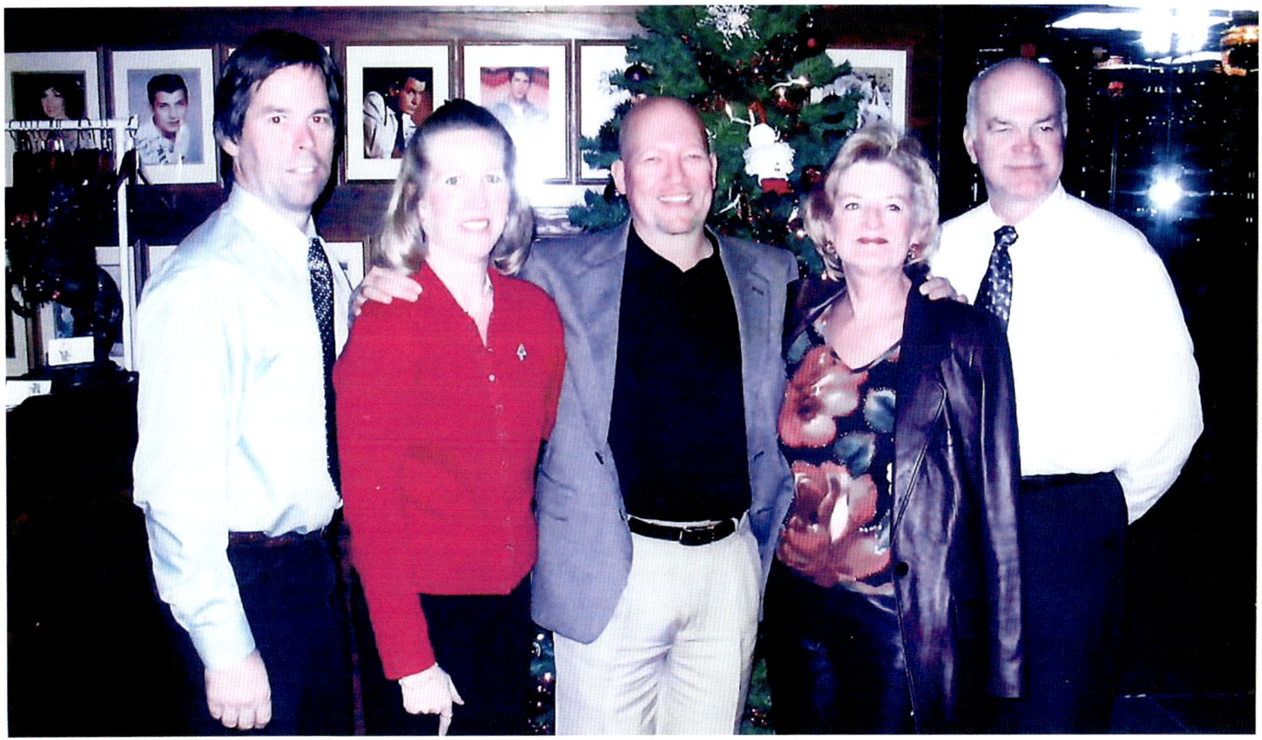

In the beginning there were five: L-R, Kent Young, Carol Womack, Tim Gollaher, Kay Sanders, and Buck Kelsey, 2003.

known now as Professor of Professional Practice, and director of the School of Nurse Anesthesia. Her full-time employment at TCU began June 1, 2003. In addition to directing Texas Wesleyan University's graduate program of nurse anesthesia from 1988 to 2002, Sanders had served the Council on Accreditation of Nurse Anesthesia Programs (COA) as an on-site visitor and was very familiar with degrees offered by other nurse anesthesia programs. She was responsible for curricular design with input from the dean and CRNA (Certified Registered Nurse Anesthetist) faculty.

Another important position was that of assistant program director. Timothy T. Gollaher, CRNA, MHS, was appointed on January 13, 2003, as associate program director. He graduated in 1995 with a master of health science degree from Texas Wesleyan and received a certificate in nurse anesthesia in 1996 from Texas Wesleyan University. He was employed by Texas Wesleyan from June 1997 through February 2003 both as an instructor and as interim assistant director in the nurse anesthesia program. Gollaher worked as a clinical instructor for nurse anesthesia students at Plaza Medical Center of Fort Worth from 1997 to 2003.

Carol Womack was hired July 28, 2003, to be the first School of Nurse Anesthesia administrative assistant to the director. On August 29, 2003, Kent Young was hired as video engineer. All four individuals (Sanders, Gollaher, Womack, and Young) still serve the SOA in their respective roles. Robert "Buck" Kelsey, MLA, CRNA, was hired June 1, 2003, to run the initial simulation labs for anesthesia practice. (He retired May 2008.)

Accreditation and Charter Class

Initial accreditation was granted in June 2003, and a class of sixty-six RNs (thirty-eight males and twenty-eight females) with the required credentials (baccalaureate degrees and critical care experience) was enrolled. After twelve months of academic work, the charter class completed sixteen months of clinical residency at sixteen hospitals in six states (Arkansas, California, Florida, Louisiana, Oklahoma, and Texas). Fifty-three graduated in December 2005 with master of science nurse anesthesia (MSNA) degrees and eligibility to sit for the national certifying examination (NCE) for nurse anesthetists. Five of the graduates earned a 4.0 GPA (Jason Breaux, Ross Castille, Donny DeSalvo, Vaughna Galvin, and Forrest Stegall). Ninety-six percent of the class passed the NCE on the first attempt (national pass rate 90 percent); 100 percent passed on the second attempt. The SOA was off to a strong start.

First Year Activities

On October 3 and 4, 2003, the SOA hosted a two-day continuing education meeting for anesthesiologists and CRNAs who practiced at SOA clinical sites. The seminar was titled Clinical Faculty Orientation and dealt with issues that face anesthesia practitioners when student nurse anesthetists are part of the anesthesia care team. The focus of the meeting was preparation of clinicians for the role of clinical teaching. The meeting was held on the TCU campus in the Kelly Center. Speakers on the program were:

- Catherine Wehlberg, PhD, Director, Center for Teaching Excellence: "Principles of Adult Education." She defined andragogy and applied Kolb's theory of adult learning styles to clinical education.
- Susan Phillips, MHS, CRNA, Clinical Coordinator, ACE Anesthesia, Texas Health Harris Methodist Hospital Fort Worth: "Orienting New Students to Your Clinical Site."
- Hylda Nugent, MHS, CRNA: "Evaluating and Counseling Clinical Students."
- Bill Hartland, PHD, CRNA, Director of Education, Department of Anesthesia, Virginia Commonwealth University: "Teaching the Teacher: Use of Simulator-Based Trigger Films to Enhance Clinical Teaching Effectiveness."

All sixty-six of the first-year students were invited to lunch to meet the clinical coordinators from TCU's eleven primary sites. The students were very excited and expressed that this informal gathering was a great stress reducer.

The First Degree: Master of Science Nurse Anesthesia (MSNA)

The SOA curriculum was designed for the registered nurse with a bachelor's degree and critical care experience. The successful completion of the curriculum led to the degree master of science in nurse anesthesia (MSNA).

The MSNA was a twenty-eight month program with twelve months of classroom and simulation lab work (phase I) and sixteen months of clinical residency (phase II). The SOA offered this degree from 2003 until 2014. A total of 460 graduates earned this degree, passed the certifying examination, and are now CRNAs.

Phase II began in the fall semester of the second year and continued through the fall semester of the third year. Sixteen months in length, phase II included a clinical residency, a series of concepts courses on advanced principles of practice, and clinical correlation conferences. Additionally, phase II classes focused on the nurse anesthesia profession and incorporated professional and practice concepts from phase I. Theoretical instruction on the perioperative foundations of anesthesia practice were taught in principles of anesthesia practice courses and reinforced in the anesthesia skills laboratory. The anesthesia skills lab included a human patient simulator, anesthesia machines, back models, and other teaching aids appropriate to nurse anesthesia education. Concept courses taught during the clinical phase included lectures, discussions, and case presentations taught via interactive video teleconferencing.

Faculty Support

TCU SOA was supportive of faculty with both academic and clinical responsibilities who wished to pursue graduate education. Several CRNA clinical coordinators without graduate degrees expressed an interest in the SOA's curriculum. To support their pursuit of graduate degrees, the *Outline to Be Used When Requesting Approval of Graduate Degrees for CRNAs (Completion Degree Programs),* was submitted to the COA in the fall of 2005 and approved by the COA in May of 2006. Mike Sadler, CRNA, Delores Padgett, CRNA, and Oscar Fimbres, CRNA, took advantage of this opportunity.

2006 Self-Study and Site Visit

In 2006 the SOA had twenty-six clinical sites in five states. On the first day of the COA visit, the reviewers visited hospitals in Louisiana (Baton Rouge and Lafayette) and in the DFW area. On the second day, the reviewers held conferences with campus officials and with all students; second-year clinical students at clinical sites outside of Tarrant County met with the reviewers over video teleconferencing. There were only two citations dealing with student communication and their understanding of their due process rights. Both issues were resolved and the nurse anesthesia program received ten years accreditation, the maximum given by the COA.

The Second Degree: Doctor of Nursing Practice

The Beginning

During October 11-14, 2005, TCU School of Nurse Anesthesia hosted Lorraine Jordan, PhD, CRNA, CAE, FAAN, Senior Director of Research and Quality, American Association of Nurse Anesthetists (AANA) as their Green Chair Professor. During her visit she met over lunch with several TCU faculty and administrators. The focus of the discussion was the future of nurse anesthesia education: the clinical doctorate. Below are the last two paragraphs of her report:

> To end my outstanding visit as the Green Chair, I had an opportunity to meet with Dr. Nowell Donovan, Provost, Dr. Bonnie Melhart, Assistant Provost, Dr. Paulette Burns, Director Harris School of Nursing, Ms. Kay Sanders, Director of the Nurse Anesthesia School, and Mr. Timothy Gollaher, Associate Director of the Nurse Anesthesia School. Summarizing the past 4 days events and learning opportunities provided an opportunity to express my impressions of TCU as an outsider.
>
> The faculty, staff, and institution are well positioned in the higher education arena as a solid academic institution willing to explore cutting-edge opportunities. The nurse anesthesia program is clearly viewed as an innovative program in the forefront of anesthesia. Her colleagues view Ms. Kay Sanders as being on the cutting-edge of education and note that her students attain high levels of academic success. It is Ms. Sanders's record of success and the TCU administration's willingness to be leaders in the nurse anesthesia education that will set TCU apart from other academic institutions. Dr. Rhonda Keen-Payne's support moving forward with investigating a clinical doctorate nurse anesthesia program is vital to the future of the program. TCU is a sound academic institution primed to consider a clinical doctorate in nurse anesthesia education. With hard work and administrative support, I anticipate only positive momentum to make the clinical doctorate in nurse anesthesia a reality at TCU. The clinical doctorate will place TCU on the map for the first clinical doctoral

> nurse anesthesia program that does not require a master's degree in nursing for entry. It is truly an exciting venture.
>
> —*Jordan, 2005*

Doctor of Nursing Practice (DNP)

Harris College initiated the postmaster's DNP in August 2007.

> The DNP is a practice doctorate designed to prepare experts in specialized advanced nursing practice. The focus is on practice that is innovative and evidence-based, reflecting the application of credible research findings and theories to improving healthcare outcomes.
>
> —*Excerpt from* New Program Proposal to TCU Graduate Council *submitted by Dr. Linda Harrington, April 2007*

Among the graduate students in the charter DNP class were several SOA faculty (Kay Sanders, Tim Gollaher, and Hylda Nugent). The first cohort completed the degree in May 2009. As her doctoral project, Kay Sanders designed the DNP in anesthesia curriculum. She stated that she appreciated input from the MSNA students.

Doctor of Nursing Practice-Anesthesia (DNP-A)

More opportunities for innovation occurred when the COA adopted standards for practice-oriented doctoral degrees in 2004. In 2007 the AANA mandated the doctoral degree by 2025 for all graduates. The SOA was the fifth program in the nation to gain accreditation by the COA to award a clinical doctorate (DNP degree in anesthesia: DNP-A), and accepted the first DNP cohort in January 2009. In December 2011 sixteen students graduated with DNP degrees, along with forty-six master's degree graduates. By 2013 the SOA admitted only doctoral students. Through 2017 there were 249 new certified nurse anesthetists that held practice-oriented doctorates from TCU in anesthesia.

The Program

The doctor of nursing practice (DNP-A) for postbaccalaureate registered nurses is an innovative, solution-focused program designed to prepare nurse anesthesia students to lead efforts in solving complex health care issues and developing new health care opportunities, specifically in the context of nurse anesthesia practice. The program builds on TCU's mission: "Learning to Change the World" (TCU Graduate Catalog, 2019).

Educational Philosophy

The Handbook for the TCU School of Nurse Anesthesia states:

> The faculty believes doctoral education should prepare an individual who exhibits qualities of mind and character necessary to live a fulfilling life. Further, such education facilitates thoughtful judgment, analytical approaches to problems, and ethical leadership and responsible citizenship. Such expectations require teaching and learning to be interactive, continuous, and conducted with the assumption faculty and students learn from each other. Teaching and learning are both casual and purposeful, and involve affective, cognitive, and psychomotor changes.
>
> Learning the professional practice of nurse anesthesia is enhanced by a safe supportive environment, high expectations, freedom to question and explore, and a diverse, challenging practice experience. The graduate must be able to integrate sound, scientific knowledge with technical and clinical skills in order to competently manage complex anesthetic care of patients. The results of the professional practice of nurse anesthesia should be the betterment of the practitioner, the profession, and society."
>
> —*Handbook for the School of Nurse Anesthesia, 2018–2019*

DNP-A Curriculum

The DNP-Anesthesia is designed for the postbaccalaureate RN who seeks certification in anesthesia and doctoral education. It is a thirty-six month program.

Innovative Strategies

Simulation Laboratory

Student-centered, experiential learning is at the heart of TCU nurse anesthesia simulation curricula and has been since the inception of the TCU nurse anesthesia program. The Human Patient Simulator (HPS) is a computer-model-driven, full-size mannequin that immerses students in a simulated, interactive operating room environment. The HPS has light-sensitive eyes, blinks, speaks, and breathes, has a heartbeat and a pulse, and will accurately respond to procedures performed on humans such as: CPR, intravenous medication, intubation, ventilation, and catheterization. Students administer all types of anesthesia responding to real-time clinical changes as they would in a real clinical setting. Scenarios are manually controlled by TCU nurse anesthesia faculty to meet specific curricular goals. TCU nurse anesthesia students practice in simulation before entering the clinical arena. During the clinical phase of the program, students prepare using hands-on experience to administer anesthesia. Advanced simulated scenarios using high-risk, low-exposure scenarios ensure that students gain experience with clinical situations they would rarely see in patients.

'Simulation Saturdays'

Roseann Diehl, Mike Sadler, and Vaughna Galvin designed and implemented an innovative educational opportunity for clinical students. Local CRNAs and anesthesiologists come to campus for continuing education and to share their expertise with the students. Students and CRNAs participate in four simulated advanced anesthesia scenarios, each lasting approximately ten minutes. Each student serves as a primary anesthesia provider and a second student stands by to help if needed.

CRNAs are granted four CEUs for participating. The CRNAs serve as "confederates" or actors to add to the fidelity of the scenario and demonstrate the dynamic environment of the operating room. For example, a typical scenario begins with a patient hand-off from a confederate CRNA. Then, within seconds to minutes, a pathophysiological scenario which is manipulated by TCU faculty plays out (e.g., laryngospasm, difficult ventilation, hypotension, emergence hypertension).

Once the scenario ends, the students assess their own nontechnical skill performance, and then a debriefing session is held in which all participants, both students and confederates, share their expertise. It is understood by all parties that this is a nonthreatening and dynamic environment where suspension of disbelief is the philosophy.

Pain Management Seminars

The SOA holds two-day seminars twice each spring for clinical students. These are presented by nonfaculty CRNAs with expertise in peripheral nerve blocks and central line placement and are held in the UNT Health Science Center Medical School Cadaver Lab. Students complete online modules prior to the seminar and participate in hands-on experiences with cadavers using two different techniques for peripheral nerve blocks (ultrasound and peripheral nerve stimulation). Seminars are very well received by students.

2016 COA Self Study and Site Visit

The SOA hosted its third on-site visit by the COA in April 2016. By then the SOA had expanded to fifty-three clinical sites. In addition to local sites, the reviewers visited hospitals in Tampa, Baton Rouge, and Houston.

The Senior Reviewer at the Exit Conference said that in his twenty years of service as a reviewer for the COA, he had never until then visited a program without at least one area of concern. Consequently, the SOA received no citations and was granted another ten years of accreditation.

Chronic/Non-Surgical Pain Management

Advanced Pain Management Fellowship—Mission and Goal

The mission of the program is to "educate Certified Registered Nurse Anesthetists (CRNAs) to be competent providers of care to patients who suffer from chronic pain. The purpose of the Advanced Pain Management program is to educate and prepare advanced pain management practitioners to deliver holistic pain management care, including comprehensive pain management interventions and patient education." (TCU Graduate Catalog, 2018-2019) Graduates from the Advanced Pain Management Fellowship Program who meet all of the National Board of Recertification for Nurse Anesthetists (NBCRNA) eligibility criteria will be able to apply for the Non-surgical Pain Management (NSPM-C) subspecialty certification exam. The NSPM credential program measures the knowledge, skills, and abilities of NBCRNA-certified registered nurse anesthetists for practice in the NSPM field (http://www.nbcrna.com/NSPM/Pages/NSPM.aspx).

The goal of this postgraduate program is to "approach pain management holistically by addressing the treatment of pain in ways that ultimately seek to restore normal homeostatic well-being." (TCU Graduate Catalog, 2018-2019) When a return to normal and healthy regulation is not possible, students will seek to provide comfort, hope, and meaning to support a patient's highest potential of human functioning.

Beginning

The American Association of Nurse Anesthetists (AANA) began delivering advanced pain management education through hands-on cadaver continuing education courses in late 2008. This was in direct response to an assessed need for quality pain management education content, accessible by and designed for the nurse anesthesia pain management community. In addition to the need for robust educational offerings for nurse anesthesia pain management practitioners, the physician chronic pain practitioners were increasingly questioning the advanced educational preparation of CRNAs relative to advanced pain management, and consequently their ability to manage, deliver, and ultimately receive reimbursement for complex and full-scope

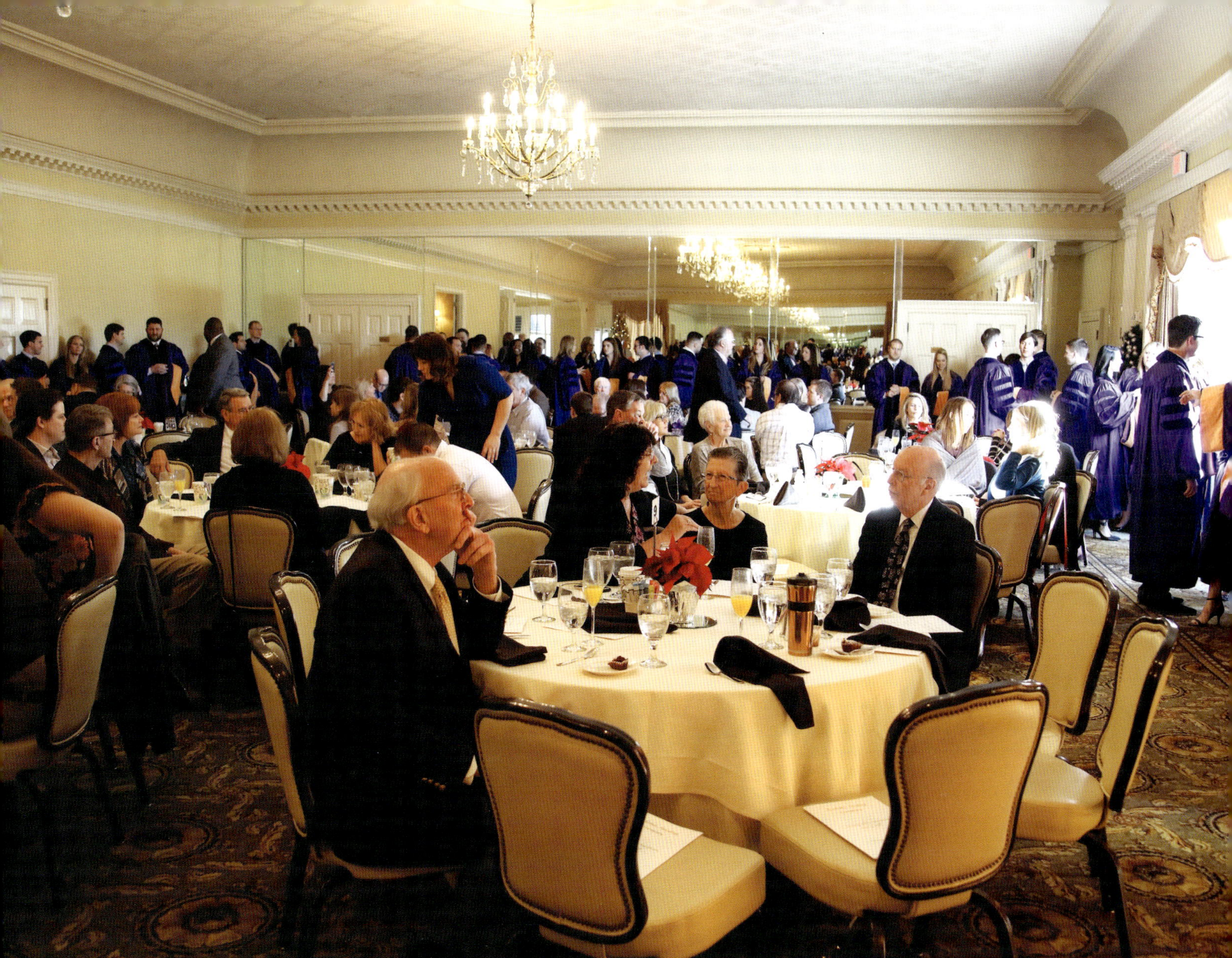

Graduates at Anesthesia's brunch and hooding ceremony, Dec. 15, 2018.

pain management services.

These needs and threats prompted AANA staff to petition the AANA board of directors to allow for the exploration and initiation of formalized graduate-level advanced pain management education for nurse anesthetists. The request was honored, and a search began for an academic partner to deliver the content. Their ideal partner was a private university which was free from state political control over curricular content. They wanted an institution with a proven track record of delivering distance education for both non-degree and degree programs. The partner institu-

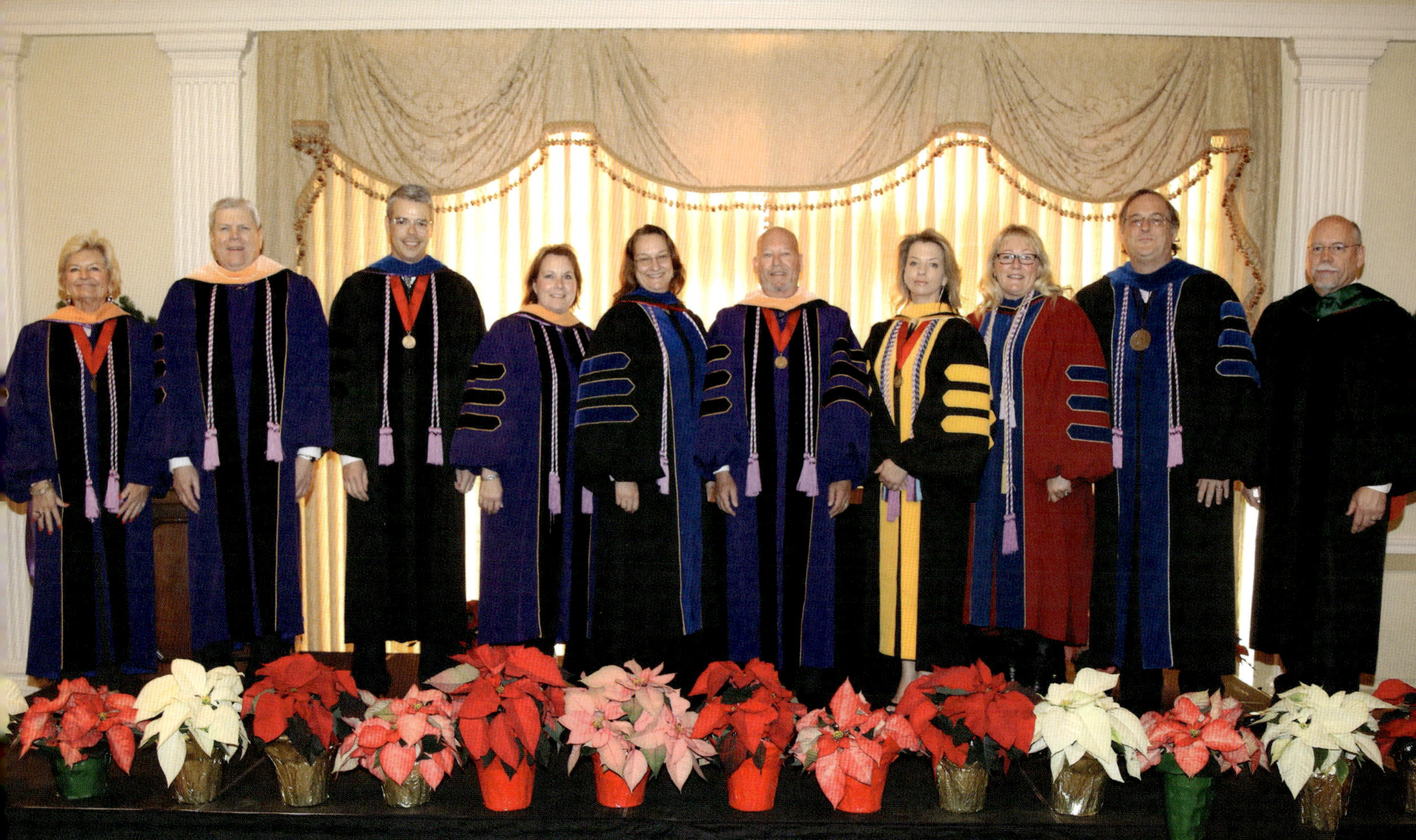

Anesthesia faculty at the hooding ceremony, Dec. 15, 2018. L-R, Kay Sanders, Mike Sadler, Dru Riddle, Hylda Nugent, Monica Jenschke, Tim Gollaher, Vaughna Galvin, Roseann Diehl, Dennis Cheek, and Ron Anderson.

tion needed to encourage innovation and be willing to partner, rather than consume, this new educational concept. Universities with medical education and graduate medical education programs might have difficulty working within these parameters. Additionally, the partner institution would need to manage any political controversy surrounding this new program.

In 2011 AANA partnered with Hamline University in Saint Paul, Minnesota to provide a university-based postgraduate certificate program in response to CRNAs' demands for formalized education in chronic pain management. AANA also worked with COA to develop accreditation standards for a postgraduate fellowship program, and the National Board of Certification and Recertification for Nurse Anesthetists (NBCRNA) for subspecialty certification in Nonsurgical Pain Management (NSPM-C).

The Hamline Pain Management Program was the first COA accredited fellowship program in the nation. CRNAs have been providing chronic pain management, including interventional pain management, since the 1990s, under the pioneering leadership of Jack Neary, CRNA. However, organized medicine had publicly challenged the validity and legality of nurse anesthetists' practice in the area of pain management and actively sought the restriction and prohibition of CRNAs' practice rights in the area of pain management. Insurers and payers were also reluctant to recognize the services provided by CRNAs without demonstrable evidence of formalized education. This innovative postgraduate fellowship program in advanced pain management graduated its first cohort in 2013. In 2015 AANA hosted the first pain management summit and convened the NBCRNA, the COA, faculty, and subject matter experts about the state of the science and education in advanced pain management. The summit concluded with the decision that AANA would seek out a new academic partner with a university-based nurse anesthesia program to align the fellowship and curriculum with the practice of nurse anesthesia. In February 2016, AANA signed a partnership agreement with TCU School of Nurse Anesthesia, under the leadership of Kay Sanders, DNP, CRNA, and welcomed the first TCU cohort in August 2016. Fifteen students completed the program in August 2017. This fellowship program has produced over fifty graduates and, to date, thirty CRNAs have obtained the NSMP-C credential. (This information was submitted by Bruce Schoneboom and John Preston, former AANA Director, Education and Professional Development.)

Chapter Nine

A Short History

The Davies School of Communication Sciences and Disorders

> There has been built up by articulate man an intricate system of language, which has a peculiar capacity for fine shadings and blendings of meaning, for subtle symbolizations. This system of language is used by man for the purpose of translating muscle and nerve into business agreements and theatrical elegance, into last wills and sonnets. It is the material out of which men make laws, deify the blue above, and win their mistresses. It is the greatest man-made power under the heavens, and without a mastery of it, one proceeds at the risk of all good things, at the risk of the grand assumption that life is precious.
>
> — *Dr. Wendell Johnson, Because I Stutter*

From the early advocacy of Edward L. Pross through the thirty years of leadership by Dorothy Mays Bell and those who followed her, the TCU Davies School of Communication Sciences and Disorders (COSD) has evolved over more than seventy years into a nationally recognized research and clinical training site for students pursuing degrees in communication sciences and disorders as well as a beacon of hope to the Fort Worth community. The following short history of COSD at TCU draws largely on Bell's 1980 book, *Development of the Speech and Hearing Clinic at Texas Christian University: A Personal Perspective.*

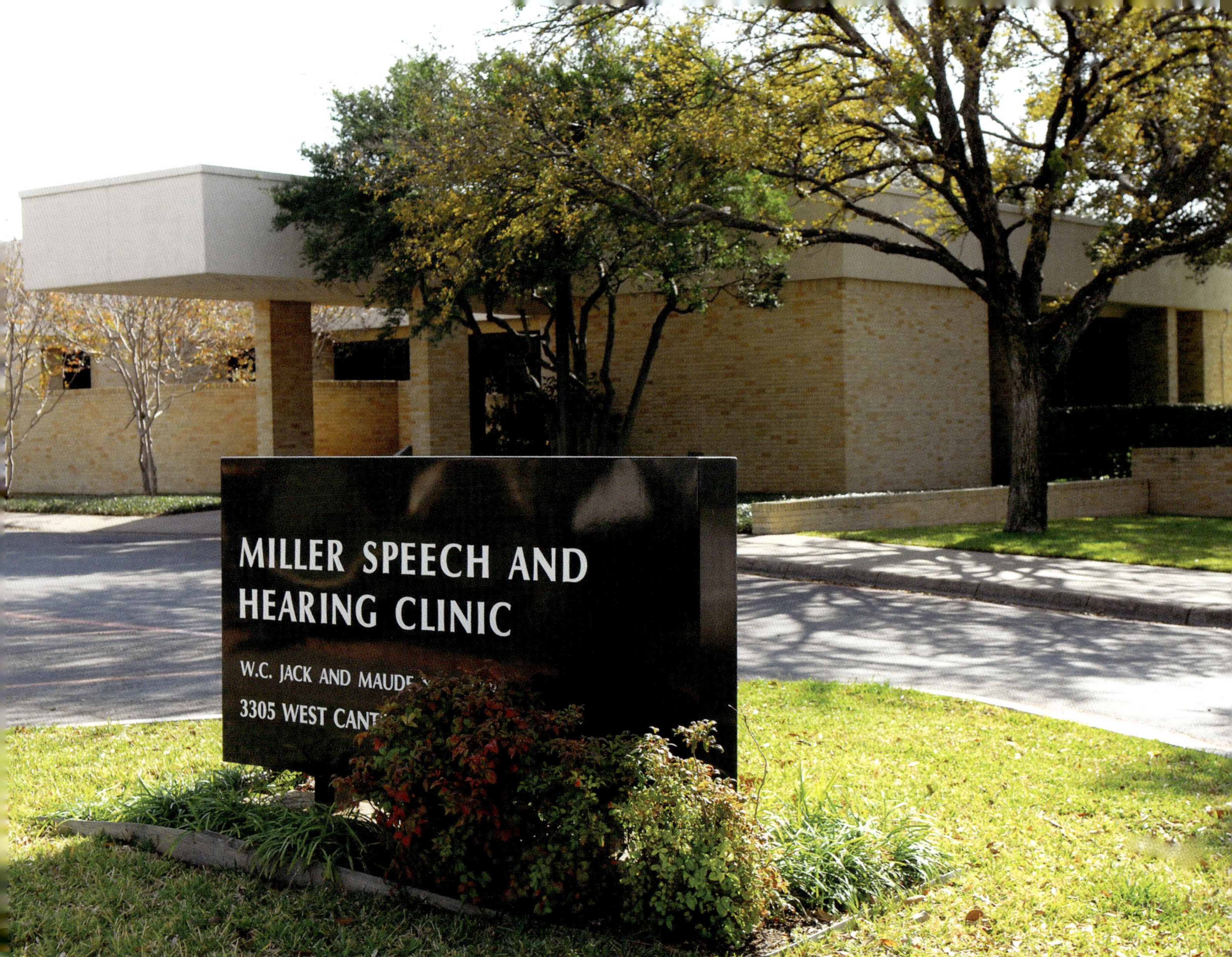

Miller Speech and Hearing Clinic.

A Personal Mission to Develop a Speech and Hearing Program at TCU

The history of COSD at TCU begins with a dream of Edward L. Pross, who arrived on the TCU campus in fall 1947 as a professor in the Department of Speech-Drama-Radio. He moved to Fort Worth with his family, which included his young son, Craig, who was diagnosed with an intellectual disability. Craig lacked the ability to use speech or language to convey his most basic wants, needs, or desires. It was the dream of Pross that his son would one day be able to talk—that Craig would be able to express his thoughts and emotions. To achieve this dream, Pross set in motion plans to develop a speech clinic at TCU where students could learn to help children such as Craig acquire speech (the oral articulation of sounds that form words) and language (a set of shared symbols that represent thoughts, feelings, and ideas).

Pross was a native of Chillicothe, Ohio. He had a passion for history, communication, and learning, and earned a PhD in history from the Ohio State University. Prior to World War II, he taught at Murray State University, the University of Nebraska, the Ohio State University, and the University of Iowa, where he suspended his academic life to serve his country as a commander in the US Navy during World War II. After the war, Pross obtained a PhD in speech at the University of Iowa. During his Iowa studies, Pross took courses in speech correction from Wendell Johnson, director of the Iowa Speech Clinic and an early leading figure in COSD. This experience had a profound effect on Pross's life.

Pross originally taught courses in speech correction to students majoring in speech, theatre, and radio, a few of whom would go on to be certified as Speech Correctionists by the Texas Education Agency. But it was the hiring of a young instructor named Dorothy Mays Bell that truly set Pross's dream in motion. Milestones in the development of COSD during Pross's tenure include:

- 1947—Pross hired by TCU as chairman of the Department of Speech-Drama-Radio.
- 1947—Classes in speech correction first offered at TCU.
- 1947—Speech correction services first offered by TCU to the Fort Worth community.
- 1949—Dorothy Mays Bell hired as instructor, began teaching speech correction.
- 1951—First dedicated therapy room—Ed Landreth Hall, room 105—created.
- 1955—First major (BA) in speech correction offered at TCU.
- 1955—TCU Speech and Hearing Clinic established preschool for the deaf and preschool for the intellectually disabled.

Founding Director of the TCU Speech and Hearing Clinic

Dorothy Mays Bell arrived at TCU in 1949 with little experience in teaching or speech correction. Nevertheless, over the next thirty years, she became responsible for the creation of what is today the TCU Speech and Hearing Clinic, laid the groundwork for the creation of Starpoint School, and improved the lives of thousands of individuals and families in Fort Worth through the power of speech, hearing, and communication.

During her time at TCU, Bell earned both an MA and PhD. She went on to lead the development of the Program in Communication Pathology and the TCU Speech and Hearing Clinic from their infancy through their establishment as icons on the TCU campus and in the Fort Worth community. Bell was officially named director of the TCU Speech Clinic in 1951. At that time, she was the only faculty member other than Pross who taught courses in speech correction at TCU. Her clinical work included both children and adults. Many TCU students with communication impairments were referred to Bell for treatment, and she helped to improve their voice and articulation abilities. She worked with children who had cerebral palsy, children with deafness or severe hearing impairment, children and adults with voice and articulation disorders—and had an immeasurable impact on all.

The year 1955 was a watershed for the TCU Speech Clinic, housed within the College of Fine Arts. It was then that Pross received a grant from the Hogg Foundation for Mental Health to study speech therapy approaches for children with intellectual disabilities—a study that Bell led. To support the study, TCU Chancellor McGruder Ellis Sadler allowed the TCU Speech Clinic to be housed in Barracks Building number six on the TCU east campus. Through the efforts of Bell and Pross, 1955 was also the first year that TCU offered an official academic major in speech correction. This was also the beginning of the Preschool for the Deaf and Preschool for Children with Language Disabilities—the latter still continuing to this day in the Early Childhood Language program at the Miller Speech and Hearing Clinic.

Through Dr. Bell's intrepid leadership, the academic program in Speech Correction and the TCU Speech and Hearing Clinic grew into the nationally ranked program and training facility we have today. Milestones in the development of TCU's COSD program during Bell's tenure include:

- 1959—First dedicated speech correction faculty hired (Telete Lawrence, Patsy Sharpe).
- 1959—Bell receives funding from Opti-Mrs. Club to continue Preschools for Deaf Children and Children with Language Impairments.
- 1960—Frank Hughes appointed Dean of Fine Arts.
- 1960—TCU Speech and Hearing Clinic moves to the "Yellow House."
- 1961—Speech correction program meets requirements for basic clinical certification by American Speech-Language-Hearing Association.
- 1962—George Tade appointed chair of the Department of Speech.

Early Childhood Language Programs

The origins of today's Early Childhood Language program lie in the spring of 1955, when Pross received a grant from the Hogg Foundation for Mental Health to study methods for teaching speech to children with intellectual disabilities. TCU students received scholarships to learn as classroom teachers, and the program grew into one of the most innovative and effective learning environments in the country for methods to treat speech and language in children with intellectual disabilities.

Bell developed innovative methods to assess articulation, hearing, and language in this population. She was one of the first professionals in speech pathology to value the role of pragmatics—the social rules for language use—which she taught to these young children. The curriculum included a focus on behavior modification, training in self-care, motor coordination, body control, and sound production. Bell also taught her unique methods to other professionals in Fort Worth through mentorship and training opportunities.

During this time, the TCU Speech and Hearing Clinic also treated adults with acquired communication disorders. As faculty were added to the program, the scope of training given to TCU students majoring in communication pathology created clinicians who were as knowledgeable and skilled as any in the country. Today, the tradition of training highly educated and skilled clinicians who become leaders in the field continues, as do the clinical programs initiated by Bell in the early 1950s. Additional milestones during the period of her tenure include:

- ♦ 1963—Laura Lee Crane brings McGinnis's approach to TCU, a multisensory phonics-based method for improving reading, writing, and oral language abilities. This served as the foundation for Wilma Jean Tade's Preschool Language Program.
- ♦ 1963—Jeannette Bell hired as the first full-time clinical supervisor.
- ♦ 1964—At the urging of M.J. Neeley, Bell visits New York, convincing Marguerite Slater to move her Starpoint School to TCU.
- ♦ 1964—Marguerite Slater treats school-age children with learning disabilities in the TCU Speech Clinic.
- ♦ 1966—Degree in communication pathology changes from BA to BS.
- ♦ 1967—First masters degree in speech pathology offered at TCU.
- ♦ 1968—TCU moves from certification of hearing therapists to teachers of the deaf and/or hard of hearing.

Chapter Nine

Preschool for the Deaf

> Then one day a call from Dean McCorkle: Could the Clinic assume responsibility for teaching speech to deaf children?
>
> —*Bell, 1980*

In the summer of 1955, the Listening Eye Preschool for the Deaf lost their language teacher and was in great need of a program to teach the children language and speech skills. T. Smith McCorkle, Dean of the School of Fine Arts, called Bell to ask if the TCU Speech Clinic could assume responsibility for teaching these children. Funded by the Opti-Mrs. Club of Fort Worth, this program led to the establishment of the Preschool for the Deaf at TCU, the precursor to today's Habilitation of the Deaf and Hard of Hearing program.

Over the next few years, resources enabling the clinic to test, teach, and habilitate the deaf and hard of hearing grew immensely. Bell oversaw the purchase of the clinic's first audiometer for hearing testing, the construction of the first hearing suite (i.e., sound booth), and the acquisition of new space for the clinic in the Barracks Building. She was also able to hire Ruby Parmalee (funded by the Opti-Mrs. Club) as teacher to the preschool deaf children.

Deaf and hard-of-hearing children attended the preschool from 9:00 a.m. to noon each morning. In the days before sign language was an accepted teaching practice for deaf children, Bell and Parmalee opened up new worlds of communication opportunities for these children through innovative habilitation and pedagogical techniques, including amplification (this was before hearing aids were widely available; the clinic utilized what today would be called FM systems), phonics, and rhythm-based activities. The incredible impact that the preschool was having on these children was recognized in the December 1958 issue of *TCU Magazine*.

In 1961, Marjorie Moore was hired as a part-time instructor for the program, and in 1966, she came onboard as the first full-time coordinator of the deaf habilitation program. Today, Teresa Gonzalez is the latest in the line of coordinators of what grew into the program for Habilitation of the Deaf and Hard of Hearing, and she carries the torch in training future professionals how to open up new worlds of communication for this population. Additional milestones in the development of COSD include:

- 1968—Elaine Freeland joins faculty as first audiologist.
- 1971—Master of arts in speech therapy changed to master of science.
- 1972—Wilma Jean Tade hired as teacher in the Preschool Language

Program.

- 1972—Marylee Norris hired as clinical supervisor.
- 1973—George Tade appointed Dean of Fine Arts.
- 1973—Ralph Behnke appointed chair of the Department of Speech.
- 1973—Speech Clinic Annex donated by Mr. and Mrs. Clarence B. Smith.
- 1976—Marjorie Moore retires.
- 1976—Paula Scott hired as coordinator for the Deaf and Hard of Hearing program.

The Legacy of the Smith Family

> Imagine anything you think that would go into the making of a functional and beautiful clinic. We had it. Imagine two people so unselfish and so charitable. We had them.
>
> —*Bell, 1980*

In 1974, Dorothy Mays Bell was asked to attend a lunch meeting with Dean George Tade and Clarence B. Smith of Fort Worth. The year before, the Smiths had given the largest gift to date to the Division of Communication Pathology in the form of the new Speech Clinic Annex, at the corner of South University Drive and West Cantey Street. Over hamburgers, the Smiths asked Bell: "What can we do for you now?" Bell, cautious not to ask too much after receiving the gift of much-needed additional space the year before, mentioned that the program would benefit from student scholarships to fund tuition. The Smiths' response: "We were thinking about an entire building—just for the Speech Clinic" (Dorothy Mays Bell, *Development of the Speech and Hearing Clinic at Texas Christian University: A Personal Perspective).*

The Miller Speech and Hearing Clinic building, named after W. C. "Jack" and Maude Miller, the parents of Mrs. Smith, opened its doors formally on April 25, 1976. At that time, it was one of the premier speech and hearing facilities in the United States, and the new clinic spurred growth in both the undergraduate and graduate programs. It also offered clinical training opportunities and services to the Fort Worth community.

Today, the Miller Speech and Hearing Clinic continues to serve as the primary clinical training facility for the Davies School of Communication Sciences and Disorders. The clinical, classroom, and research spaces within the clinic building serve as a proud testimonial to the value and service the Smith family saw in the training of future speech-language pathologists and habilitation of the deaf majors.

Over the years, thousands of speech-language pathologists have been trained in the Miller Speech and Hearing Clinic and have gone on to serve children and adults with communication impairments. Graduates of the Habilitation of the Deaf and Hard of Hearing program continue to teach and habilitate children with hearing loss locally and throughout the state of Texas, while undergraduate and graduate speech-language pathology students have represented TCU throughout the world.

The Miller Speech and Hearing Clinic continues to serve as a cornerstone of the TCU campus and as a representation of how philanthropy can help to change lives. Milestones in the development of COSD at TCU include:

- 1974—The Smiths met with Dean Tade and Dr. Bell and offered to fund the creation of a new building for the TCU Speech and Hearing Clinic.
- 1975—Groundbreaking ceremony held for the new clinic.
- 1976—Grand opening of the state-of-the-art Miller Speech and Hearing Clinic.
- 1977—After thirty years of leadership and service, Dorothy Mays Bell retired.
- 1977—Joseph Helmick appointed new director of the Division of Communication Pathology.
- 1983—Division of Communication Pathology housed the first federally funded bilingual speech pathology training program.
- 1995—New Department of Communication Sciences and Disorders was formed.

A New Era

Throughout the 1980s and 1990s, the programs in speech-language pathology and habilitation of the deaf and hard of hearing continued to grow at TCU. As infant survival rates and the aging population increased, so too did the need for trained speech-language pathologists and habilitators of the deaf in the United States. The new millennium thus brought on rapid growth in the number of students seeking COSD degrees. With the added growth came a need for resources to support the educational and clinical training needs of undergraduate and graduate students.

As COSD at TCU entered the new millennium, student growth continued to expand. By 2015, the total number of undergraduate and graduate COSD majors exceeded two hundred students. During this period, the graduate program in speech-language pathology grew from twenty-four to forty students across two cohorts. This growth was supported by new faculty lines. Between the years 2008 and

2015, COSD added two tenure-track faculty lines and three professional-practice faculty lines. The faculty who filled these positions brought further distinction to COSD through their innovative research programs and clinical expertise.

In the 2000s, the Davies family of Houston provided transformational support for COSD. Marilyn Davies is the proud mother of Morgan, a 2012 graduate of the Habilitation of the Deaf and Hard of Hearing program. Marilyn Davies was grateful for the mentorship that her daughter received from Teresa Gonzalez, who served as Morgan's primary adviser and instructor. In 2013, Davies saw how the substantial increase in student numbers, especially in the graduate program, was impacting the student experience in COSD. To alleviate pressures created by the larger student population, Davies provided a gift that supported the construction of the Davies Graduate Workroom, an addition to the Miller Speech and Hearing Clinic; the workroom was opened to graduate students in fall 2014. Davies quickly realized that the space added by the graduate workroom was a small part of a larger, much-needed solution to the challenges facing COSD. She understood that COSD needed resources that would support its growth into the distant future. In 2014, she established the Davies School of Communication Sciences and Disorders with a transformative gift. This endowment supports students and faculty and has allowed COSD to provide innovative, state-of-the-art learning experiences in the undergraduate and graduate academic programs. In 2018, COSD joined other academic units in Harris College to develop a new PhD program. The Davies endowment will also help to support graduate students seeking research doctorates with emphases in COSD. These future leaders will go on to change the world.

Chapter Ten

Kinesiology

The Development of a New Discipline at TCU

Joel B. Mitchell was a candidate for an assistant professor position offered by the Department of Physical Education at TCU in 1988. His interview schedule included a meeting with the university provost at the time, William Koehler. Koehler held the title of both provost and vice chancellor for academic affairs and had worked his way up the administrative ranks from the Chemistry Department. To a wet-behind-the-ears PhD, as Joel put it, he was an imposing figure, and his familiarity with the natural sciences gave him some understanding of the publication titles that he read in Mitchell's curriculum vitae. As an exercise physiologist coming out of a progressive exercise science doctoral program at Ball State University, Mitchell had been involved in projects that reflected the contemporary trends in that subdiscipline. He was the author or coauthor of papers that involved work with blood analysis, muscle biopsies, and other measures that required invasive procedures on human research subjects. The TCU Department of Physical Education, then a member of the School of Education, had never had a faculty member who conducted this kind of research.

"This is an impressive list of work you have been involved in," Koehler told Mitchell, "but if you are offered a position here and decide to accept it, you will not be able to continue with this type of research." Mitchell was taken aback and saw this attitude as a dealbreaker; apparently, this conservative private school was not ready to move forward in the world of exercise science. Mitchell felt he would have to take his job search elsewhere. In the exit interview, the standard question was presented to him: "Based on your day of meetings, what questions do you have of us?" Foremost on his mind was the significant concern that Koehler's declaration had raised, so he asked what vision the department had for their new faculty in the area of exercise science and whether he would be able to develop a research agenda based on

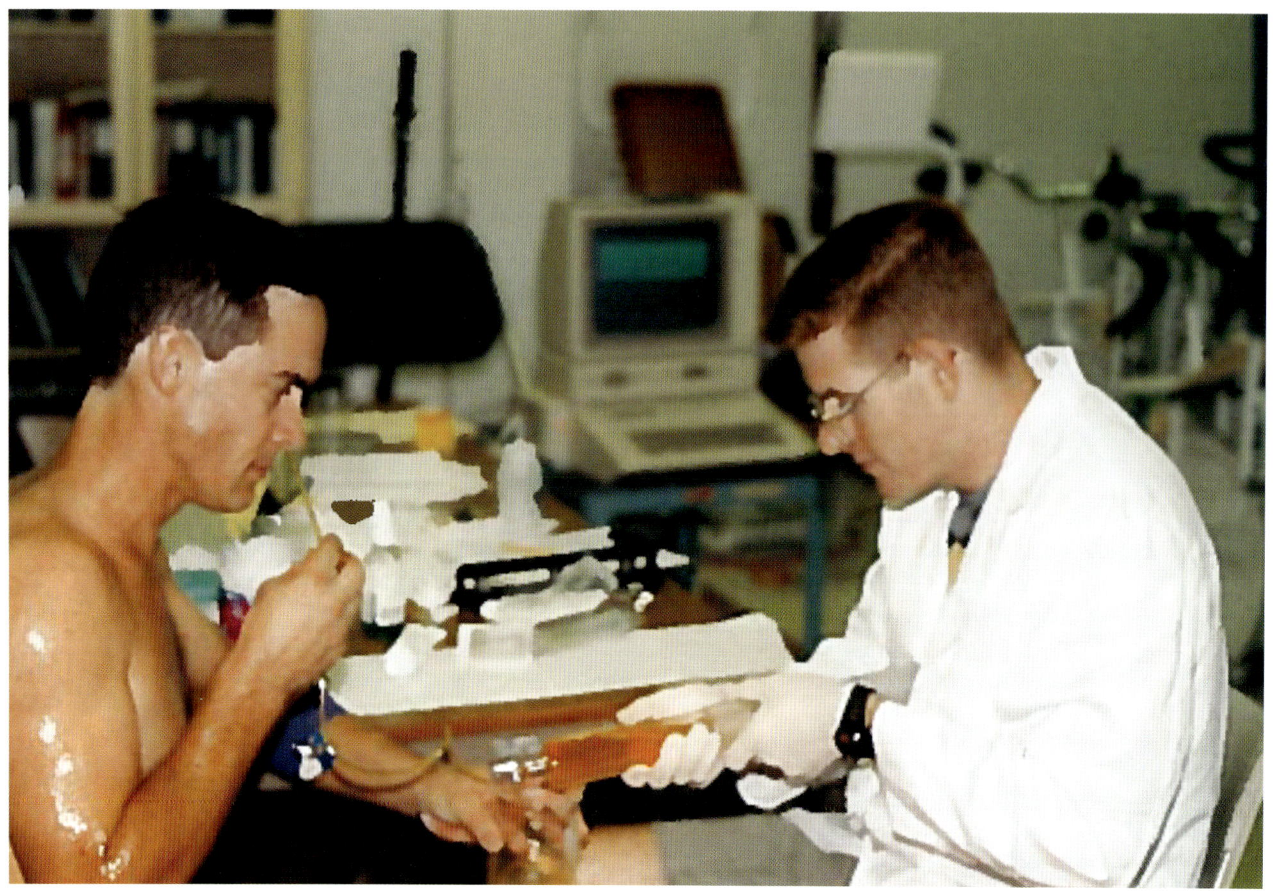

Kinesiology Lab.

his doctoral training. Doug Hastad, the department chair and interim dean of the School of Education, was quick to respond: "Don't worry about Koehler. We'll educate him about the kind of research we need going on in this department." "It may not have been a wise decision on my part," Mitchell said, "since it could have meant a futile battle to change the culture in the department and beyond, but I decided to put my trust in Hastad and others in the university." Joel Mitchell accepted the position when they called several days later with an offer. Doug Hastad was a physical educator by training, but he was savvy enough about the direction that contemporary programs were taking to recognize that for a department to stay current, new hires with new skills and perspectives were needed.

In 1988, the Department of Physical Education had already undergone a number of changes that represented the new direction that departments of this type were experiencing across the nation. Ten years prior, when the chair of the department retired, a group of forward-thinking faculty members made a commitment to a new approach. The new chairperson, Gerry Landwer; new faculty, including Dan Southard, a motor control specialist; and existing faculty adopted a departmental philosophy and a core curriculum that emphasized kinesiology. This was a significant departure from the decades-old departmental focus. Historically, as part of the School of Education, the department defined its mission as preparing teachers of physical education and offering courses that met the university core requirements for physical activity. The new curriculum supported majors in what was called movement science, with biokinetic and sociobehavioral tracks. The philosophical change and new curricular emphasis resulted in a name change to the Department of Kinesiological Studies.

Progressive kinesiology departments, like the one formulated by this group of faculty, included formalized subdisciplines representing study that focused on all aspects of human movement. These four areas of study are based on the traditional sciences, with adaptations to explain the function of the moving human body. Biomechanics uses the principles of physics to describe the body as a moving machine with forces and torques measured as kinetic variables, and velocities and angular changes in body segments analyzed to produce kinematic variables. Exercise physiology, based on the principles of biology, biochemistry, and biophysics, describes the metabolic changes that occur in the body with acute and chronic exercise. Motor behavior is an umbrella subdiscipline that includes motor control, motor learning, and motor development. Its roots are found in a combination of neurophysiology, neuropsychology, and learning theory. Sport psychology is a subdiscipline that relies on traditional psychological theories and emphasizes the importance of understanding the psychological aspects of human performance in sport and other competitive undertakings. Exercise psychology, a more recent outgrowth of sport psychology, uses many of the same principles but deals largely in the noncompetitive realm. Underpinning all of these four subdisciplines is a sound understanding of the structure and function of the human body that is found in the traditional study of anatomy and physiology.

Members of kinesiology departments do not all agree on the full extent of the subdisciplines that should be included in their departments—or even what constitutes a subdiscipline; suffice it to say, there are multiple facets to human movement. This is reflected in the variety of subjects represented in a contemporary department, some of which may not have their own foundational body of knowledge; rather, they rely on the principles of the primary subdisciplines. For instance, adapted physical education, based on the idea that traditional forms of sport and physical activity must be modified to accommodate those with innate or acquired disabilities, is an important applied aspect of kinesiology. Similarly, sport nutrition, founded on nutritional and physiological principles, is another topic studied in kinesiology departments. Health, wellness, fitness, and strength and conditioning are also specializations found under the umbrella of kinesiology. An additional and important piece of the puzzle is athletic training, the misnamed clinical area of preparation that deals with the care and prevention of athletic injuries—misnamed because the term suggests that these professionals are responsible for training athletes for competition when, in fact, they are sports medicine practitioners. Educating physical education teachers is, of course, a remaining specialty in most contemporary departments.

The faculty who converted the Department of Physical Education to the Department of Kinesiological Studies were ahead of their time. They understood that a new emphasis on studying human movement was underway, but they were not successful in getting others to understand how their ideas and the biokinetic and sociobehavioral emphases that they developed could actually be used by students selecting these areas of study as a major. Aside from the general idea that these were legitimate areas of study to expand our knowledge of human function and to provide students a foundation for graduate study, there was a disconnect with the professional preparation focus that had been, and still was, present in the School of Education. Across the nation, kinesiology was studied as an applied science, covering a spectrum from athletic performance on one end to clinical sciences on the other. Sport scientists were interested in maximizing performance using all the biomechanical, physiological, and psychological principles at their disposal. For the general population, these same principles could be used to promote health and well-being in hospital-based settings. The emphasis on health and well-being is captured effectively in the American College of Sports Medicine's lobbying effort to the US Congress that promotes "exercise as medicine." Proponents of this approach argue that exercise should be considered a "vital sign" that every physician should incorporate into the health assessment of a patient and that federal funding provided to the National Institutes of Health should be earmarked for exercise science research. In the middle of the spectrum is applied health and fitness, with professionals carrying out their practice in fitness centers, corporate wellness facilities, hospital-based cardiac rehabilitation programs, and other semiclinical and clinical settings. Athletic training has also consistently fallen in the middle of the spectrum as an applied profession that uses all the principles of kinesiology and medicine to deal with athletic injuries.

Despite the progressive decisions made by TCU faculty in the late 1970s, over the course of the next five to eight years, practical and political realities within the department, school, and university coalesced, leading to the undoing of their efforts. Declining enrollment and new leadership at the school and department levels led to a reversion to what was comfortable to the university administration as a whole. Jerry Mangiri, the dean of the School of Education, and Hastad, the new department chair, were teacher-preparation specialists, and part of their marching orders was to fix the problems that the university saw in the department. As a result, in 1985, the department name was changed back to the Department of Physical Education, and the traditional emphasis on teacher preparation was given greater priority.

When Joel Mitchell arrived in the department in fall 1988, what was called movement science had been pared down from its former dual biokinetic and sociobehavioral emphases. There was, of course, physical education, and added to the mix was a new major in sports and recreational leadership. The latter was a major that had been added to the department at the insistence of upper administration, presumably as a "soft major" for less academically proficient students and student athletes. Historically, the department had always battled the stigma of physical education as an easy major for those not at the top of their classes. Outsiders seemed to think that all department faculty did was teach students how to teach others to play games, and someone in the upper administration did not see any harm in adding a major with a recreation emphasis that didn't even have the minimum GPA requirement needed for admission to the School of Education's teacher-certification program. On and off campus, the stereotypes associated with a physical education department were strong. Mitchell tells a story that illustrated the problem: when he explained to an electrician who came to his house to make a repair that he worked in the Department of Physical Education at TCU, he replied, "I bet you really enjoy teaching in the gym with all those cute girls wearing shorts." "It would have taken more time than I had to correct his misperception," Mitchell said, "so I let it go, but I realized that his response summed up what the general public thought of our department." On campus, although expressed in a more politically correct way, the attitudes and misunderstandings were really not that much different. As faculty developed their laboratories, requesting funding for expensive instruments, they often had to deal with comments like, "Why do you need a gas analyzer? Don't you guys just need bats and balls to do your work?" Colleagues were often surprised to find laboratories tucked away in the Rickel Building that looked a lot like what they would expect to see in biology or chemistry departments.

Hastad's and Mangiri's push to return to the past in promoting physical education as a major departmental emphasis seemed in contrast to Hastad's recognition that exercise science should also be supported. There were strong exercise scientists like Dan Southard in the department, and even before Mitchell's arrival Hastad had begun to purchase some of the equipment necessary to outfit an exercise physiology laboratory. What this signaled was that physical education and kinesiology could coexist, or more accurately, as history would show, kinesiology could serve as an umbrella to encompass physical education in combination with other areas of study related to human movement.

In 1988 the Department of Physical Education had nine faculty members, representing various areas of study within exercise science. In larger programs in universities across the country, "old guard" versus "new guard" factions were clearly established, creating considerable departmental discord. Newer faculty struggled to move these departments forward while still recognizing the value of training physical education teachers and respecting the foundation that long-standing members of the department had built. Because the department at TCU was small and because of the personalities involved, the disagreements in approach did not create the kind of conflict that plagued many departments in the field. Several of our faculty members had been at TCU for over thirty years; they had been part of—and had survived—the changes in the department's name and emphases that newer approaches to kinesiology had brought about.

Billie Sue Anderson epitomized the old-guard physical education teacher. She was a TCU alum who had earned a physical education degree from the department in the 1960s and then done a stint in the public schools before returning to TCU to earn her master's degree. Upon completing her graduate degree, she was hired by the department and went on to complete a forty-year career teaching physical education methods, recreation, and health courses. She was a stereotypical Texan, beginning with her name and including her heavy drawl and her use of quaint country sayings. When Mitchell returned to the office dripping wet from a quick trip across campus in the hot September sun, "Miss A," as everyone affectionately called her, pointed out his lack of familiarity with the Texas environment. "Young man, you're going to have to learn to amble," she advised him. "When it's one hundred degrees out, you can't go racing around at full speed like that or you'll melt." In the 1980s, despite her age and the crippling effects of rheumatoid arthritis, she could still beat even the most athletic young men in the badminton class she taught every semester. George Harris and Betty Sue Benison had a similar longevity in the department and taught courses in the same general areas as Miss A: health, recreation, and physical education. Harris was a physical educator with an emphasis in outdoor activity who was an expert in canoeing, rock climbing, orienteering, and other recreational activities. He regularly collaborated with Campus Recreation, taking groups on weekend trips to show students the wonders of nature and how to survive in the wild. Benison was a health educator who taught multiple sections of the enormously popular course in human sexuality. Some of her courses had little to do with kinesiology, but, as holdovers from the days when health and physical education were paired, they served a need as electives for the general student body.

The courses based on the exercise science subdisciplines were taught by the newer faculty who came to the department with research-based doctoral degrees and strong foundations in the natural and social sciences. Their courses in biomechanics, motor control, and exercise physiology were rigorous, and their research was published in top-tier journals in their fields. Their research programs were not, however, conducted without their overcoming significant obstacles. The development of state-of-the-art laboratories required space and resources. Although the university gradually provided some of these resources, new faculty were not given the large start-up packages that the research-intensive universities were providing new hires so they could outfit research labs. As a result, faculty had to be patient and innovative; they improvised by acquiring refurbished equipment, doing their own computer programming, seeking external funding, and even building some of the needed instruments. Dan Southard was able to keep a motion analysis system running well beyond its expected life span, using what he called a "duct-tape-and-baling-wire" approach. With support from the university for major pieces of equipment to outfit the Exercise Physiology Lab, Mitchell supplemented those pieces and stretched his research dollars by modifying cycle ergometers and other pieces of equipment in his garage and by building computer interfaces with what would now be considered glacially slow Apple IIe computers.

A second obstacle that was actually more significant than lab development was introducing the department's work to, and getting approval from, the Institutional Review Board (IRB). This effort addressed the reluctance in allowing the invasive human subjects research that Provost Koehler had initially expressed to Mitchell during his interview. The first project Mitchell proposed was a fluid replacement study in which he would be conducting maximal oxygen uptake testing, taking blood samples, and doing nasogastric intubation to measure rates of gastric emptying. He had been trained in these techniques as part of his graduate education. The IRB had received some warning from the director of sponsored projects, Jan Fox, that a new guy in the Department of Physical Education was going to be submitting a protocol for review that was unlike anything they had reviewed previously. Despite this warning, many IRB members were still incredulous that someone in "PE" would be conducting these kinds of procedures. It was the "bats and balls" view of our department that generated this kind of skepticism. It was not that faculty in the department did not do research, since Southard, Allan Lacy, and others had ongoing research agendas; instead, it was the fact that their work did not involve higher risk, invasive measures. The motor control and pedagogical studies that they conducted could be approved through expedited review, without attracting the attention and concern brought on by blood sampling, intubation, maximal exercise testing, exposures to extreme heat, and other methods common in exercise physiology.

"It was an educational process for all involved," Mitchell declared. "I was attempting to educate my fellow faculty from the varied departments represented by the committee membership, and in the process, I was being educated on the approach needed to allay fears and obtain approval for this type of work." To prepare for his first protocol review, a meeting he was required to attend, he gathered letters of support from colleagues in health science centers, the United States Olympic Committee, and research-intensive universities, explaining that these techniques were common in exercise science research, and the kinds of questions he wanted to address were contemporary in the field. The exercise protocols and data-collection methods he proposed to use were not without risk, but they did not contain the level of risk that the IRB conjured up. A long-standing member of the Department of Philosophy suggested that Mitchell was practicing medicine without a license, a conclusion he arrived at because he had undergone a maximal exercise stress test as part of a clinical workup, and he saw the exercise testing as a similar procedure. Mitchell pointed out the difference between a test performed on an older, at-risk individual for diagnostic purposes and data collection on a young, highly trained endurance athlete.

Hastad had kept his word as he simultaneously worked behind the scenes with Jan Fox, Associate Provost Larry Adams, and even Koehler himself to help Mitchell educate the IRB. Eventually, making sure that adequate safety measures were in place and that those conducting the procedures had appropriate training, the IRB gave Mitchell approval to move ahead with his first study. This represented a significant step forward in gaining the credibility and respect that would help the department become recognized as more than a traditional physical education department. Additional exercise physiologists would be hired in the coming years, and the work conducted by other faculty in the various subdisciplines would become more sophisticated, requiring higher levels of IRB scrutiny and approval.

In the early 1990s, another milestone that served to alter the internal and external perceptions of the department was the designation of the movement science major as the accepted pre-physical therapy (PT) plan of study on campus. Similar to other preprofessional courses of study like premed or prelaw, physical therapy schools do not mandate a specific major that students must follow; rather, there is a set of prerequisite courses, primarily in the traditional natural sciences, that students must complete to be eligible for admission. Students can choose any major as long as they meet the prerequisites; however, because human movement is the basis for PT and because movement science already requires many of the biology, chemistry, and physics prerequisites, it is a logical major for pre-PT. The benefit to the department was that the pre-PT designation gave the department something that the rest of the university and even the general public understood, and it carried with it a certain amount of credibility, especially as it related to the clinical world. "The irony was that no department faculty were trained as physical therapists, so we spent our educational efforts training students for a profession that, although related to our subdisciplines, had a very different application than what we were interested in," Mitchell pointed out. "Very few of our students go on to become academicians or professionals with specific expertise as biomechanists, exercise physiologists, or sport psychologists. Nevertheless, along with the national trend of growth in kinesiology departments, the inclusion of pre-PT as part of our focus contributed to a three- to fourfold increase in our undergraduate enrollment over the next two decades." In comparison to the enrollment of approximately one hundred undergraduate students in the 1980s, the department achieved a plateau of between 300 and 350 students by 2010. Students who have graduated with the high grade point averages necessary to gain admission to PT school have been successful in pursuing their doctorate of physical therapy in some of the best schools in the nation.

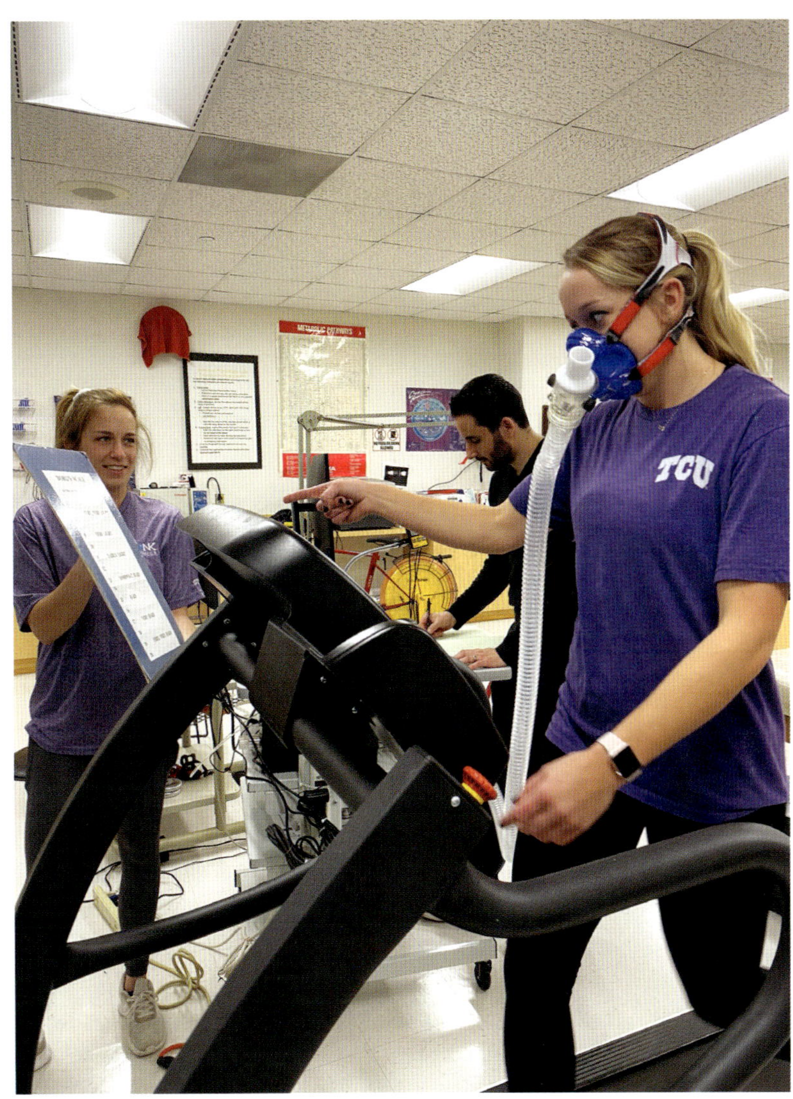

L-R, Ashlynn Williams, Andreas Kreutzer, and Brianna Barnhill in the Kinesiology Lab, January 2020.

Another factor that contributed to the department's increased enrollment was the addition of a major in applied fitness, originally titled "fitness promotion" and later changed to "health and fitness." This major was designed to prepare students for careers in the health and fitness industry, which included personal training, corporate fitness, strength and conditioning, and other professions that use kinesiological principles to improve the general function of those who engage in physical activity to improve their health or enhance athletic performance. In the latter part of the 1990s, the department also added a major in sport psychology to prepare students to pursue graduate education to become certified as practicing sport psychologists. Although this major has not produced many candidates for graduate study in sport psychology, it is a popular major for those who want to study the psychological aspects of human movement and athletic performance without the heavy immersion in the natural sciences that the movement science major requires.

Other curricular changes involved eliminating the sports and recreational leadership major and the coaching classes. The latter were part of the athletic eligibility system in which coaching classes for football, basketball, baseball, and track and field were all taught by the coaching staff. In the faculty's view, those classes represented a conflict of interest, and lacked any academic rigor, with classes that met for five to ten minutes per session and grade rosters that contained nothing but As. The coaching classes and the recreational leadership major only served to perpetuate the harmful stereotype that the department faculty spent endless amounts of energy trying to dispel.

As these changes took place, and as new faculty with strong backgrounds in the different areas of kinesiology were hired, the issue of "what's in a name" continued to dog the department. Despite its growth and the increasing sophistication of the exercise sciences, the persistent stigma of physical education as an undemanding area of study was a liability in attracting strong students, establishing community relationships, obtaining external research funding, and so forth. In 1996, Provost Koehler agreed to allow the department to change its name to the Department of Kinesiology and Physical Education, with the possibility of dropping "Physical Education" at a later date. Koehler had been provost in the 1970s during our earlier effort to rename the department, and he reminded Mitchell, now department chair, that "I have a strong negative memory of the failure and political discord that accompanied that change the first time around, so you are going to have to really prove yourselves this time." As a result of his hesitancy, the change was set up on a two-year trial basis; long-term approval—and the possibility of further streamlining the name—depended on avoiding the decline in enrollment that had accompanied the earlier use of kinesiology in the department name. Because enrollment actually continued to increase during this period and because Koehler and other administrators recognized that we were following a national trend, in 1998 the provost approved a final name change to simply the Department of Kinesiology.

One course that came out of the changes experienced in the 1980s was "Physical Education: An Evolving Discipline." It provided students with a basic foundation of kinesiology and introduced them to the varied opportunities that existed in the field. This title, although somewhat contrived, did capture the idea that departments like this one were truly undergoing substantial change. The department instituted a kinesiology core for all undergraduate majors, regardless of their focus and professional intent. At the heart of this core were four courses that have provided a common foundation for all of the majors and established a level of rigor such that students would not find an easy way through the study of kinesiology. The core consisted of anatomical kinesiology, motor behavior, exercise physiology, and biomechanics. The anatomical course has served as a gatekeeper for the department, since, if students cannot manage the content of this course, it is a good indication that they are not suited to pursue a major in the Department of Kinesiology.

A consistent activity throughout all of these changes has been the preparation of athletic trainers, a joint venture between TCU Athletics and the Department of Kinesiology. Elmer A. Brown was the first head athletic trainer hired by TCU, and he established the Athletic Training Education Program (ATEP) in 1952. The ATEP, initially approved by the National Athletic Trainers' Association (NATA) in 1972, has been approved or accredited by various accrediting bodies since that time. From 1972 until Brown's retirement in 1976, the faculty and staff consisted of Brown and one assistant athletic trainer. In 1978, after several years of interim leadership, T. Ross Bailey was promoted from assistant to head athletic trainer, a position he held until 2000, with a dual role as ATEP director. Up until 2003, students studying to become athletic trainers typically majored in movement science or physical education, and the clinical courses needed to pass licensure and certification exams were taken as coursework that was structured like a large minor. Their clinical training was accomplished via immersion with assignments to the varsity sports programs at TCU, where they assisted the professional staff in caring for the athletes. In 2003, athletic training was established as a full major with more extensive course offerings to meet the content delivery and accreditation standards set by the Commission on Accreditation of Athletic Training Education (CAATE). That same year the ATEP director position was separated from TCU Athletics and established in the Department of Kinesiology, and in 2006, a clinical coordinator position was added. This position is responsible for developing clinical sites on and off-campus and ensuring that students are receiving the clinical experience necessary for licensure and certification. These two positions represented a new approach in the department since they were defined as professional practice (not tenure-track) positions, paralleling the faculty structure found in Harris College, particularly in nursing. In developing the major and dedicating two faculty lines to athletic training, the Department of Kinesiology took greater ownership of the ATEP, although it is still a collaborative effort with athletics. The professional staff in athletics still serve important roles as preceptors supervising the clinical experiences of student athletic trainers, and they occasionally teach as adjuncts in formal courses. In 2005, TCU began employing a full-time team physician for athletics. In addition to teaching in the ATEP, this individual also serves as medical director for the ATEP, a position required by CAATE.

Athletic training is the only major in the department that requires a secondary admissions process. Students must first be admitted to the university before they apply and are interviewed for one of the sixteen spots available for each entering cohort. The program has consistently graduated students who are admitted to graduate programs where they pursue master's degrees and serve as graduate assistant athletic trainers in university settings. Students who do not want to practice at the college level usually obtain teacher certification as double majors with physical education so that they can be hired in middle and high schools.

In 2000, the university-wide rearrangement of schools and colleges initiated by

Chancellor Michael Ferrari led to one of the most significant historical events in the department. The Department of Kinesiology left the School of Education and joined three other departments to form the College of Health and Human Sciences, now the Harris College of Nursing & Health Sciences (HCNHS). The majority of the faculty believed that they needed to leave the School of Education since our interests and focus no longer aligned well with its emphasis on teacher certification. The department also had the choice of joining the College of Science and Engineering, a move that would have been logical given the parallels with biology, chemistry, physics, and psychology that existed. In the end, however, aligning with health sciences represented a good middle-ground position for us since health science was a common theme among many of our areas of study; we had a connection with the accredited professional preparation focus in Harris College; and we did not want to compete for resources with the doctoral-granting programs in science and engineering. As a professional program preparing students to practice in a clinical setting, athletic training is the program that most closely parallels the accredited clinical programs found in the other units in Harris College: Communication Sciences and Disorders, Social Work, and Nursing. As a professional program that prepares students to become certified as teachers, physical education does not have the same health care emphasis as the other units in the college; however, there are some similarities in the general approach to training students. In contrast, movement science as a preprofessional major is not bound by external accreditation and does not have clinical proficiencies as primary content delivered in the coursework. The same is true for the health and fitness and the sport psychology majors.

On balance, Harris College has been a good fit for the Department of Kinesiology, especially given the politics of college alignment and the deans who have overseen the college. The original concern among faculty and leadership in the non-nursing units was that because of their size and the fact that the deans have all come from nursing, there would be an unbalanced emphasis on the needs of nursing to the detriment of the smaller units. However, when the Department of Kinesiology joined the college in 2000, Rhonda Keen-Payne was the dean, and she fostered a culture of inclusion and balance. When Keen-Payne stepped down, Paulette Burns continued the culture of inclusion and made extra efforts to ensure that the needs of all units were represented and met by her office. In the second decade of the new millennium, after the tragic loss of Burns, Susan Weeks has continued to provide the leadership that reinforces the faculty's belief that they made the right decision in choosing the Harris College as their home.

As the curriculum in the undergraduate program changed to reflect the development in the general field of kinesiology, the graduate program mirrored these changes to a large extent; however, over the past several decades, there has been greater stability in the graduate program. Research is a common theme in the department, and undergraduate students are engaged in senior research projects, but at the graduate level, as one would expect, research is the essence of the program. With the growth of the department's scientific emphasis, research activity also increased, and successful graduate students have embraced the process. Although the graduate program is small, with approximately twenty students enrolled, the department has attempted to select students who are ready to spend two years of their lives immersed in the exciting process of generating knowledge. Those with curiosity and drive, who relish hours in the lab rather than simply performing in the classroom, are our success stories and have provided the student backbone of our graduate program. Over the years, approximately half of these students have gone on to pursue doctoral study.

Exercise physiology has been the graduate emphasis that has attracted and graduated the greatest number of students. There have been half a dozen faculty engaged in exercise physiology research over the past three to four decades; they have mentored dozens of master's students who have gone on for doctoral degrees in preparation for jobs in academia or taken positions as research associates or found other interesting niches in the professional world of exercise science. The latter have included unique opportunities like US Air Force flight-training specialists, exercise science research and development jobs in the private sector, competitive sport performance coaches, and researchers for pharmacological corporations.

Beginning with its roots in physical education, and continuing with the contemporary areas of emphasis, the study of human movement has had a foundation as an applied science. Correspondingly, applied learning, a teaching method that has recently become more popular in many disciplines, has always been a mainstay as an educational tool in kinesiology. Those who have spent their careers working with students in laboratory, clinical, and educational settings see the current trend as an articulation of what they have been doing for decades. Whether at the undergraduate or graduate level, there is no more effective way to teach than to roll up your sleeves and dive in with students as teammates in the problem-solving process. The research laboratories and other learning environments in the Department of Kinesiology have been settings for applied learning, with sometimes poignant or, as in the following case, humorous results.

The environmental chamber used for studies examining the influence of temperature on various thermoregulatory and hydration responses during exercise was known for being a bit temperamental. For a study examining the influence of environmental temperature on immune function, a graduate research assistant and Joel Mitchell needed to hold the temperature in an eight-by-twelve-foot insulated box near 0°C, but the chiller was not up to the task. The student had the idea of going across campus to chemical stores to get some blocks of dry ice and run a fan across them to help bring the chamber temperature down to the desired level. It seemed like a reasonable approach, and temperature-wise, it worked. Mitchell himself was the research subject for the trial that day, and as he and the student began the preparations for what was supposed to be an hour-long exposure, things did not feel quite right. Even though Mitchell had not begun exercising yet, he started hyperventilating in response to a simple pre-exercise baseline data collection protocol. Surprisingly, the student researcher was experiencing the same symptoms. The two looked at each other, and without a word, both gestured in the direction of the door, realizing they needed to vacate the chamber. Looking at the gas analyzers monitoring the chamber, they immediately found the reason for their difficulties: the carbon dioxide levels were in excess of 10 percent (compared to normal ambient levels of 0.03 percent). It was a forehead-thumping moment as it dawned on these researchers that dry ice gives off carbon dioxide as it "melts." Although not a moment that Mitchell is particularly proud of, since he and the student should have seen this as a problem from the outset, it is a classic example of students and their mentors working together to generate new knowledge and learning from their mistakes.

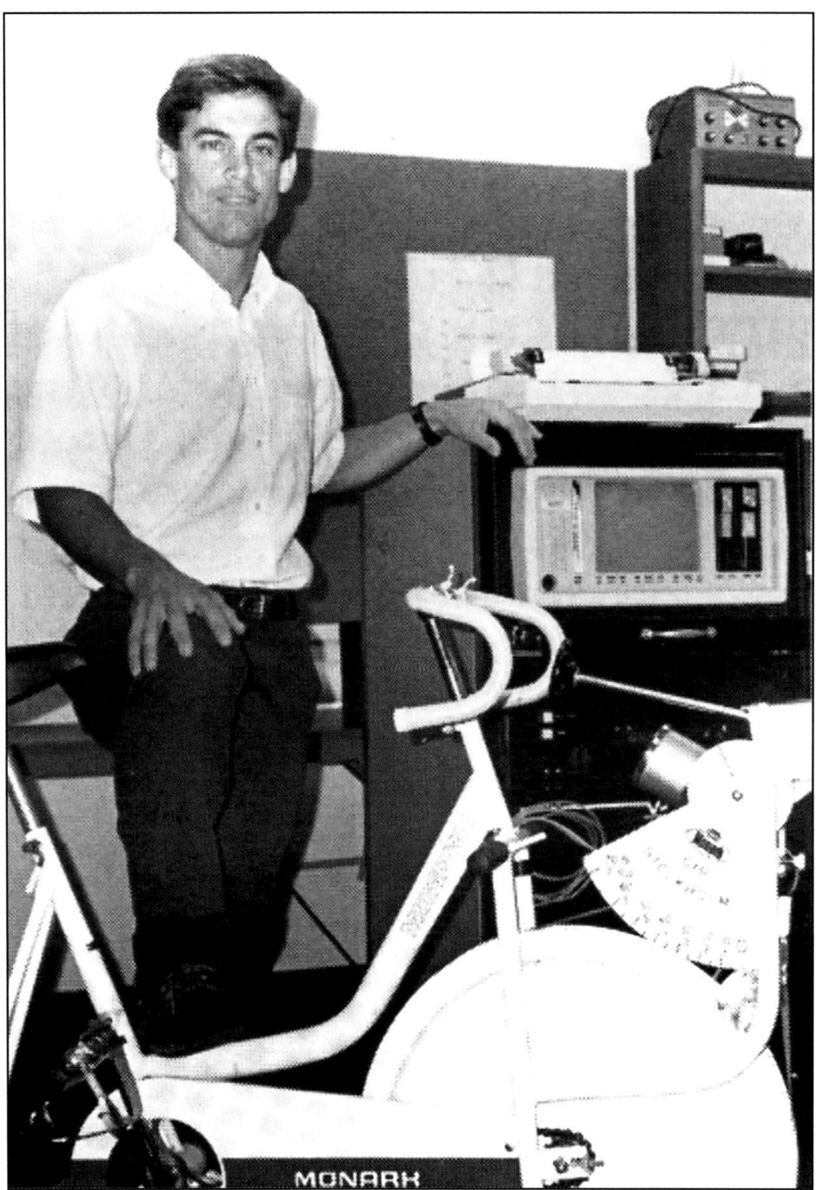

Joel Mitchell in his laboratory in the Rickel Building.

The other areas of emphasis in the graduate program—motor control, sport psychology, nutrition, and physical activity—have also attracted students who have gone on for further graduate study or have found employment in movement-related professions. Recently, the department has added one more graduate emphasis, this one in exercise psychology, that builds upon Debbie Rhea's work in public schools following her 2012 sabbatical trip to Finland to study their education system and physical education practices. The exercise psychology emphasis is based on a unique approach to physical education that Rhea has captured in what she calls the LiiNK (Let's Inspire Innovation 'N Kids) Project.

To fully understand the LiiNK Project and later the development of the LiiNK Center, it is necessary to go back to 1999, when Rhea was hired to fill the position being vacated by the retirement of Billie Sue Anderson. When Rhea arrived at TCU, the number of physical education majors had dwindled to single digits. This was due to a combination of factors: the increased emphasis in the other areas of kinesiology, the high cost of tuition with a relatively low return on the investment for physical education teachers, and the need for someone to come in and breathe new life into the program. For the first decade of the new millennium, Rhea's leadership helped to build the physical education major up to the point of viability, but it was an arduous task. A significant educational trend in public schools has been the elimination of physical education and recess breaks as forms of unstructured physical activity, resulting in fewer available positions in physical education for graduates. The irony of this trend, obvious to anyone paying attention to Americans' health, is that we are now facing an epidemic of obesity, at least partially brought on by young people's inactive lifestyles. Finland, a world leader in educational rankings, has done just the opposite; in fact, they incorporate multiple recess breaks into the school day, a practice that is at least partially responsible for their lower rates of obesity and possibly their educational successes.

After her sabbatical in Finland, Rhea saw that if we adopted some of their principles into our educational practices, it would not only improve health and learning but also be an effective way to give new credibility and importance to the teaching of, and the practices associated with, physical education. With this seed idea in mind and with shoestring funding, she ventured into the school systems in the Dallas–Fort Worth area. With her infectious enthusiasm and energy, she was able to convince several private and public schools to allow her to implement the Finnish principles into their classrooms. She added multiple recess breaks, along with an important character development component, starting with first-grade students and adding a grade level with each successive year of the project. The LiiNK Project has been very successful, showing improved academic and social performance among those students at participating schools. A number of graduate students have benefited from their involvement as research assistants in the LiiNK Project, and upon graduation, have been hired back into the project to help meet the demand from school systems across Texas and the region. Clearly, physical activity, regardless of how it is implemented, is an important aspect of the development of human beings: we are meant to move.

Other collaborations have helped members of the Department of Kinesiology engage in work that is meaningful in promoting health, further emphasizing the good fit of the department in Harris College. In the early 2000s, Dr. James Barbie, a local physician who directed the John Peter Smith Sports Medicine Fellowship Program, approached members of the Department of Kinesiology seeking a collaboration that would allow their fellows to gain the research experience required for their specialization. It was an ideal partnership, since the physicians gave us both the medical oversight necessary to carry out many of our higher-risk procedures and access to funding to support clinically relevant projects. In return, we provided the fellows with a research experience that was not available in their hospital system. Studies involving the use of exercise as a means of reducing the risk of cardiovascular disease and type 2 diabetes in older, at-risk populations would not have been possible without this collaborative effort. When Dennis Cheek was hired in nursing, he joined with Joel Mitchell and Melody Phillips in the exercise physiology group to bring his expertise in endothelial function as an important new component in understanding cardiovascular disease. Studies based on using exercise to reduce the risk of disease have also included collaborations with members of the biology and psychology departments, as we have incorporated principles of immunology to investigate the role of systemic inflammation as a modifiable risk factor. As a result of this work, the Exercise Physiology Lab has evolved to the point that, along with the usual treadmills and cycle ergometers, at least half of its square footage is dedicated to instrumentation that can also be found in biology, chemistry, and biochemistry laboratories. Again, graduate students have been heavily involved in the research conducted in collaboration with all of these medical professionals and academic colleagues.

Shortly after his arrival in 2013, and continuing until his departure in 2019, Jonathan Oliver joined forces with physicians, physical therapists, and clinical researchers at the Ben Hogan Sports Medicine Center, a group working under the umbrella of Texas Health Resources. Their studies dug into the very contemporary topic of sport-related concussions, attempting to understand how nutritional interventions, concussion recovery protocols, and specific diagnostic procedures can reduce the adverse effects of this serious brain injury. In addition, they evaluated various resistance exercise protocols to determine how variations from traditional approaches can improve adaptation and enhance clinical outcomes. The collaboration with these outside groups led to the development of The Sports Performance Center at TCU, which opened its doors in 2018. Interestingly, one of the key players in this collaboration, Craig Garrison, a physical therapist with a doctorate in clinical biomechanics, is a 1990s alum of the Department of Kinesiology.

Meena Shah was hired in 2000 to fill the health position after Betty Benison's retirement, and with a PhD in nutrition, she too represented a change in the background and emphasis of kinesiology faculty members. Shah is interested in how nutritional interventions can affect human health, especially in the realm of cardiovascular disease, diabetes, and other metabolic disorders. In addition to conducting nutritional intervention studies in her Metabolic Lab, Meena Shah has maintained a strong research relationship with a group of colleagues at UT Southwestern Medical Center. This collaboration has allowed her access to funding and clinical research support in her area that is not available at TCU. As in the case of all of such collaborations, students have benefited from being involved in research that exposes them to clinical researchers in the broader community.

Gloria Solomon led the sport psychology emphasis at the graduate level until her retirement in 2019. During her time in the department, she also included a large contingent of undergraduates in her research team. She has completed two stints at TCU, first arriving as an assistant professor in 1995 before leaving for an eight-year appointment at California State University, Sacramento, in 2001, and then returning in 2009 as a full professor. Her work focused on the coach-athlete relationship, with a particular emphasis on how coaches' expectations that are based on an athlete's prior accomplishments impact coaches' behaviors as they interact with their athletes. More recent work also included the concept of mental toughness and its impact on sport performance. Unlike other areas of kinesiology, sport psychology research is not equipment intensive because most data are collected using questionnaires. Regardless of the nature of the data-collection methodology, the same progression and sophistication of approach that has been observed in the other subdisciplines has taken place in sport psychology.

Over a thirty-five-year career beginning in 1980, Dan Southard represented the heart and soul of the department. He had been among the progressive group that had driven the early initiative to move heavily in the direction of kinesiology; during his six-year term as department chair, he implemented many curricular changes, and through it all, he was a true kinesiologist. With a specialization in motor control, he was interested in understanding how motor patterns change, how practice facilitates that change, and how dynamic systems theory explains neuromuscular function. Southard was in kinesiology heaven one fall when we moved the treadmill and our metabolic analysis system down the hall to his lab to collaborate on a project to examine the biomechanical and physiological correlates of fatigue during prolonged running. With a happy look on his face, he remarked, "This is true kinesiology when we attempt to explain human movement using multiple approaches from the various subdisciplines."

Although students benefited tremendously from his instruction and research supervision, his purist view was such that he was not overly interested in the application of the knowledge he produced and conveyed; rather, his efforts were geared toward increasing our understanding of how human movement is controlled, regardless of how that information might be used. He used biomechanical principles to explain motor control; thus, in a small department where faculty had to teach courses outside their immediate specialty, along with motor behavior courses, he also taught the biomechanics course. Using dynamic systems theory as the basis for his motor behavior classes and classical physics as the foundation for biomechanics, Southard did not make his classes easy. Students were happy to survive his courses and somewhat affectionately, or maybe out of a sense of awe and respect, called him "Dr. Death," a title that he not only didn't mind but actually delighted in.

The description of the current Department of Kinesiology provides a sharp contrast to the department's culture and practice in the 1970s and 1980s. If the same conversation Mitchell had with Provost Koehler during his 1988 interview were to take place in 2019, there would have been no question that his qualifications were a good fit for the department. In fact, the kind of background shown in his curriculum vitae would be a requirement even to be considered for a position. Teaching exercise science courses, conducting scientifically and clinically relevant research, and preparing students to make a difference in people's lives by incorporating physical activity lie at the core of a contemporary and progressive department. Although earlier physical educators had many of the same objectives, their approach was different, and the field has clearly evolved to the point that if any of them from the mid-twentieth century were to visit our department today, they would have difficulty recognizing it as their own. Some tend to look down on physical educators as lesser academicians; however, given the need to deal effectively with the obesity epidemic, this is a dangerous judgment. Even some of the most accomplished exercise biochemists, many of whom had their initial training in physical education, will insist upon the importance of teaching children and young adults the value of maintaining a physically active lifestyle.

CHAPTER ELEVEN

TCU Social Work

A History of Service

Background of the Social Work Profession

Social work as a profession in the US began in the 1800s with two significant organizations leading the way. The Charity Organization Society (COS) was founded in 1877 to provide centralization of poverty programs. The settlement house movement began in 1886, focusing on providing aid within communities, particularly for immigrant families. Both organizations emphasized training of workers in order to provide effective service. This training was provided through supervision at the agencies until 1898, when the New York School of Philanthropy was begun as a three-month training program for social workers. It became affiliated with Columbia University in 1904 to provide an eight-month university-level graduate training course (Day 1989). For almost a century, most education in social work was on the graduate level.

During the 1930s, the social work profession began an MSW accreditation process that included a requirement for educational content to be delivered within colleges and/or universities (Shaefor 2014). While several programs across the country offered social work courses and/or emphases on the undergraduate level, accreditation was only for graduate programs, and the profession did not recognize baccalaureate graduates as first-level professionals. In 1952, the Council on Social Work Education (CSWE) was founded to provide consistency for educational standards across the United States and allow programs to be accredited based on those standards. The National Association of Social Workers (NASW), the largest professional association of social workers, was founded in 1955, bringing together several smaller, specialized organizations to represent the profession as a whole and to ensure societal sanction and job placement. It also opened the door for the profession to assess and determine the need for professionally prepared baccalaureate social workers (Popple and Leighninger 1990).

Over the next two decades, with the War on Poverty and its many programs supported by the federal government, particularly the US Department of Health, Education, and Welfare (HEW), the demand for social workers in all areas of social welfare and health care increased. As HEW began to implement these programs during the 1960s, the agency found that there were not enough social workers graduating from MSW programs to meet the staffing demands of those programs. Many MSW-trained social workers were more interested in clinical social work than in working in government poverty programs. HEW required applicants for positions to have academic preparation that included the knowledge and skills to deliver services to vulnerable groups. This required a professional rather than the purely academic focus found in psychology or sociology programs. Based on this awareness, HEW and the federal government created financial support for universities and colleges to develop undergraduate social work programs (Karger and Stoesz 1990). Many universities began to offer more courses on the baccalaureate level and to develop programs that included internships to prepare students for professional practice.

Administrators of the government programs recognized that if those hired to staff the programs did not have a degree that was professionally recognized, the success of the programs would be undermined (Shaefor 2014). NASW began to address the divisive issue of recognition of social workers with baccalaureate degrees during the 1960s. This led to an intense debate between MSW graduates and educators and those teaching undergraduates and seeking to staff agencies. The pressure on NASW to "designate graduates from bachelors-level social work education programs as first-level professional social workers" (Shaefor 2014, 198) led to a call for a referendum on the issue. In 1969, in a close and surprising vote, the referendum passed, recognizing baccalaureate social workers as first-level professionals. As a result the CSWE had to develop separate accreditation standards for undergraduate programs in order for them to offer social work degrees. In 1974, the first standards for BSW education were published. The number of programs quickly expanded across the US as the demand for the degree grew. Many of those programs were within sociology departments.

Development of Social Work at TCU

At TCU, the chair of the Department of Sociology, Dr. Larry Adams, saw in the early 1970s that many of the sociology majors at TCU were interested in social work as a profession. He was aware of the developments in social work education and the availability of money from Title XX of the Social Security Act to develop undergraduate social work programs. Although there was some opposition to the development of a social work program within the department, he applied for a Texas flow-through grant for Texas universities to build programs. He was awarded approximately $250,000, allowing the department to hire a director and begin the hiring process to establish a social work program within the Department of Sociology. Dr. Arthur Berliner, a social worker in the Federal Correctional Institution in Fort Worth who had worked on drug research with the TCU Institute for Behavioral Research, was Dr. Adams's choice to direct the program (Larry Adams, pers. comm., January 3, 2018).

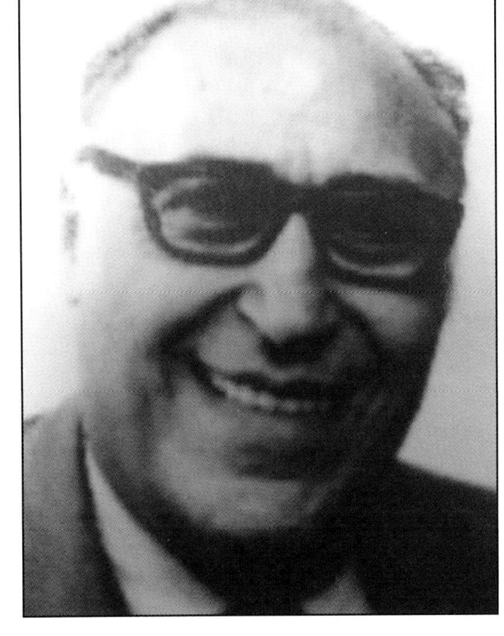

Dr. Arthur Berliner.

In 1975, the Social Work Program began with a major in social work, offering courses in social work based on accreditation standards. Part of the mission of the program had been to develop a curriculum that could be accredited as quickly as possible. For two years, Berliner taught all courses and worked with a part-time field coordinator to develop internships. In 1977, the program hired the first full-time field coordinator, Linda Moore. Together the two faculty members developed the curriculum and submitted the self-study for accreditation. The real building of the undergraduate program began in 1978, when it achieved full accreditation from the Council on Social Work Education (CSWE), retroactive to 1975. After being reaffirmed in 1983, the program continued to be reaffirmed on the CSWE eight-year cycle (1991, 1999, 2007, and 2015) and is fully accredited today (CSWE n.d.).

During the 1980s the Social Work Program remained a part of the Department of Sociology under the direction of Chair Jim Henley. Larry Adams became Dean of Graduate Studies in 1980 and later assumed the position of associate provost. Enrollment in social work courses continued to grow, and efforts to have courses fit university core requirements were successful. The program developed the junior evaluation process to emphasize the gatekeeping role of the faculty to protect the profession. Students were required to apply for admission to field education, the internship component of the program. They were interviewed by the faculty to determine their fit with the values of the profession and their knowledge and skills for practice. This was a successful process and led to affirmation from the community and the profession (Moore and Irwin 1990; 1991).

Strong community relationships were developed as students placed in human service agencies successfully completed their internships. Many graduates were offered employment within those agencies based on their strong performance as interns. As enrollment in the program grew, student efforts that engaged community support led to a third full-time faculty position being added to the program. In 1986 Moore presented the first proposal to begin an MSW program at TCU, but the university declined due to lack of resources. After receiving many awards, including recognition as the Texas Social Work of the Year, Dr. Berliner retired in 1988, although he returned in 1992 to teach the Social Work ethics course (TCU 360, 2013). Charlene Irwin was appointed director of the program in 1988. When she resigned to take another position, Linda Moore was appointed as director in 1991.

The 1990s were a decade of strengthening undergraduate social work education. At TCU, this led to significant changes in faculty and status. Two new faculty members were hired: David Jenkins and Tracy Dietz as field director. The three faculty oversaw two decades of change and growth. The number of agencies with which the program worked grew; a Professional Advisory Committee was established with responsibility for program evaluation; and the faculty increased its national service efforts and its campus and community recognition. Faculty served as members of CSWE Commissions and committees and the National Association of Social Workers, Texas (NASW/TX), officers of the Texas Association of Undergraduate Social Work Educators (TAUWSE), the Texas Association of Social Work Deans and Directors (TASWDD), the Texas Field Educators Consortium (T-FEC), the Association of Baccalaureate Program Directors (BPD), and CSWE, making the program visible nationally. Faculty were also a part of these organizations in order to support and further develop the mission of undergraduate social work education both nationally and at TCU.

The faculty also increased its publication rate. Moore and Irwin had written two seminal articles on gatekeeping. Dietz and Jenkins worked with Moore to produce three more articles to the lexicon of gatekeeping, as well as several presentations at national meetings. Moore and Dietz, along with Alan Dettlaff, who joined the faculty in 2001, also began significant work on the use of the Myers Briggs Type Indicator as a tool for understanding different learning and personality styles in the educational setting, including field education. This led to publications, presentations, and a teaching module for field instructors to help them understand differences in student performance in the agencies. This became a significant instrument for helping students develop tools for working with clients and peers and for increasing self-awareness (Dettlaff, Moore, and Dietz 2006; Moore, Dettlaff, and Dietz 2004).

In the 1990s, issues within the society included increased focus on spouse abuse leading to internships with police departments and the criminal justice system. School social work gained increased attention, and students were placed in several local school systems working with a variety of clients and issues. In 1980, the Bureau of Labor Statistics indicated that growth in the profession would be significant and demand for the program strong, and their projections were borne out (Alpert and Auyer 2003).

Independence

During the 1990s, the ongoing modification of accreditation standards led to issues for TCU's accreditation process. The self-study was due in 1998, but CSWE now required program autonomy, a difficult issue for a program within another academic discipline. Discussion with the dean of AddRan College of Arts and Sciences, Michael McCracken, and Provost William Koehler led to the development of the Department of Social Work, separate from the Department of Sociology, in 1998. Linda Moore was elected as the first department chair. The Department of Social Work was reaffirmed in 1999 by CSWE as a separate entity within the AddRan College.

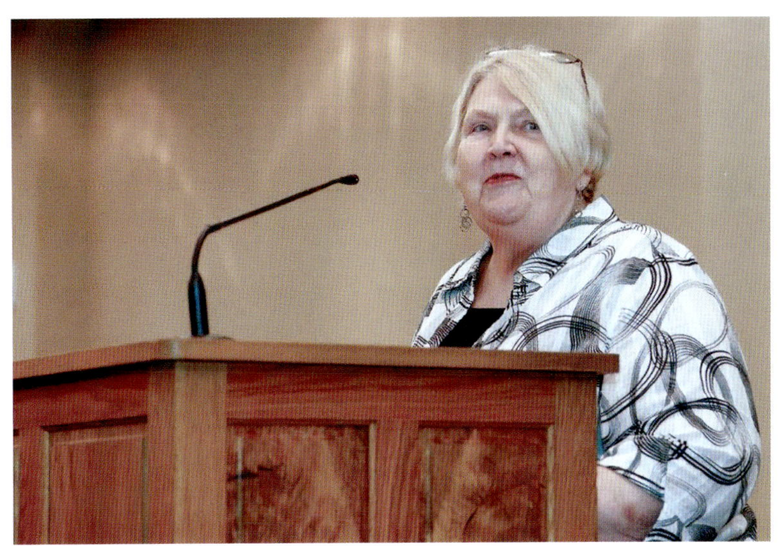

Linda Moore, former chair of the Department of Social Work, at Social Work's Annual Banquet, April 21, 2016.

During the first decade of the 2000s, the country was facing many problems resulting from combat overseas and the fear of terrorism at home. A greater societal focus on issues facing veterans led to more attention to mental health issues. Social justice, always a program focus, demanded more attention as instances of exclusion and oppression surfaced. The changes in the legal rights of the LGBTQ community led to an increased emphasis on policy issues facing clients and society and an increase in agency placements. Homelessness, an ongoing societal concern, was addressed through internships and academic offerings (Zastrow 2016).

The beginning of a new century also brought about significant change in the academic landscape of TCU. University planning efforts led to the reorganization of colleges and departments. Harris College of Nursing became the College of Health and Human Sciences with a focus on professional programs. The departments of Social Work, Communication Sciences and Disorders, and Kinesiology each left another college to join nursing to form the newly named college. Social Work moved out of the trailer in which they had been housed for twenty years and into the Bass Building, thus allowing closer communication with nursing. A fourth faculty member was added in 2001 when Alan Dettlaff, a graduate of the program, became director of field education. Tracy Dietz was elected department chair in 2001 and served until 2004. Dr. Moore again resumed the chair position, serving until 2007, when David

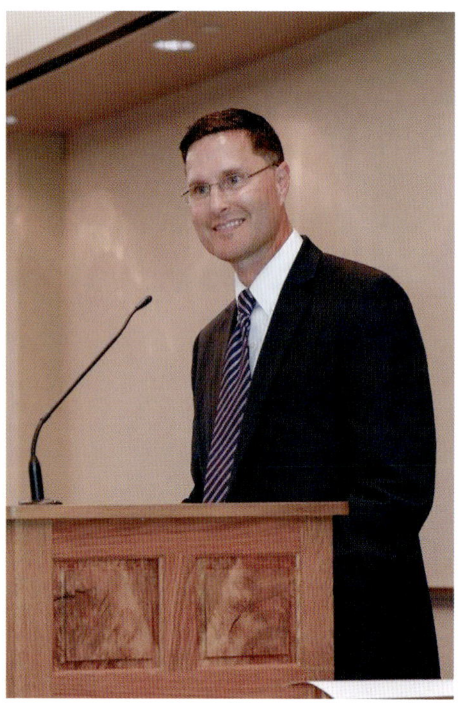

David Jenkins, former chair of the Department of Social Work, at Social Work's Annual Banquet, April 21, 2016.

Jenkins was elected chair.

Over the first three years of the new college, concerns about the name of the college and its impact on external financial support were raised and debated. In 2005, the college was renamed Harris College of Nursing & Health Sciences, reflecting the several departments and their contributions to professional health education. Harriet Cohen, an assistant professor of social work at TCU, joined the faculty in 2006. Much of the focus during the first decade of the new century was the development of a Master of Social Work (MSW) program. Under the leadership of Dean Rhonda Keen-Payne, consultants were hired to study and provide justification for this effort, and supported the efforts to develop the MSW program. The hiring of Dr. Paulette Burns as dean of Harris College of Nursing & Health Sciences in 2006 and the increased focus of the board of trustees on expanding graduate education led to the final approval of an MSW program in 2012. James Petrovich was hired in 2010 to help support the development of the MSW program; he also served as director of field education during the 2011-2012 academic year. He resumed full-time teaching when Lynn Jackson was appointed in 2013 to direct field education for both programs. The MSW Program admitted its first students in 2013 and was fully accredited by CSWE in 2015 (retrieved from https://socialwork.tcu.edu/msw/).

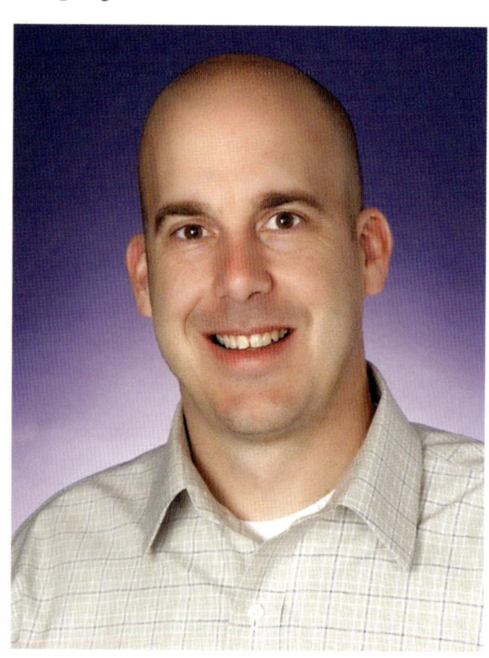

James Petrovich, chair of the Department of Social Work, August 15, 2010.

In 2016 significant changes occurred in the department. After the hiring of Nada Elias-Lambert in 2013 and Aesha John in 2015, Cohen, Dietz, and Moore retired, and Jenkins moved to another university, leaving a large void in the department. To fill this void, James Petrovich was named chair of the department and seven new faculty were hired over the next three years. These new faculty included Tee Tyler and Jennifer Martin in 2016, Katie Lauve-Moon and

Brandi Felderhoff in 2017, and Samantha Bates, Mary Twis, and Sh'Niqua Alford in 2018. Beyond simply replacing prior faculty, these new faculty support an intentional departmental emphasis on expanding its research capacity with new faculty investigating areas such as interpersonal violence, intellectual and developmental disabilities, homelessness, reproductive rights, social identity transitioning, gender-based discrimination in faith-oriented organizations, human trafficking, positive youth development, and more. Using their research to inform their teaching and through the department's increased use of students as research assistants, the program continues its historical commitment to TCU's Teacher-Scholar model.

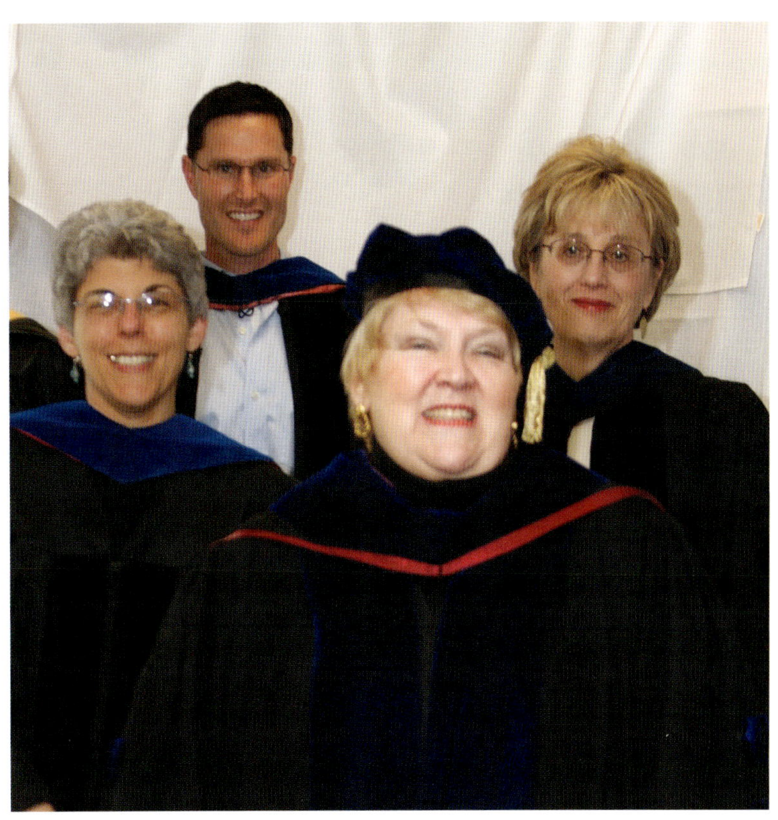

Social Work faculty: L-R, Harriet Cohen, David Jenkins, Tracy Dietz, and Linda Moore, 2017–2018.

In addition to an increased emphasis on research, the present faculty has developed a strategic plan that includes five values necessary for effective social work education and practice. They are excellence, student-centeredness, collaboration, community engagement, and social justice. Additionally, the department has completed the development of a strategic plan that focuses on four strategic initiatives. These four initiatives are:

1. Excellence in teaching and scholarship,
2. Recruiting and retaining outstanding students, faculty, and staff,
3. Transformational community engagement,
4. World-class learning environments.

With the departmental strategic plan being well integrated into and aligned with

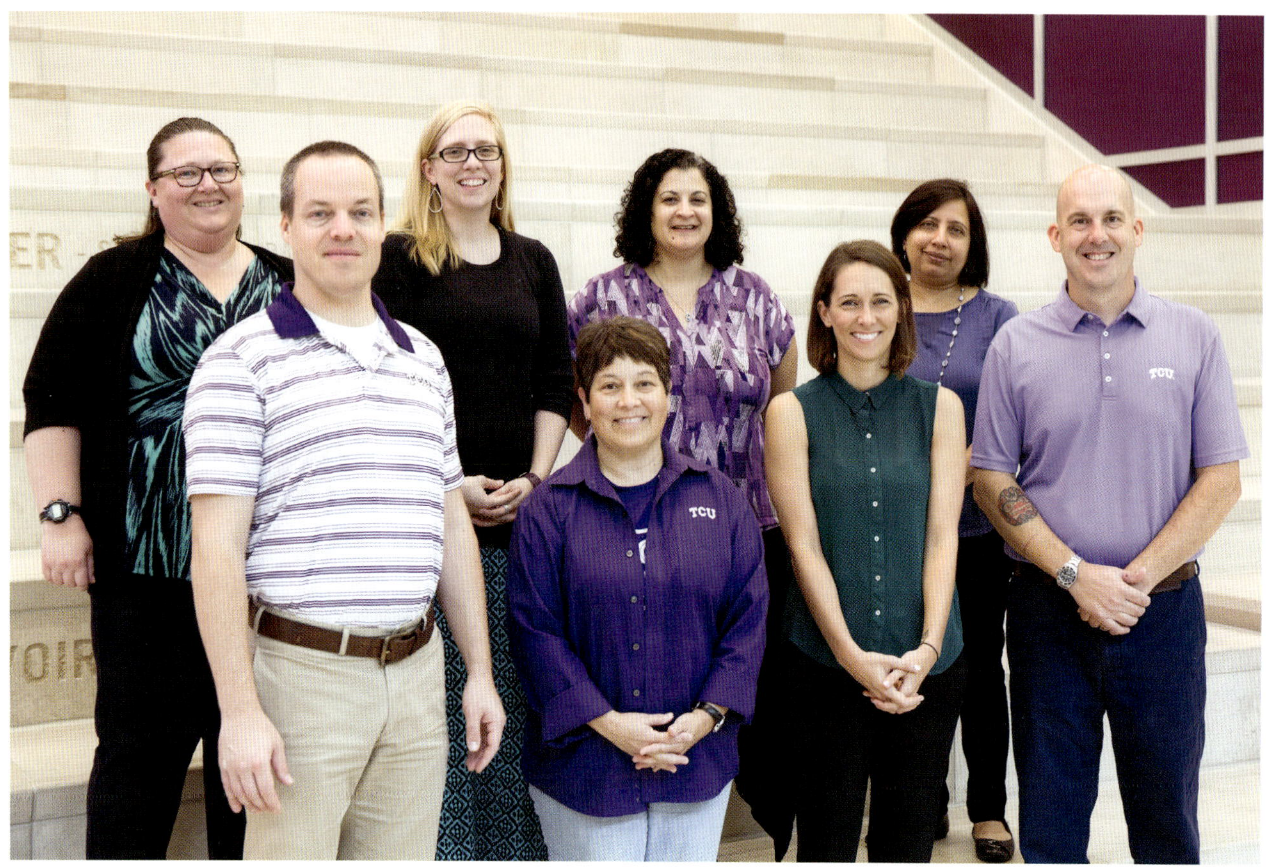

Social Work faculty: L-R (back row) Jennifer Martin, Brandi Felderhoff, Nada Elias-Lambert, and Aesha John; (front row) Tee Tyler, Lynn Jackson, Katie Lauve-Moon, and James Petrovich, 2017–2018.

plans developed by the college and university, the department is poised to continue its long history of commitment to TCU's mission and values. Stemming from the strategic plan and new departmental values is an emphasis on the development of leadership skills for faculty and students and an emphasis on teaching students to use the scientific method to validate and improve their practice. The department remains responsive to new issues in the profession and will focus particularly on sensitivity to trauma with the adoption of trauma-informed care. Faculty are examining the strengths and limitations they face and how to infuse discussion of these into the curriculum (J. Petrovich, pers. comm., January 9, 2018). Despite differences over the decades, the abiding value is the development of competent and ethical social workers able to confront serious social issues currently facing the global community, the hallmark of the department since 1975.

Appendix I

Excerpts from the Dean's Report to the Harris College of Nursing Board of Directors

November 8, 1948

In my September report I called attention to the fact that the Harris Hospital nursing department was greatly understaffed. The situation has now become acute. There are few registered nurses working evenings and nights, and the director of nursing has attempted to solve the problem by changing student assignments and using students to fill these vacancies. Students are being exploited, their educational program is being interrupted and in at least one instance a student's health was jeopardized.

The following are illustrative of the situation:

Students are assigned to the nursery for a period of four weeks for experience in caring for the normal newborn, as well as the premature infant. Of the last two students who were assigned for this experience, one spent three weeks on night duty, and one day 2:30 to 11:00, in the premature nursery. She was then assigned to care for postpartum patients. It was only after strong protest on my part that this student had the remaining four or five days care for normal newborn infants.

The other student had one day, one evening and one night caring for the normal newborn; a few hours one day in the formula room and the remainder of the time was assigned to the care of premature infants.

Another student has been on night duty since August 18, a total of two months and 21 days, except for 6 days and 10 afternoons. Still another student has worked at night since September 15, except for two days 7:00 to 3:30 and five days 2:30 to 11:00. Students on night duty must get up for class during the day, and therefore do not have unbroken rest as do employees.

Another student was allowed, upon approval of her physician, to go on duty on her nineteenth post-operative day following an appendectomy. She was placed on night duty, but I refused to allow her to work these hours, not only because of the recent appendectomy but because within the last year she had chest surgery for a tuberculous condition.

I should like to call your attention to paragraph five on page two of the contract between the Hospital and the College of Nursing, which reads as follows: "Said Hospital agrees to maintain a nursing service that meets current best practices, and if there is an unusually large service, then to provide enough graduate nurses and auxiliary workers to maintain this service over and above the needs of the College of Nursing. The faculty of such College of Nursing in conjunction with hospital authorities shall determine the length of time each student shall spend on a service, but it shall be according to current best practice."

Students' assignments have been made twenty-seven months in advance and in keeping with this agreement. The nursing departments knows well in advance how many students will be assigned to each service.

I am calling attention to this problem because (1) in case of criticism by accrediting bodies, I want the Board to know we have tried to meet standards set up by those organizations. Unless corrections are made, there is great danger of losing accreditation by the Texas State Board of Nurse Examiners and by the National League of Nursing Education. (2) We are operating a school of nursing and are graduating young women who are expected to have a certain degree of proficiency in caring for all kinds of patients and yet we are denying them the experience necessary to develop this proficiency. Further, because graduate nurses do not wish to work evenings and nights, students are assigned for those hours a large portion of the time. One reason registered nurses refuse evening and night duty is that after two years of it as students, they never want to do it again. We are paying the salary of clinical instructors who want to teach the student how to nurse by supervising her at the bedside. There is no better way to teach nursing, but we are unable to carry the plan through because the student is so rarely on day duty.

Head nurses who have sufficient personnel to assign students to day hours have done so and haver further cooperated with instructors in selecting patients for student assignments on the basis of student needs. When this has been done, the student cares for fewer but for sicker patients and under the direct supervision of the instructor. The student does no less work by this method of assignment, and is able to give and to learn to give good nursing care.

Under present conditions we shall be graduating nurses who do not know how to give good nursing care and are likely to not even know what good nursing care is because they so rarely see it. A young student cannot be thrown into a complex nursing situation for which she is not ready and be expected to learn how to give good nursing care without supervision. Too often the student who is conscientious becomes discouraged and withdraws from the school, as did a sophomore student when given responsibility for the care of thirty patients from 11:00 p.m. to 7:00 a.m. Many of these patients were on the urological service and she had been given no instruction in the care of such patients. She had been assigned to that division for surgical patients and had received some instruction for this experience. After a week she could bear the situation no longer and withdrew, stating that she did not like nursing. This student was persuaded to return after a lengthy conference, in which she admitted that she loved nursing and wanted to be a nurse, but that she could not be responsible for more than she could do and for carrying out procedures for which she had been given no instruction.

Appendix 2

Letters from Physicians Following the October 26, 1960, Meeting with the Harris Hospital Medical Staff

FIRST LETTER

October 27, 1960

Dear Board Chairman:

I wish to clarify and summarize my discussion last evening at the joint meeting of the Medical Staff of Harris Hospital and the Board of Directors of the Harris College of Nursing.

The Medical Staff feels that the original purpose of the Harris Hospital sponsoring a School of Nursing was not only to educate nurses but also to improve nursing care of the patients of Harris Hospital.

As it now exists, many of the Staff feel that the nursing school is only a department of T.C.U. and is of very little benefit to the patients of Harris Hospital. Let it be remembered that all material assistance given to the school by the hospital is paid for by the patients and as such, is a sacred trust.

Dr. Sealy asked me how this relationship could be improved. May I make two suggestions:

First the Board of Directors think first of patient care at Harris Hospital; Second, the Board of Directors avail itself of conferences with committees of the Medical Staff. There is one, the *Patient-Care Committee,* that has made exhaustive studies in all phases of this relationship. Their reports are available to you.

We appreciate the opportunity the Board granted us to appear before them. We recognize your unselfish devotion to the education of nurses.

May we assure you of our sincerity and deep concern for the welfare of our patients at Harris Hospital.

Sincerely,

(Name withheld) M.D.

SECOND LETTER

November 2, 1960

Dear Board Chairman:

The meeting of October 26 was in my opinion very informative and helpful. The panel handled itself very well. I am sure that the doctors present have a clearer concept of the Harris College of Nursing as a result of the facts brought out.

I was impressed by the following ideas that were developed:

1. The essential difference between the Diploma Program and the Degree Program is one year of Academic work. The nursing instruction is practically the same.
2. The two, however, for reasons that appeared not too clear, are incompatible and cannot run concurrently.
3. The college is under contract to Harris Hospital to offer a diploma course, but we are told that said course has been abandoned because of so few applicants. Such as apply are referred to other nursing schools.
4. The "atmosphere" of the Harris College of Nursing is such that applicants for the Diploma Program have been made to feel

unwelcomed and unwanted and even inferior to Degree Students. The expressed preference is toward the Degree Student. The question arises: if the "climate" were more favorable to Diploma Students would the above mentioned incompatibility be an insoluble problem?

The fact remains that the expanding Harris Hospital needs competent Registered Nurses, and the Harris College of Nursing should be in a position to attract and to train capable young women who are interested in becoming nurses. Experience of other local nursing schools indicates a considerable demand for the Diploma Program. (St. Joseph freshman class has 42 living in dormitory—Peter Smith freshman class has 52 living in dormitory.)

It is reasonable to assume that many capable prospects, unable financially to undertake the longer course leading to a degree, may well be able to manage the shorter Diploma course, and after working a while return for a degree. These people should not be turned away. Careful review of the policy of the Harris Hospital College of Nursing may reveal areas of compatibility between Degree and Diploma Programs that have been assumed to be non-existent.

Yours truly,

(Name withheld) M.D.

THIRD LETTER

November 9, 1960

Dear Board Chairman:

As a member of the staff of the Harris Hospital, I am writing this letter to you for two purposes. First, to thank you and the other people on the Board of the Harris College of Nursing for your interest, time, and efforts in carrying out your responsibilities for the development of nurses within our community. My second purpose is to pass along observations and impressions, again as an interested surgeon who practices primarily within the Harris Hospital. I am unable to speak from the standpoint of statistical facts, but I am able to speak as a physician who is interested in the care of patients.

DEPTH OF COMPASSION VS. DEPTH OF EDUCATION: A definition of compassion is extremely difficult, but in my opinion includes interest, sympathy, gentle attention and kindly attitude towards the patient's discomfort (physical as well as emotional), necessary treatment, and future recovery. In my opinion, our present system of nursing encourages the factor of interest more in the direction of medical and pathological points of interest, but less and less in the direction of emphasizing compassion. They are thus becoming a "technician" and not a true "nurse." I agree that education and depth is a desirable, but at the present time it is overemphasized and most emphatically at the expense of the former points.

a. In years gone by a student nurse worked hard and without question. The hours were long, duties numerous, and responsibilities placed upon shoulders at an early age. "Repetitive duties" were frequent, but these helped shape a nurse to become proficient in practically all phases of nursing function. Having experienced an arduous training program in postgraduate surgery in which "repetitive duties" were numerous, I know of the monotony that can occur. But the experiences, though monotonous, developed habits and attitudes which to me have become an invaluable part of my present way of life. As the years have gone by, I have more completely understood the rationale behind so many of the undesirable features of our training system. I still believe that hard work, application of "elbow grease," closer contact with patient's nursing needs, and even occasionally moving a "bedpan" can be helpful in forming better nurses and doctors. I cannot help but feel that the attitude on [the] part of the various instructors and the administrative head of the nursing service of the Harris Hospital is based somewhat upon the occasions of ruffled feelings that invariably come about from any system that involves intensive effort. I am sure too, that with this feature, nurses have developed a resentment towards teaching physicians and now that there is a shortage of nurses, the opportunity for expression via the present curricula has become more apparent.

b. Personal contact with the patient has been changed and I would be more than willing to accept a change if such were conducive to maintaining and improving the patient care. It is my impression that the nursing care has now become more impersonal, that more of the contact with the patient has been transferred to the hands of different types of personnel, including L.V.N.'s and nurse aides. The majority of the latter group of people are well intentioned individuals, mostly in the middle ages of life and some in the latter ages of life, who try to the very best of their abilities to perform their duties. They have not been able to have as extended an education as nurses have had in the past, nor are they in an age group to be able to readily adapt to patients under the stress of sickness and on some occasions to the stress of physical effort in caring for the sick. A young woman can, however, be instructed in an efficient manner to learn to carry out these functions; without question, she is able to absorb, coordinate, practice, and become proficient. It is the younger women who go into professional nursing schools and are the ones more susceptible to being taught these important points. We have, I believe, shifted these duties to an older aged group of people and who are unable to meet the standards that have been set up by previous nursing schools.

c. "Coldness." Since the beginning of my practice ten years ago it has frequently been repeated by lay people in my own personal contact that the attitude of the nursing service and student nurses in the Harris Hospital when compared with nurses of other hospital institutions within our city, is one of aloofness and coldness. I fear that this attitude has come about with the apparent de-emphasis of patient contact and assumption of patient responsibility.

In my own observation among the professional student nurses on the floors, the current student does not respond as quickly to an order. Too frequently she is indifferent towards commonly accepted courtesies. At the present, grasping a problem is not done with the ease and dispatch that I have more frequently found in the past. Graduates of the present schools appear to be more primarily concerned with the dispatch of paper work. They are not as well informed with the patient's latest condition and progress.

Sincerely yours,

(Name withheld) M.D., FACS

FOURTH LETTER

December 8, 1960

Dear Board Chairman:

This letter is in reply to your request that I write you in regard to our discussion on November 10, 1960, relative to Harris College of Nursing, and nursing care at Harris Hospital.

My interest is no different than should be the interest of any individual associated with Harris Hospital or any other hospital, namely good patient care. We all have a direct responsibility to the patients to make every effort to see that they receive good, competent, and complete medical care. The attending physician is also equally responsible to the patient for negligent acts or negligent omissions of a nurse attending that patient in the hospital. This is under the "loaned servant doctrine," and is discussed in a letter from the attorney for Harris Hospital to the Administrator several years ago.

I still believe that Harris Hospital in general gives the best nursing care in the community, but I would not say that overall it is adequate. When a night nurse in charge of a floor does not see a paralyzed patient for three nights, that is not good patient care. When two patients in a ten day time receive medication ordered for someone else, and especially when the medicine is given by a student nurse who is being supervised by an instructor of the College of Nursing, then this is doubly poor patient care. These instances are occurring every week, and therefore patient care cannot be good under these circumstances.

Shortage of graduate nursing personnel is probably the greatest reason for inadequate nursing care. Now if Harris College of Nursing is to be associated with Harris Hospital, and use the patients of Harris Hospital for instruction purposes, then the College of Nursing should attempt to fulfill the nursing needs of Harris Hospital.

I have been a member of the Medical Staff of Harris Hospital for over twelve years, and have served several years as a member of the Committee on Patient Care. In October 1959, this committee made several recommendations on the staffing segment of the nursing service. The following is part of that report:

"Toward the procurement of adequate nursing personnel considerable study should be made in the *utilization of the students* of the affiliated School of Nursing in direct patient care other than that for pay, or as students as part of supervised teaching. A diploma program of nursing requires less cost and time than a degree program. The Dean of Harris College of Nursing stated: 'The diploma student, when graduated, would not be qualified for Public Health Nursing.' Public health nursing is not given to patients in this hospital, so let us train nurses by the diploma training program in greater volume, and in less time, and at less expens[e] than the degree program. A general education including: History, English, Religion, Government, etc., is wonderful for everyone, but the additional time, and expense does not make a better bedside nurse, and prevents some girls from even entering nursing training.

"Requiring diploma students to work for the hospital for six to twelve months after completion of training, and before getting a diploma, would furnish additional trained personnel for the hospital. The hospital could furnish room, board, and laundry for this service. This service to the patient would be in the form of repayment to the patient for their participation in nurses training.

"Let us train our nurses for good beside nursing, and not for administration and supervision. Supervision of good bedside nursing and patient care requires the ability of the supervisor to personally be able to render that service herself. Training for administration and supervision can come later in the form of post graduate training, for those who desire it.

"More effective supervision could be obtained by assigning the supervisors under the Director of Nursing Service directly to the floors concerned, as occurs with the Operating Room, and Delivery Room Supervisors."

I am convinced that the trend of nursing education for a degree rather than a diploma has very definitely resulted in shortage of nursing personnel, and thus inadequate patient care. If the Medical Education trained all doctors to be specialists, and there were no general practitioners, then medical care by the doctors would be far from adequate. (I am a specialist.)

What Harris Hospital, and all hospitals I know of, need, are more nurses who can and will give good beside nursing to the patient.

Briefly, my recommendations, other than those above are:

1. Establish, promote, and encourage a Diploma School of Nursing rather than the degree School of Nursing. If a nurse then desires to get a degree, let her take the additional one to two years training to obtain this nursing degree.
2. Have all instructors who teach practical nursing in the hospital be nurses who are actively practicing bedside nursing in the hospital.

Very Truly yours,

(Name withheld) M.D.

Appendix 3

Excerpts of the Dean's Presentation to the Harris Hospital Medical Staff, October 26, 1960

I asked to come before you in order to discuss a problem which makes it extremely difficult for the faculty to do the job we believe we are obligated to do.

Before discussing the problem and asking for your help, I would like to (1) explain what we as a faculty believe to be our responsibility, (2) give the source of our authority and responsibility, and (3) explain what we are trying to do and the reasons for doing them, that is, describe the sequence of learning experiences for a typical student during four years in Harris College of Nursing.

The Charles H. Harris Trust Fund Indenture specifically states:

1. "It is the Primary purpose of the Party of the First Part (Dr. Charles H. Harris) to establish a college of nursing."
2. "It is the purpose and necessary to the proper establishment and operation that said college be affiliated with a hospital and a college or university."

A Board was appointed by Dr. Charles H. Harris and authorized to make the above arrangements. Arrangements with a university and with a hospital were made at the request of and were approved by Dr. Harris.

Contracts with Texas Christian University and with Harris Hospital which were prepared under the guidance of Dr. Charles H. Harris state that:

"The Harris College of Nursing when chartered as provided for in the Charles H. Harris Foundation shall at the earliest possible time set up, organize, and conduct such a College of Nursing as will meet the requirements for accreditation by the National League of Nursing Education. Said College of Nursing in affiliation with an accredited college or university shall offer courses leading to the degree of Bachelor of Science in Nursing."

The faculty interprets these actions as mandates to conduct a collegiate program in nursing which leads to the degree of Bachelor of Science in Nursing, and which meets requirements for national accreditation.

The Board apparently made the same interpretation, since we received full support in financing and carrying out what we believe to be our responsibility.

We as a faculty are criticized by medical and hospital personnel who know practically nothing about our program.

I do not object to criticism if it is given to help rather than to destroy and if it is given to the appropriate persons. I dislike intensely having persons tell students the program is no good and that they will not know how to nurse when they are graduated.

Some who are most critical fail to observe the first principle necessary in solving a problem. They fail to get the facts.

The faculty is criticized and the school is criticized in the presence of students by persons who do not even know there is a difference between an educational program and a department of nursing service and assume that objectives of the two are identical.

I would like to discuss the program of a typical student:

1. She is responsible for her own room and board and pays $2400.00 in tuition for the program.
2. Approximately half of her program in semester hours is in general education, most of which is completed the first two years.
3. She has twenty-four months nursing experience in addition to

one semester in the sophomore year when she practices various nursing procedures basic to all nursing.

4. She has more practice in caring for patients than do students in diploma programs under the new curriculum prescribed by the Texas State Board of Nurse Examiners.
5. During the last twenty-four months a typical week for the student consists of 12 hours class; 12 hours faculty guided nursing experience; and 16 hours work for the hospital for which she is paid.

I have been greatly concerned, and I know that you have about relationships between medical and nursing staffs and Harris College of Nursing. Comments attributed to various members of these groups indicate a lack of understanding of the purposes and the programs of the College of Nursing.

Criticisms which have been particularly harmful are those made to young students who when faced with the responsibility of giving nursing care are already insecure. When faculty members are with these students they give them the needed help and encouragement. It is when the student is without guidance during work days that she is told that the College of Nursing is not offering a sound program [and] that she will not know how to nurse when she is graduated.

By the time students have reached mid-semester of their senior year, they have developed sufficient competence in nursing and have gained enough self-confidence to make their own judgments, *even to analyze reasons some people make derogatory remarks about the college.* The sophomores or young junior student is put in an indefensible position. In addition to a feeling of personal inadequacy, she is forced to listen to criticism of her school while trying to carry out the nursing assignments.

The aspect of the whole thing which concerns me most is the effect an environment created by distrust may have on students and on recruitment. Will students now enrolled recommend nursing to other students? How will parents of these students feel about nursing and how many will be willing to suggest to other parents that nursing is a good field for their daughters?

It seems to me that more good could be accomplished if we all worked together to try to help students and increase enrollment. Perhaps if we look together at some of the facts we might find a way to work together.

Nursing education has for the most part been outside the educational system of the country. In recent years, however, junior and senior colleges have begun to assume responsibility for conducting educational programs in nursing. At present approximately 150 senior colleges and universities are offering programs in nursing. Many junior colleges throughout the country are providing instruction in academic courses for diploma programs and a few are conducting two-year programs in nursing. The Kellogg Foundation has given money to develop additional programs in junior colleges.

The Harris College of Nursing is one of 150 schools offering a baccalaureate program in nursing and one of 90 holding national accreditation. The program was developed at the request of the late Dr. Charles H. Harris. The curriculum was discussed with him over a period of four years before it was presented to and approved by Texas Christian University. During development of the curriculum the faculty availed itself of consultation services in efforts to establish a sound program.

The relationship with Texas Christian University was planned by Dr. Harris and executed by his representatives. The faculty of Harris College of Nursing is endeavoring to carry out the purposes for which Dr. Harris established the program. The College is not fully supported by the $1,000,000 Charles H Harris Trust Fund, but the income is gradually increasing and will continue to do so, as 10% of the income is added to the capital each year. Success of this program will mean less expense to the Hospital and to patients who provide income for the Hospital. The Trust Indenture directs that income from the Trust Fund be used for an educational program in another field in case there should be no baccalaureate program in nursing.

Without getting into the merits of collegiate in comparison to a non-collegiate education in nursing, I would like to point to a few facts which have considerable bearing on recruitment to schools of nursing. Between the years 1942 and 1955 there was a decrease in the number of girls graduating from high school annually. By 1955 the number was back up to the 1942 level. At the same time there were many more opportunities for girls in business, in industry, and in teaching.

Between the academic years 1954–1955 and 1958–1959 there was a 35% increase in the number of girls graduating from college in one year. Considering the decrease in the number of girls graduating from high school these figures take on added significance. College enrollment of girls is steadily increasing and at a rate higher than the increase in graduates from high school.

The point I want to make is that colleges and universities are going to have an increasingly high number of girls admitted. Many of these girls will be interested in nursing and if given encouragement will undoubtedly choose nursing as a field of study.

Recruitment is a job for all of us. All of us should be working together to increase enrollment in all schools of nursing. The student and her parents will decide on the type of program they want. Some will choose diploma programs, others will choose collegiate programs. There must be a choice available if we want to interest college-minded people in nursing. There is a place for all graduates we can produce from all kinds of programs.

Another factor which influences recruitment is that of finance. At least fifty percent of our students are receiving some financial assistance. Dr. W. W. Ward must be given credit for providing opportunities for many students who would not otherwise be in school. He is providing more than $5000.00 per year for scholarships. Texas Christian University is giving an additional $6000.00 for nursing students. If we had more money to help students we could enroll more students.

Appendix 4

President Sadler's Letter of Appreciation to Members of the Harris Hospital Medical Staff

November 1960

Dear Sir:

The Board of Trustees of the Harris College of Nursing joins with me in expressing our very deep appreciation for the most constructive help you are giving to the students in this important unit of our program. The kind of guidance which you provide is indispensable in the preparation of these young people, and we are extremely grateful to you. Mr. Joe Clarke, Chairman of the Harris College Board, most heartily endorsed the suggestion in the last Board meeting that we express to you and to the other physicians the appreciation which we feel for the constructive service you are rendering.

The demand for the graduates of the Harris College of Nursing assures us that this type of highly professional training is needed. The type of informal, yet direct, teaching which you and the other physicians give is not only indispensable but it is a type of instruction which no others could possibly give.

Thank you very much,

M. E. Sadler

Chancellor

Appendix 5

Ruth Eloise Sperry Award Recipients, 1981–2014

DATE	RECIPIENT	DATE	RECIPIENT
1981	Monette Graves	2000	Marinda Allender
1985	Peggy Mayfield	2001	Carolyn Cagle
1988	Katy Nichols	2002	Diane Hawley
1988	Billie Hightower	2003	NA
1988	Willadean (Williams) Ball	2004	Kris Riddlesperger
1989	Rhonda Keen-Payne	2005	Jimmie Borum
1990	Danna Strength	2006	Phyllis Allen
1991	Frances Richardson	2007	Pam Frable
1992	Linda Curry	2008	Suzy Lockwood
1993	Marinda Allender	2009	Linda Martin
1994	Carol Stephenson	2010	Dennis Cheek
1995	Susan Wilson	2011	Diane Hawley
1996	Rhonda Keen-Payne	2012	Jimmie Borum
1997	Linda Curry	2013	Kathleen White
1998	Danna Strength	2014	Jodie Weatherly
1999	Susan Weeks		

Appendix 6

Fellows of the American Academy of Nursing (FAAN)

FELLOWS
FACULTY
Kathy Baker (Director, Nursing Research and Scholarship)
Kathy Baldwin (retired)
Carol Howe (Associate Professor and Paula R. and Ronald C. Parker Endowed Professor)
Virginia Jarratt (former Dean)
Suzy Lockwood (Interim Dean, HCNHS and Associate Dean, TCU Nursing and Nurse Anesthesia)
Dru Riddle (anesthesia faculty)
Susan Weeks (former Dean; current Vice Provost for Academic Affairs, TCU)
Cathy Young (retired)

BSN ALUMNI	DNP ALUMNI
Mindi Anderson	Gary Brydges, DNP, CRNA
Mary Lou Bond	Joan Clark, DNP
Vivian Littlefield	Cole Edmonson, DNP
Virginia A. Lynch	James Walker, DNP, CRNA
Ainslie Taylor Niebert	Anne Dabrow Woods, DNP

Appendix 7

Letter from Chancellor Moudy to Dean Virginia Jarratt

October 20, 1977

Dr. Virginia R. Jarratt
Dean, Harris College of Nursing

Dear Virginia:

Heartiest congratulations on your being named a Fellow of the American Academy of Nursing. Is there a higher honor? In this life? I imagine the answer is "no" to both.

You have our very best wishes as well as our profound admiration.

Cordially yours,

J. M. Moudy, Chancellor

tn

cc: Dr. Wilsey
Dr. Brewer

Appendix 8

Lucy Harris Linn Institute Speakers

YEAR	NAME	TITLE	UNIVERSITY	TOPIC
1976	Dr. Madeleine Leininger	Dean and Professor of Nursing and Anthropology	College of Nursing, University of Utah	Culture Shock and Change in Nursing
1977	Dr. Marlene Kramer	Professor of Nursing (author, *Reality Shock: Why Nurses Leave Nursing*)	University of California, San Francisco	Reality Shock in Nursing
1978	Dr. Helen Creighton (a lawyer)	Professor of Nursing	University of Wisconsin, Milwaukee	The Law, the Nurse, and the Individual Nurse
1979	Dr. James J. Lynch	Psychologist and author of *The Broken Heart: The Medical Consequences of Loneliness*		Loneliness is a Fatal Disease
1980	Dr. Ingeborg G. Mauksch	Professor of Nursing	Vanderbilt University, Nashville, TN	Nursing: Heading for the 21st Century
1981	Dr. Mila Ann Aroskar	Associate Professor	School of Public Health, University of Minnesota	Ethical Dilemmas: Does Your Opinion Count?

YEAR	NAME	TITLE	UNIVERSITY	TOPIC
1982	Dr. Barbara Stevens	Director of the Division of Health Services, Science and Education	Teachers College of Columbia University, New York City	The Nurse as Executive
1983	Dr. Barbara Redman	Author and Consultant; Former National Coordinator for patient health education	Veterans' Administration, Washington, DC	Current Trends in Patient Education
1984	Sister Rosemary Donley	Dean, School of Nursing	Catholic University of America, Washington, DC	The Image of Nursing: Strategies for Change
1985	Dr. Hurdis Griffith	Founder and Vice President of *The Legislative Network for Nurses, Inc.*		Nursing's Legislative Report Card: An Update on the 99th Congress
1986	Dr. Patricia Donahue	Associate Professor (author, *Nursing: The Finest Art*)	College of Nursing, University of Iowa	Change in Nursing . . . Our Past, Our Future
1988	Dr. Anne DuVal Frost	Assistant Professor of Nursing	College of New Rochelle, NY	Marketing Nursing as Essential Expertise
1989	Dr. Barbara Joyce	Clinical Nurse Specialist in Psychiatric and Holistic Nursing	Columbia Greene Medical Center, Hudson, NY	Holistic Nursing Practice: A New Meaning
1999	*Suspended*			
2000	Dr. Peter Buerhaus		School of Nursing, Vanderbilt University	Nursing Tomorrow: Shortages, Solutions, Opportunities

Appendix 9

Vital Signs, Spring '98

Harris College of Nursing's

Vital Signs

"Where your talents and the world's need cross, there lies your vocation."

VOLUME 1 NUMBER 1 SPRING 1998

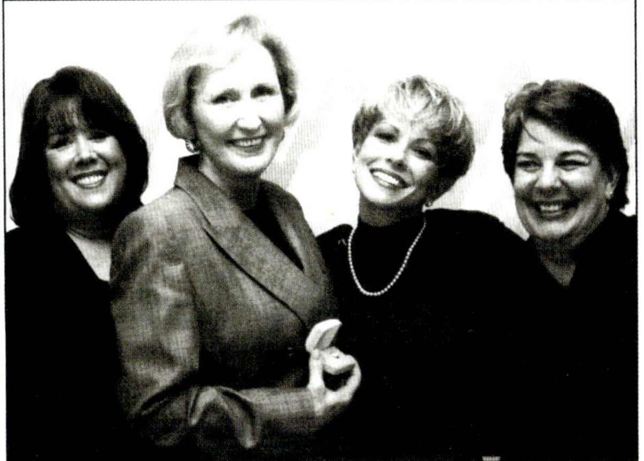

Left to Right: Dr. Kathleen Bond, Dean and Professor of HCN; Charolette Hilley Pierce, 1998 Outstanding Alumna; Connie Koehler '74 and President, HCN Alumni Association; and Dr. Rhonda Keen-Payne '78 and Professor of HCN.

Dealing In Healing: 1998 Harris College of Nursing Outstanding Alumna Charlotte Hilley Pierce '63

IT JUST DIDN'T MAKE SENSE to Charlotte Hilley Pierce '63.

Expectant mothers in the throes of labor needed the expertise of registered nurses, not just aides, as they prepared to deliver their babies. But in the late '70s, it wasn't done that way.

But that's the way it should be done, decided Pierce, then the assistant director of women's services at Harris Methodist Hospital. Within a month the change was made and, as one of Pierce's nurses at the time tells it, the staff members thought it was their idea.

"Charlotte respects theory and research," said Nursing Prof. Rhonda Keen-Payne, friend and mentee of Pierce. "But when necessary, I have seen her dismiss the soundest theory as bunk and unnecessary."

Pierce's compelling blue eyes sparkle at the retelling. "Rhonda likes to say that my favorite saying is that it's easier to ask forgiveness than to get permission, but I don't always think that. I certainly do believe in planning, but you can waste a lot of time and energy planning. I like to act, not spend a lot of time on something that is pretty obvious."

It's that sort of "just do it" attitude that has taken this year's Harris College of Nursing Outstanding Alumna award recipient (a mother of three and active community volunteer, by the way) to the top of her profession and beyond. For the past seven months, Pierce, the administrative director for patient services at Harris Methodist Southwest and Northwest, has served as head administrator at HMSW.

It's an interim position she didn't ask for and she's "quite happy, thank you" to hand back that stethoscope. "I guess the most reward I get from my job is to see someone develop and grow and take risks," she said of her position as nursing administrator. "I believe people really want to succeed and do the right thing. You just have to believe in them and give them the opportunity."

That's a way of life she learned growing up as the only girl in an East Texas family with "very dominant male forces." Her father and brother and cousins who seldom tolerated any "little princess" attitude instilled the belief that she could do, and be, anything she wanted.

Not that there were many open doors. Back then, she said, women had three choices—teacher, nurse or home economist. Nursing won.

Good thing. During her 35 years of teaching, leading and mentoring, the lively, determined nurse made a difference.

"When I was in nursing school, it was important to make sure you squared the corners, had a tight bed," she said. "I wanted to know why. At home I had contour sheets, why not at the hospital?"

Indeed, questioning has caused Pierce to implement many wide-ranging changes that have improved healthcare, at least among the patients she touches each day. And when making those changes, say those around her, she does so with a radiant smile and a healthy dose of dry wit.

"I just believe you've got to enjoy what you do and if you don't, you've got to figure out why," Pierce said, a sly smile creeping in. "You can make your day fun or you can make it miserable. It's your choice.

"I go for the light side." ■ —*NB*

Appendix 10

Curriculum/Degree Plan for Bachelor of Science in Nursing

(Harris School of Nursing. Appendices. Self-Study Report, 2000: 69.)

69

TEXAS CHRISTIAN UNIVERSITY-HARRIS SCHOOL OF NURSING
DEGREE PLAN FOR BACHELOR OF SCIENCE IN NURSING

EFF: 95F

NAME ______ SS# ______

RN: AD____ DIP____ LVN____ OTHER______ ADM DATA: SAT V____ M____ T______

TRANSFER: TCU___OTHER______ ACT ______ OTHER______

HOME ADDRESS: ______ ADM GPA: JR COL ______ SR COL ______

TRANS CR: JR COL ______ SR COL ______

FTW ADDRESS: ______ DATE OF BIRTH: ______

DATE ENTERED TCU: ______

HOME PH# ______ TCU PH# ______

INITIAL ADVISER ______ DATE ______ CURRENT ADVISER ______

UCR	PREREQ	GRADE	TRANS	TCU	C/S*	UCR	NSG COURSES	GRADE	TRANS	TCU
PS-L	BIOL 20204 AandP I									
PS-L	BIOL 20214 AandP II					W	N30013 HIST/CONT PERSPECT			
PS-L	BIOL 20233 MICRO						N30023 CULTURAL and ETHICS			
PS	PSYC 10213 INTRO						N30033 TEACHING STRATEGIES			
	NURS 10303 GandD									
SS	SOCI 20213						N30012 THEORETICAL BASIS			
HS-U	HIST 10603/10613					HC	N30013 CONC: NSG/HLTH PROM			
M	MATH 10043						N30183 PRAC: HLTH ASSESS			
							N20612 PHARMACOLOGY			
OR CONCURRENT										
	NTDT 10403						N30632 CONC: GERONT			
	SPCO 30153/20113/20193						N20713 CONC: ADULT NSG I			
CONCURRENT WITH NURS 20713							N20783 PRAC: ADULT NSG I			
	NURS 30353						N20813 CONC: PSYC MNTL HLTH			
UNIV CURRICULUM							N20882 PRAC: PSYC MNTL HLTH			
WW	FRESH COMP 10803									
WW	SOPH COMP 20803						N40213 CONC: MATERNAL-CHILD			
RS	RELI						N40283 PRAC: MATERNAL-CHILD			
FA	FINE ARTS						N40713 CONC: ADULT NSG II			
FL							N40783 PRAC: ADULT NSG II			
FL										
SS	ELEC					CI-W	N40303 CI-HC DELIVERY			
	EXPL ELEC						N40813 CONC: COMM HLTH			
	FREE ELEC						N40882 PRAC: COMM HLTH			
UD	NON NSG ELEC**						N40912 CONC: NSG MGMT			
UD	ELEC						N40983 PRAC: NSG MGMT			
							OR N40100/40500 NSG ELEC**			
	TOTALS									
OTHER COLL ATTENDED (DATES) AND COURSES TAKEN					S HR		N30330 SPEC PROB			
							N30002 JUNIOR HONORS SEM			
							N40003 SENIOR HONORS SEM			
							TOTALS			

GRADUATION SUMMARY:

NON NSG/EXAM		* NSG BY CBE	
NON NSG/TRANS		NSG BY TRANS	
		HSN NSG CR HRS	
NON NSG AT TCU		TOT. NSG HRS	
NON NSG AT GPA		TOT. NON NSG HRS	
HSN NSG GPA		**TOTAL GRAD HRS**	

* CULURAL SELECTIVE (C/S)—MAY BE SATISFIED BY COURSE IN RELI, EXPL ELEC, FREE ELEC, FA, SS ELEC OR UDE. INDICATE WHICH COURSE SATISFIES C/S REQUIREMENT.

**STUDENT WILL TAKE EITHER THE NON-NURSING UPPER DIVISION OR A NURSING ELECTIVE.

APPROVED FOR GRADUATION:

MINOR ______

DEAN ______
Rhonda Keen-Payne, R.N., Ph.D.

GRADUATION DATE ______

DATE ______

STATE BOARD RESULTS ______

MBW/AL/sm **R 11/9/99**

Appendix 11

Rankin Lectureship Speakers

DATE	SPEAKER	TOPIC
1998	Susan Dadakis Horn	The Impact of Managing Care Rather than Cost-Containment Strategies
2002	Faiga Jamaldin-Qudah	Financial Management to Achieve Healthcare Goals
2003	Diane Schull	Clinical Nurse Specialist Role: Past, Present, Future
2005	Barbara Holtzclaw	Fever Revisited: Applying Nursing Science
2006	Rhonda Keen-Payne	Can a Pandemic Be Managed? Lessons from 1918
2009	Lisa Hopp Leslie Rittenmeyer	A Global Community of Evidence-Based Practice: Implementation Science and the Joanna Briggs Collaboration
2010	Susan Hassmiller	The Future of Nursing and Healthcare
2011	Ronda Hughes	Proactive Approaches to the Changing Landscape of Healthcare
2012	Bobbie Berkowitz	Promoting Health Equity: Evidence-Based Programs in Public Health
2013	Gwen Sherwood	Transforming Healthcare: The New Science of Quality and Safety
2014	Brenda Zierler	Inter-professional Education and Collaborative Practice
2015	Madeline Schmitt	Inter-professional Health Practice
2016	Linda Harrington	Cognitive Technologies: The Game Changers in Digital Health
2017	Virginia Lynch	Forensic Nursing Science and the Global Agenda in Contemporary Health Care
2018	Terry Jones	Unfinished Nursing Care: State of the Science & Future Directions
2019	Maureen "Shawn" Kennedy	Is Nursing's Legacy Coming Full Circle?
2020	Jane Barnsteiner	Quality and Safety Education for Nurses in an Amazon World

Appendix 12

Sample Degree Plan: Bachelor of Science in Nursing

(Harris College of Nursing & Health Sciences—Nursing. Appendices for Standards I–IV—Texas Christian University Baccalaureate Nursing Program. Self-Study Report, Fall 2010: 16.)

Appendix III-A-5
Texas Christian University- Harris College – Nursing
Sample Degree Plan: Bachelor of Science in Nursing

Freshman Semester I	**Freshman Semester II**
BIOL 20204 (Anat & Phys) (NSC)....4 ENGL 10803 (Freshman Comp) (WCO)....3 PSYC 10213 (General Psychology)....3 NURS 10043 (Survey of Prof Nsg) (CA)....3 Humanities elective (HUM)....3 Total credit hrs....16	BIOL 20214 * (Anat & Phys) (NSC)....4 NTDT 20403 (Nutrition)....3 Religious Traditions (RT)....3 SOCI 20213 (Introductory Sociology) (SSC, CA)..3 NURS 10303 (Human Development) (SSC)....3 Total credit hrs....16
Sophomore Semester I	**Sophomore Semester II**
BIOL 20233 * (Microbiology) (NSC)....3 ENGL 20803 (Sophomore Comp) (WCO)....3 Historical Traditions (HT)....3 MATH 10043 ** (Elem Statistics) (MTH)....3 NURS 20033 (Teaching Strategies) (OCO)....3 Humanities Elective (HUM)....3 Total credit hrs....18	NURS 20041 (Genetics/Genomics in Nursing)....1 NURS 20163 (Pharmacotherapeutics)....3 NURS 20224 (Fund/Assess: Concepts)....4 NURS 20284 (Fund/Assess: Practicum)....4 Free Elective....3 Elective #....2 Total credit hrs....17

Junior Semester I	Junior Semester II
NURS 30714 (Adult Nsg I: Concepts)........................ 4	NURS 30313 (Mat/Wom Hlth Nsg: Conc)............3
NURS 30783 (Adult Nsg I: Practicum)........................ 3	NURS 30382 (Mat Nsg: Practicum).......................2
NURS 30813 (Psyc-MH Nsg: Concepts) 3	NURS 30413 (Pediatric Nsg: Concepts)...............3
NURS 30882 (Psyc-MH Nsg: Practicum) 2	NURS 30482 (Pedi.Nsg: Practicum).....................2
Humanities elective (HUM) 3	NURS 30632 (Gero Nsg).....................................2
	Fine Arts elective (FAR).......................................3
Total credit hrs.. 15	Total credit hrs...15

Senior Semester I	Senior Semester II
NURS 40053 ## (Crit Inq in Hlth Care Del) (SSC,GA) 3	NURS 40813 ## (Com Hlth Nsg: Concepts) (CSV)..3
NURS 40114 (Adult Nsg II: Concepts)........................ 4	NURS 40882 (Com Hlth Nsg: Practicum).............2
NURS 40183 (Adult Nsg II: Practicum)...................... 3	NURS 40913 (Role Dev & Nsg Mgmt: Conc) 3
NURS 40632 (Res & Theory in Nsg Prac).................. 2	NURS 40984 (Role Dev & Nsg Mgmt: Pract) 4
Literary Traditions (LT)... 3	
Total credit hrs.. 15	Total credit hrs..12

* The following courses will satisfy the TCU CC requirement for Natural Sciences (NSC) Human Experiences and Endeavors: BIOL 20214 and 20233; applies to NURS-BSN only

** MATH 10023 is a prerequisite to MATH 10043 if lacking two years high school algebra

\# Choice of elective will depend on other choices made in the HMVV and HEE

\## Writing Emphasis Course (WEM)

Total Graduation Requirements – 124 semester hours; 69 Nursing, 55 Non-Nursing

Appendix 13

Curriculum Comparison of Traditional and Accelerated Tracks

(Harris College of Nursing & Health Sciences—Nursing. Appendices for Standards I–IV—Texas Christian University Baccalaureate Nursing Program. Self-Study Report, Fall 2010: 39–40.)

Appendix III-C-1

Curriculum Comparison of Traditional and Accelerated Tracks

Traditional BSN Track (TBT)	Accelerated BSN Track (ABT)
FRESHMAN YEAR	SUMMER I ***Theme:* Human responses to disease and disability**
NURS 10043 (Survey of Prof Nsg)	NURS 20163 (Pharmacology) *NURS 39113 (Discipline & Practice of Prof Nsg)** *NURS 39123 (Fundamentals of Prof Nsg)** *NURS 39184 (Reflective Practice & Cl Inquiry I)**
SOPHOMORE YEAR	FALL ***Theme:* Personal and social impact of medicalizing normal life transitions, such as birth and death**
NURS 20033 (Teaching Strategies) NURS 20041 (Genetics/Genomics) NURS 20163 (Pharmacology) NURS 20224 (Fund/Assess: Concepts) NURS 20284 (Fund/Assess: Practicum)	NURS 20041 (Genetics/Genomics) NURS 30714 (Adult Nsg I: Concepts) NURS 30813 (Psyc-MH Nsg: Concepts) NURS 30313 (Mat/Wom Hlth Nsg: Concepts) NURS 40632 (Res & Theory in Nsg Practicum) *NURS 39285 (Reflective Practice & Cl Inquiry II)**

JUNIOR YEAR	SPRING ***Theme:* Dynamic interface between advanced biomedical and information technologies and vulnerable client populations**
NURS 30714 (Adult Nsg I: Concepts) NURS 30783 (Adult Nsg I: Practicum) NURS 30813 (Psych-MH Nsg: Concepts) NURS 30882 (Psych-MH Nsg: Practicum) NURS 30313 (Mat/Wom Hlth: Concepts) NURS 30382 (Mat/Wom Hlth: Practicum) NURS 30413 (Pediatric Nsg: Concepts) NURS 30482 (Pedi Nsg: Practicum) NURS 30632 (Gero Nsg Concepts)	NURS 40114 (Adult Nsg II: Concepts) NURS 30413 (Pediatric Nsg: Concepts) NURS 40813 (Com Hlth Nsg: Concepts) NURS 30632 (Gero Nsg Concepts) *NURS 49285 (Reflective Practice & CI Inquiry III)**
SENIOR YEAR	SUMMER II ***Theme:* Controversies in contemporary nursing practice with emphasis on hospital-as-culture**
NURS 40053 (Crit Inq Hth Care Del) NURS 40114 (Adult Nsg II: Concepts) NURS 40183 (Adult Nsg II: Practicum) NURS 40632 (Res & Theory in Nsg Prac) NURS 40813 (Com Hlth Nsg: Concepts) NURS 40882 (Com Hlth Nsg: Practicum) NURS 40913 (Role & Mgmt: Concepts) NURS 40984 (Role & Mgmt: Practicum)	NURS 40913 (Role & Mgmt: Concepts) *NURS 49488 (Prof Nsg Residency)**

*Denotes courses designed specifically for the ABT. For example, ***NURS 39113: Discipline and Practice of Professional Nursing*** subsumes concepts taught in 3 TBT courses (NURS 10043, 20033, 40053), which contain overlapping content. Essential student outcomes, e.g. teaching projects, are woven through ABT practicum courses, demonstrating increased complexity and competency.

Appendix 14

Harris College Deans

YEARS	DEAN	TITLE	DECEASED DATE
1942–67	Lucy Harris	Dean & Professor, Harris College of Nursing	May 27, 1981
1967–79	Virginia Jarratt	Dean & Professor, Harris College of Nursing	June 17, 2006
Jan. 1980– July 31, 1980	Joan Goe	Interim Dean	
1980–95	Patricia Scearse	Dean & Professor, Harris College of Nursing	April 5, 2011
1995–96	Rhonda Keen-Payne	Interim Dean & Professor, Harris College of Nursing	
1996–99	Kathy Bond	Dean & Professor, Harris College of Nursing	
1999–2000	Rhonda Keen-Payne	Dean & Professor, Harris College of Nursing	
2000–05	Rhonda Keen-Payne	Dean & Professor, College of Health & Human Sciences	
2005–06	Rhonda Keen-Payne	Dean & Professor, Harris College of Nursing & Health Sciences	
2006–14	Paulette Burns	Dean & Professor, Harris College of Nursing & Health Sciences	Dec 12, 2014
Dec. 2013– March 2015	Susan Weeks	Acting Dean & Professor, Harris College of Nursing & Health Sciences	
2015–18	Susan Weeks	Dean & Professor, Harris College of Nursing & Health Sciences	
April 2018– May 31, 2019	Suzy Lockwood	Interim Dean, Harris College of Nursing & Health Sciences; Associate Dean & Professor, TCU Nursing	
June 1, 2019– present	Chris Watts	Dean, Harris College of Nursing & Health Sciences; Professor, Davies School of Communication Sciences & Disorders	

Appendix 15

Harris College of Nursing & Health Sciences Pillars

OUR VISION
To transform global health.
OUR MISSION
To enhance global health through education, scholarship, and innovation.
OUR PILLARS
Preparing Global Citizens—Harris College prepares globally minded human change agents who transform lives.
♦ Equipping human change agents: preparing graduates who are clinically capable and ethically motivated to lead others in transforming care.
♦ Growing mind and character: teaching that leverages a world view, public interest, and industry leadership.
♦ Multi-layered approach: respected academic institution dedicated to improving lives through innovative education, research, and community outreach.
♦ Metroplex connection: vast professional opportunities and partnerships to leverage and experience.

Community of Growth—Harris College is a supportive, compassionate community dedicated to holistic growth.
♦ Mentoring relationships: internationally renowned faculty have a vested interest in students' personal growth.
♦ Small class size: a supportive, challenging learning environment that nurtures growth.
♦ Well-rounded preparation: liberal-arts foundation with real-world application, ensuring students have the tangible skills and holistic perspective to thrive.
♦ Spirited belonging: united by our passion and purpose, we are motivated to learn from one another.
♦ Interdisciplinary approach: we are bringing disciplines together to create team-oriented, collaborative leaders
Excellence with Integrity—Harris College has a strong reputation for producing responsible leaders who act with excellence and integrity.
♦ Leading-edge learning: faculty, students, and staff are eagerly embracing opportunities for innovation and improvements in health care as the system of the future is evolving.
♦ Proven excellence: producing graduates who excel in their professions and confirm the excellence of our programs.
♦ Outstanding faculty: students learn from faculty who are practitioners, researchers, and teachers with a vested interest in providing the knowledge and skills to make a difference in a variety of health care settings.
♦ Values-centered leadership: fulfilling our purpose for the greater good with both excellence and integrity.
OUR STRATEGIC INITIATIVES
Excellence in Teaching and Scholarship.
High Quality Students, Faculty and Staff.
Transformational Community Engagement
World-class Learning Environment .

Dean's Office 9-10-2018

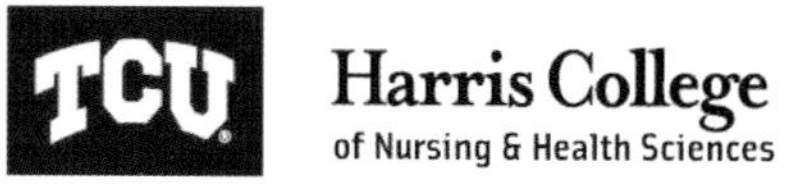

Appendix 16

Harris College Current Faculty, 2020

NAME	RANK	SINCE
TCU NURSING		
Lavonne Adams PhD, RN, CCRN	Associate Professor	2004
Gina Alexander PhD, RN, MPH, MSN	Associate Professor	2010
Marinda Allender MSN, RN, CPN	Assistant Professor	1990
Amy Anderson DNP, RN, CNE	Assistant Professor of Professional Practice	2017
Kathy Baker PhD, RN, ACNS-BC, FAAN	Associate Professor	2007
Dorothy Bartell MSN, RNC-NIC, MAT	Assistant Professor of Professional Practice	2016
Lisa Bashore PhD, RN, CPNP, CPON	Associate Professor	2013
Lori Borchers MSN, RN, IBCLC, CNE	Instructor	2014
Karen Breitkreuz EdD, MSN, RN	Associate Professor	2019
Vicki Brooks DNP, APRN, FNP-BC	Assistant Professor of Professional Practice	2018
Suzanne Bryant MS, RN	Instructor	2006
Sharon Canclini MS, RN, FCN, CNE, APHN	Assistant Professor of Professional Practice	2005
Dennis Cheek PhD, RN, FAHA	Professor	2003
Glenda Daniels PhD, RN, CNS, CGRN, CWOCN	Associate Professor	2009

NAME	RANK	SINCE
Caitlin Dodd MSN, RN, CNE, CNL	Assistant Professor of Professional Practice	2010
Kathy Ellis DNP, APRN, ANP-BC	Associate Professor of Professional Practice	2015
Donna Ernst DNP, RN, CNL, CGRN	Assistant Professor of Professional Practice	2015
Stephanie Evans PhD, APRN, CPNP, CLC	Assistant Professor	2014
Susan Fife DNP, RN, CNM	Assistant Professor of Professional Practice	2014
Pamela Frable ND, RN	Associate Professor	2000
Ashley Franklin PhD, RN, CCRN, CNE	Assistant Professor	2014
Sheila Griffin MSN, RN, CWON	Instructor	2012
Kirstin Guinn MSN, RNC-OB	Assistant Professor of Professional Practice	2017
Diane Hawley PhD, RN, CCNS, CNE	Associate Professor of Professional Practice	1998
Tracy Hicks DNP, APRN, PMHNP-BC, FNP-BC	Assistant Professor of Professional Practice	2020
Carol Howe PhD, RN, CDE	Assistant Professor	2014
Lynnette Howington DNP, RN, WHNP-BC, CNL	Associate Professor of Professional Practice	2007
Linda Humphries DNP, RN, ACNS-BC, CCRN	Assistant Professor of Professional Practice	2014
Hope Jackson PhD, RN	Assistant Professor	2016
Oteka Jackson-Cenales DNP, MSN, RN	Assistant Professor of Professional Practice	2018
Ann Johnson PhD, RN	Assistant Professor	2017
Rhonda Keen-Payne PhD, RN	Professor	1982
Michelle Kimzey PhD, RN	Assistant Professor	2017
Suzanne Lockwood PhD, RN, OCN, FAAN	Professor	1997
Kenneth Lowrance DNP, RN, APRN, FNP-BC, CNS, DCC, CNE	Professor of Professional Practice	2011
Miriam Marshall MSN, RN-BC	Instructor	2012
Shirley Martin PhD, RN, CPNP, CPON	Assistant Professor	2018
Lea Montgomery MS, RN	Assistant Professor of Professional Practice	2001

NAME	RANK	SINCE
Angela Njenga PhD, RN, MHA, BScN	Assistant Professor	2018
Eunduck Park PhD, RN	Assistant Professor	2018
Jodi Patterson PhD, MN, RN	Assistant Professor	2019
Kim Posey DNP, RN, AGPCNP-BC	Assistant Professor of Professional Practice	2017
Brenda Reed DNP, RN, FNPBC	Assistant Professor of Professional Practice	2011
Janie Robinson PhD, RN, CNE	Associate Professor	2009
Lisette Saleh PhD, RNC-OB	Assistant Professor	2012
Ashlie Seale MSN, RN-BC	Assistant Professor of Professional Practice	2016
Cari Selzer DNP, RN, ACNP-BC	Assistant Professor of Professional Practice	2018
Melissa Sherrod PhD, RN, NE-BC	Professor	2004
Marie Stark MSN, RN, RNC-OB	Assistant Professor of Professional Practice	2015
Laura Thielke MS, RN, CNL	Assistant Professor of Professional Practice	2009
Charles Walker PhD, RN	Professor	2001
Danielle Walker PhD, RN, CNE	Assistant Professor	2009
Jodie Weatherly MSN, RN, CPN	Assistant Professor of Professional Practice	2007
Susan Weeks DNP, RN, CNS, FNAP, FAAN	Professor	1994
Jo Nell Wells PhD, RN, RN-BC	Professor	1998
Leslie Zimpelman MSN, RN, RNC-NIC	Instructor	2014
DAVIES SCHOOL OF COMMUNICATION SCIENCES & DISORDERS		
Danielle Brimo PhD, CCC-SLP	Associate Professor	2012
Tracy Burger MS, CCC-SLP, CCC-A	Assistant Professor of Professional Practice	2013
Teresa Drulia PhD, CCC-SLP	Assistant Professor	2017
Lynn Flahive MS, CCC-SLP	Assistant Professor	1991
Teresa Gonzalez MS	Assistant Professor of Professional Practice	1998
Karen Hennington MS, CCC-SLP	Instructor	2014
Emily Lund PhD, CCC-SLP	Assistant Professor	2013
Laurel Lynch MS, CCC-SLP	Instructor	2013

NAME	RANK	SINCE
Irmgard Payne MS, CCC-SLP	Assistant Professor of Professional Practice	2012
Ahmed Rivera Campos PhD, CCC-SLP	Assistant Professor	2017
Jean Rivera Perez PhD, CCC-SLP	Assistant Professor	2017
Jennifer Watson PhD, CCC-SLP	Professor	1982
Christopher Watts PhD, CCC-SLP	Professor	2008
Lynita Yarbrough MS, CCC-SLP	Assistant Professor of Professional Practice	2012
DEPARTMENT OF KINESIOLOGY		
Roina Baquera MS	Instructor	2016
Todd Castleberry PhD	Lecturer	2018
Philip Esposito PhD	Assistant Professor of Professional Practice	2012
Stephanie Jevas PhD	Professor of Professional Practice	2012
Adam King PhD	Assistant Professor	2016
Melody Phillips PhD	Associate Professor	2004
Debbie Rhea PhD	Professor	1999
Meena Shah PhD	Professor	2001
Benjamin Timson PhD	Assistant Professor of Professional Practice	2015
Robyn Trocchio PhD	Assistant Professor	2019
SCHOOL OF NURSE ANESTHESIA		
Ron Anderson MD	Associate Professor of Professional Practice	2008
Dennis Cheek PhD, RN, FAHA	Professor	2003
M. Roseann Diehl PhD, DNP, CRNA	Professor of Professional Practice	2010
Vaughna Galvin DNAP, CRNA	Assistant Professor of Professional Practice	2014
Linda Harrington PhD, DNP, RN-BC, CNS	Lecturer	2002
James Holcomb DNP, CRNA	Assistant Professor of Professional Practice	2017
Monica Jenschke PhD, CRNA	Associate Professor of Professional Practice	2012
Hylda Nugent DNP, CRNA	Professor of Professional Practice	2004
Jennifer Oakes DNAP, CRNA	Associate Professor of Professional Practice	2020

NAME	RANK	SINCE
J. Dru Riddle PhD, DNP, CRNA	Associate Professor of Professional Practice	2012
Jackie Rowles DNP, MBA, MA, CRNA, ANP-BC, FNAP, DAIPM, FAAN	Associate Professor of Professional Practice	2020
Mike Sadler DNP, CRNA	Associate Professor of Professional Practice	2009
Kay K. Sanders DNP, CRNA	Professor of Professional Practice	2003
Robyn Ward PhD, CRNA	Associate Professor of Professional Practice	2019
DEPARTMENT OF SOCIAL WORK		
Sh'Niqua Alford LCSW	Assistant Professor of Professional Practice	2018
Samantha Bates PhD, LMSW	Assistant Professor	2018
Nada Elias-Lambert PhD, LMSW	Associate Professor	2013
D. Lynn Jackson PhD, LCSW, ACSW	Associate Professor of Professional Practice	2013
Aesha John PhD, LMSW	Associate Professor	2015
Katie Lauve-Moon PhD, MSW, MDiv	Assistant Professor	2017
Jennifer Martin PhD, LCSW	Assistant Professor of Professional Practice	2016
James Petrovich PhD, LMSW	Associate Professor	2010
Mary Twis PhD, LMSW-AP	Assistant Professor	2018
Tee Tyler PhD, LCSW	Assistant Professor	2016

Appendix 17

Harris College Current Staff, 2020

NAME	TITLE	SINCE
DEAN'S OFFICE		
Amanda Duvall	Career Consultant	2013
Sharon Hudson (PT)	Administrative Assistant	2002
Susan Moore	Administrative Assistant	1982
June Seely	Assistant to the Dean	2015
Chelsea Turner	Coordinator, Regulatory and Compliance	2017
Jocelyn Warren (LiiNK Project)	Administrative Assistant	2018
Sybil White	Assistant to the Dean	2003
Jeannie Bales	Administrative Assistant, Development	2006
Charles Dewar	Coordinator, Information Technology	2012
Laura Patton	Director of Development	2015
ACADEMIC RESOURCE CENTER		
Sandi Barr	Administrative Assistant	2008
Trudy Conner	Academic Advisor	2020
Stacy Dissinger	Academic Advisor	2018
Xavier Flowers	Academic Advisor	2020
Zoranna Jones	Director and Academic Advisor	2002

NAME	TITLE	SINCE
TCU NURSING		
Angela Cantrell	Administrative Program Specialist	2001
Shelley Clonts	Learning Center Associate	2018
Rose Davis	Administrative Program Specialist	2014
Kimberly Graham	Learning Center Associate	2017
Cathy Hughes	Administrative Assistant	2013
Beth Janke	Academic Program Specialist	2015
Landon Lamb	Simulation Specialist	2016
Jamie Martinez	Learning Center Technician	2014
Cheryl Mathison	Learning Center Associate	2014
Mary Morton	Administrative Assistant	1996
Catherine Serrano	Learning Center Coordinator	2014
Kristina Wigington	Administrative Assistant	2018
DAVIES SCHOOL OF COMMUNICATION SCIENCES & DISORDERS		
Janet Matzen	Administrative Assistant	2012
Sheila Speak	Administrative Assistant	2010
DEPARTMENT OF KINESIOLOGY		
Andreas Kreutzer	Instructional Lab Coordinator	2015
Elizabeth Pettijohn	Academic Program Specialist	2007
SCHOOL OF NURSE ANESTHESIA		
Kimberly Bowen	Administrative Assistant	2018
Sharlotte Crawford (PT)	Administrative Assistant	2011
Carol Womack	Executive Assistant to the Director	2003
Kent Young	Video Engineer	2003
DEPARTMENT OF SOCIAL WORK		
Rubi Orozco	Academic Program Specialist	2020
Susan Rahrovi	Administrative Assistant	2019

Appendix 18

Harris College Emeritus Faculty—Current and Deceased

NAME	EMERITUS
CURRENT	
TCU NURSING	
Kathy Baldwin	Associate Professor
Willadean (Williams) Ball	Associate Professor
Patricia Bradley	Associate Professor
Carolyn Cagle	Professor
Linda Curry	Professor
Gail Davis	Professor
Anne Lind	Assistant Professor
Peggy Mayfield	Associate Professor
Debra McLachlan	Associate Professor
Alison Moreland	Instructor
Carol Stephenson	Associate Professor
Danna Strength	Associate Professor
Susan Wilson	Associate Professor

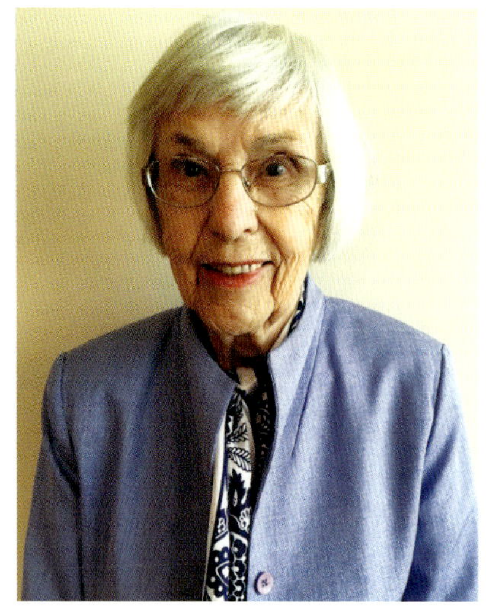

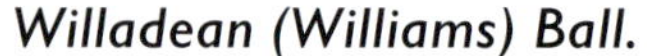

Willadean (Williams) Ball.

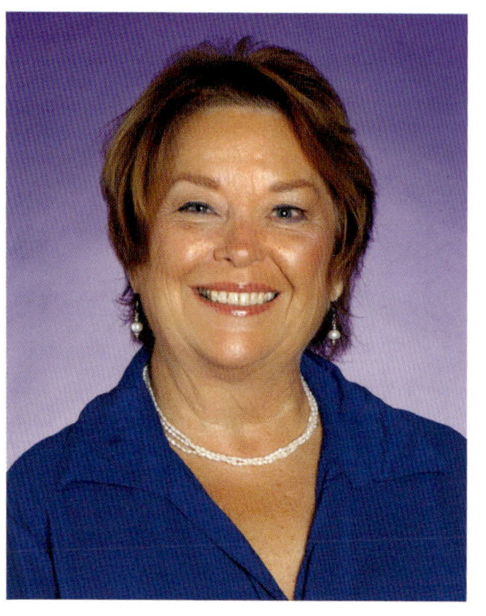

Linda Curry.

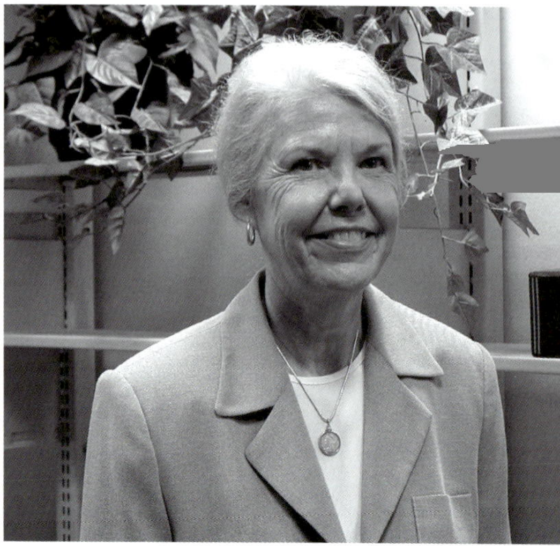

Gail Davis.

Harris College Emeritus Faculty

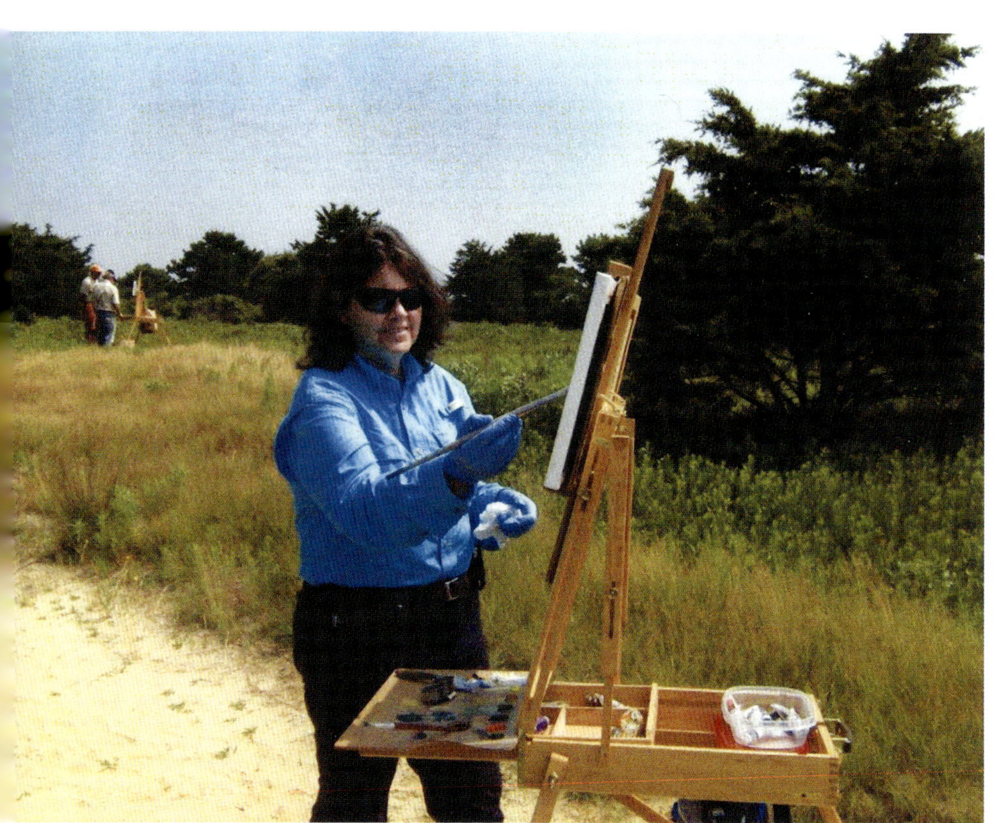

Debra McLachlan.

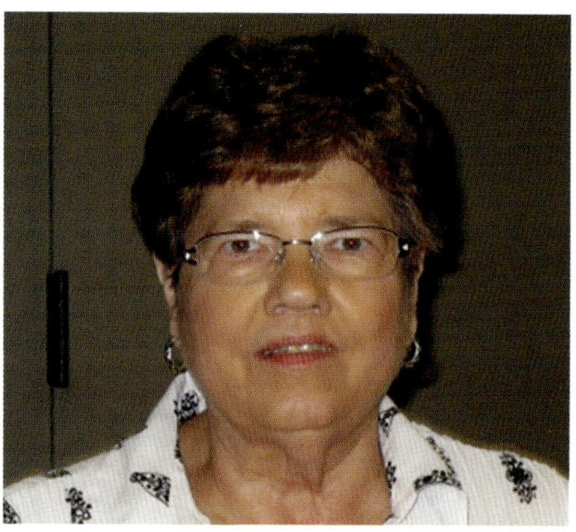

Carol Stephenson.

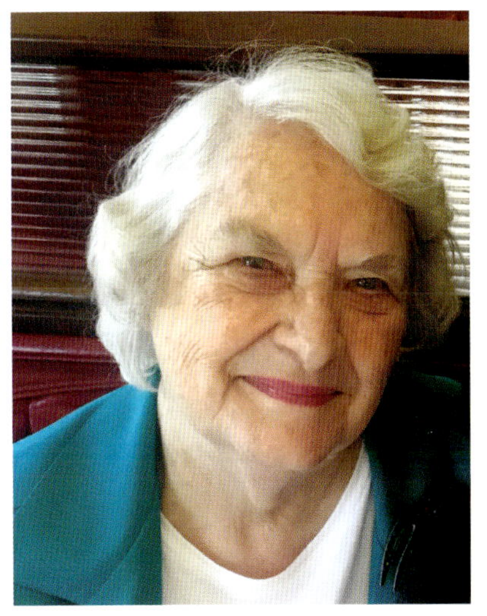

Anne Lind.

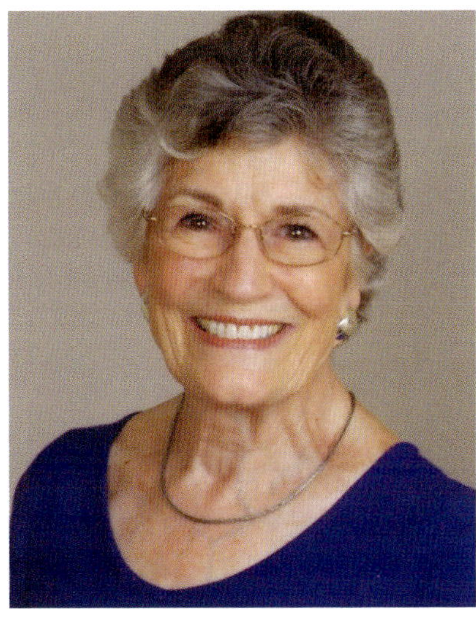

Alison Moreland.

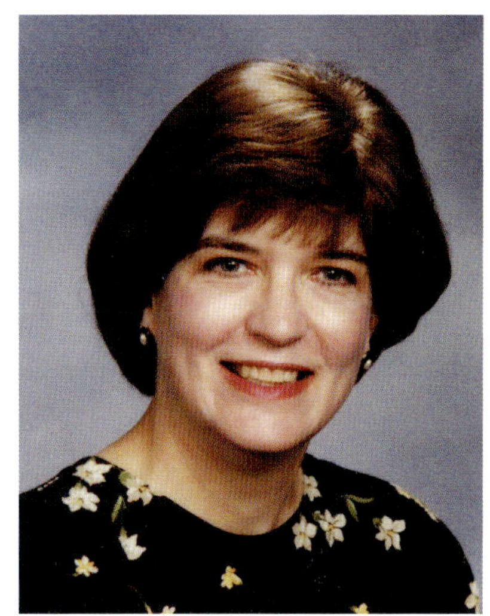

Susan Wilson.

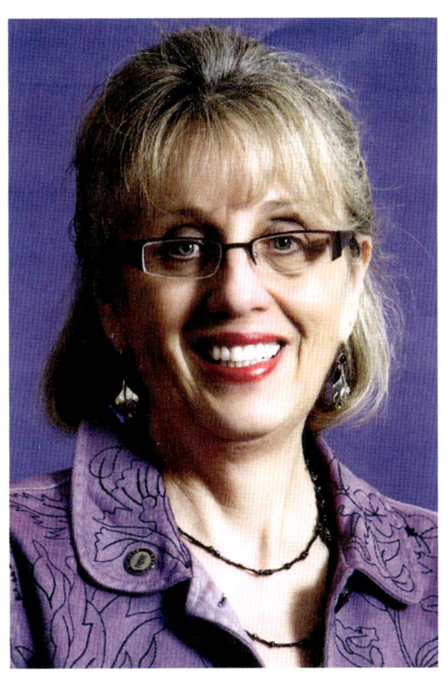

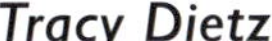

Tracy Dietz.

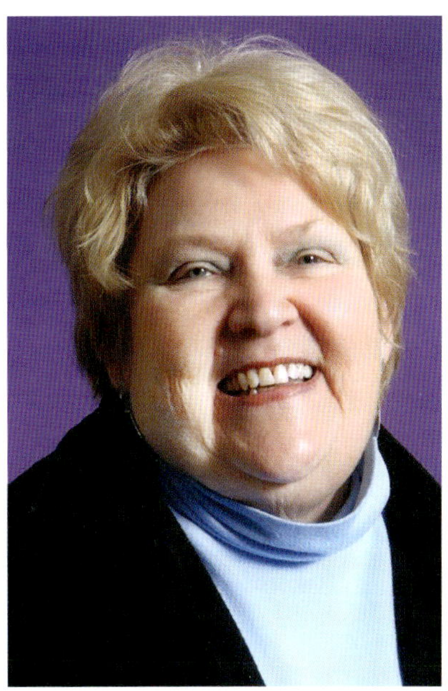

Linda Moore.

NAME	EMERITUS
CURRENT	
NURSE ANESTHESIA	
Wayne Barcellona	Associate Professor
SOCIAL WORK	
Tracy Dietz	Associate Professor
Linda Moore	Professor
DECEASED	
TCU NURSING	
Jimmie Katherine Bratton	Professor
Paulette Burns	Professor
Katy (Nichols) Cairns	Associate Professor
Lucy Harris	Professor
Billie Hightower	Assistant Professor
Mildred Hogstel	Professor
Lucille Houston	Associate Professor
Monette Graves	Associate Professor
Allene Jones	Assistant Professor
Vera Phillips	Assistant Professor
Nancy C. Sayner	Associate Professor
Patricia Scearse	Professor
Ruth Eloise Sperry	Professor
COMMUNICATION SCIENCES & DISORDERS	
Bill Ryan	Professor
SOCIAL WORK	
Art Berliner	Professor

References

"Alma Matters." 2005. *TCU Magazine.* (Spring): http://www.magarchive.tcu.edu/articles/2005-01-am.asp?issueid=200501.

Alpert, Andrew, and Jill Auyer. 2003. "The 1988-2000 Employment Projections: How Accurate Were They?" *Occupational Outlook Quarterly* (Spring): 2–21; https://www.bls.gov/careeroutlook/2003/spring/art01.pdf.\.

American Association of Colleges of Nursing. 2002. "Hallmarks of the Professional Nursing Practice Environment." *Journal of Professional Nursing* 18 (5): 295–304; doi:10.1053/jpnu.2002.12923.

American Association of Publishers. 2006. *Teaching and Writing.* http://myemail.constantcontace.com/Honor-Virginia-Lynch-.html?-soid=1101938584617&aidRt S2VfBlLE.

American Journal of Nursing. 1990. "New OSHA Rules under Fire from All Angles." 90, no. 1: 18, 22.

American Journal of Nursing. 1985. "News: LPNs are Facing Harder Ties with Trend towards RN-Only Staffing." 85, no. 10: 1165, 1180–4.

ANA (American Nurses Association). 1980. *Nursing's Social Policy Statement.* Washington, DC: ANA.

Andreoli, Kathleen G. 1992a. "Total Quality Management—A New Culture." *Journal of Professional Nursing* 8, no. 2 (March–April): 72.

Andreoli, Kathleen. 1992b. "Primary Nursing for the 1990s and Beyond." *Journal of Professional Nursing* 8, no. 4 (July–August): 202.

Arnold P. Gold Foundation. 2018. "White Coat Ceremony." The Arnold P. Gold Foundation. Retrieved from www.gold-foundation.org/programs/white-coat-ceremony 2018.

Axinn, June, and Hal Levin. 1975. *Social Welfare: A History of the American Response to Need.* New York: Harper and Row.

Bashore, Lisa, and Joyce Bender. 2017. "Benefits of Attending a Weekend Childhood Cancer Survivor Family Retreat." *Journal of Nursing Scholarship* 49, no. 5: 521–8.

Bell, Dorothy Mays. 1980. *Development of the Speech and Hearing Clinic at Texas Christian University: A Personal Perspective.* Self-published.

Benner, Patricia. 1984. *From Novice to Expert: Excellence and Power in Clinical Nursing Practice.* Menlo Park, CA: Addison-Wesley.

Board of Visitors. 2008. *TCU Harris College of Nursing & Health Sciences Board of Visitors Charter.* Texas Christian University, Fort Worth, TX.

Bowers, Donna. 2001. "The Health Insurance Portability and Accountability Act: Is it Really All that Bad?" *Baylor University Medical Center Proceedings* 14, no. 4: 347–48.

Bullough, Bonnie. "Influences on Role Expansion." *American Journal of Nursing* 76(9), 1476-81. doi: 10.23071240.

Clark, Joan, and Kathy Baker. 2014. *Sustaining CNL Academic-Practice Partnerships: Challenges & Success.* Clinical Nurse Leader Summit, Anaheim, CA, January 16–18, 2014.

Clark, Joan, and Susan Weeks. March 18, 2017. *Academic Practice Partnerships: Workforce Planning.* Presentation at the American Association of Colleges of Nursing Conference, Washington, DC.

Council on Social Work Education (CSWE). (n.d.). Directory of Accredited Programs. Retrieved from: https://www.cswe.org/Accreditation/Directory-of-Accredited-Programs.aspx.

Daniels, Glenda, and Jo Nell Wells. 2012. Lambda Eta Alpha Beta. Texas Christian University, Fort Worth, TX: Shutterfly.

Day, Phyllis J. 1989. *A New History of Social Welfare.* Englewood Cliffs, NJ: Prentice Hall.

Detlaff, A.J., Moore, L.S., and Dietz, T.J. 2006. "Personality Type Preferences of Social Work Students: Enhancing the Educational Process through Self-Awareness and Understanding of Personality Variables." *Journal of Baccalaureate Social Work,* 11, 88–101.

Detmer, Sarah S. 1986. "The Future of Health Care Delivery Systems and Settings." *Journal of Professional Nursing* 2, no. 1 (January–February): 20–27.

Dolansky, Mary A., and Shirley M. Moore. 2013. "Quality and Safety Education for Nurses (QSEN): The Key is Systems Thinking." *Online Journal of Issues in Nursing* 18, no. 3 (September).

Eggenberger, Terry, Rose O. Sherman, and Kathryn Keller. 2014. "Creating High-Performance Interprofessional Teams." *American Nurse Today* 9, no. 11: 12–14.

Elsevier. Retrieved from http://wwwconfidence connected.com/blog/2014/05/02virginia-lynch-pioneer-in-forensic-nursing (Retrieved 2-1-2018).

Farason, Holly. October 24, 2017. "Nursing Student Makes Her Mark in D.C." *TCU News & Events.* https://newsevents.tcu.edu/nursing-student-makes-her mark-in d-c/.

———. December 14, 2017. "Nursing Student Represents TCU during WHO Internship." Harris College of Nursing & Health Sciences. https://harriscollege.tcu.edu/news/nursing-student-represents-tcu-during-who-internship/.

Field, Lucy, and Elizabeth Hahn Winslow. 1985. "Moving to a Nursing Model." *American Journal of Nursing* 85, no. 10: 1100–1101.

Foley, Mory. 2004. "Health and Safety: Update on Needlestick and Sharps Injuries." *American Journal of Nursing* 104, no. 8 (August): 96.

Fort Worth Chamber of Commerce. 1978. "Nursing Has Caught Up with the Times." *Fort Worth* 54, no. 8 (August): 28-31.

Franklin, Ashley E., Paula Gubrud-Howe, Stephanie Sideras, and Christopher S. Lee. 2015. "Effectiveness of Simulation Preparation on Novice Nurses' Competence and Self-Efficacy in a Multiple-Patient Simulation." *Nursing Education Perspectives* 36: 324–25. doi:10.5480/14-1546.

Gastroenterology Nursing. Retrieved from https://journals.lww.com/gastroenterologynursing/pages/default.aspx, April 12, 2018.

Grady, Patricia A. 2016. *The NINR Strategic Plan: Advancing Science, Improving Lives.* National Institute of Nursing Research, Bethesda, MD.

Grove, Susan, Jennifer R. Gray, and Nancy Burns. 2014. *Understanding Nursing Research: Building an Evidence-Based Practice.* 6th ed. New York: Elsevier.

Hamby, Donna Leake, and Robin Christian. 2015. "The Clinical Effectiveness of a Nurse Practitioner versus a Non-Nurse Practitioner on Hospital Admissions of Older Adults Residing in Skilled or Long-Term Care Facilities: A Systematic Review Protocol." *The JBI Database of Systematic Reviews and Implementation Reports* 13, no. 5 (May): 24–35.

Harris College / TCU Nursing. November 10, 2017. "Nursing Student Reunites with Navy Family."

https://harriscollege.tcu.edu/news/nursing-student-reunites-with-navy-family/.

Harris College Magazine. 2015. Texas Christian University, Fort Worth, TX: 14, 16.

Harris College of Nursing Archives. Texas Christian University, Fort Worth, TX.

Harris College of Nursing & Health Sciences. 2018. *Harris College of Nursing & Health Sciences & TCU-Nursing Strategic Initiatives 2013–2018: Excellence in Teaching and Scholarship.* Texas Christian University Fort Worth, TX.

Harris College of Nursing & Health Sciences. 2018. Texas Christian University. Retrieved from https://harriscollege.tcu.edu on April 15, 2018.

Harris College of Nursing & Health Sciences & the Center for Healthy Aging. 2009. *Spirituality and End of Life Care: Compassionate Response to Essential Needs.* Texas Christian University, Fort Worth, TX.

Harris, Lucy. 1973. *The Harris College of Nursing: Five Decades of Struggle for a Cause.* Fort Worth: TCU Press.

Hessels, Amanda, Linda Flynn, Jeannie Cimiotti, Suzanne Bakken, and Robyn Gershon. 2015. "Impact of Health Information Technology on Quality of Patient Care." *Online Journal of Nursing Information* 19.

Hogstel, Mildred. 1979a. "Nurses' Attitudes toward Care of Elderly Hospital Patients—Can In-service Education Bring About Positive Change?" *Nursing Research* (June): 6.

Hogstel, Mildred. 1979b. "Use of Reality Orientation with Aging Confused Parents." *Nursing Research* (May–June): 161–65. https://socialwork.tcu.edu/msw/.

Hunt, Deborah Dolan. 2017. *Fast Facts about the Nursing Profession: Historical Perspectives in a Nutshell.* New York: Springer Publishing Co.

Huston, Carol. 2013. "The Impact of Emerging Technology on Nursing Care: Warp Speed Ahead." *Online Journal of Issues in Nursing* 18, no. 2.

Institute of Medicine. 1997. *Approaching Death: Improving Care at the End of Life,* edited by M. J. Field and C. K. Cassel. Washington, DC: The National Academies Press.

Institute of Medicine. 2001. *Crossing the Quality Chasm: A New Health System for the 21st Century.* http://www.nationalacademies.org/hmd/~/media/Files/Report %20Files/2001/ Crossing-the-Quality-Chasm/Quality%20Chasm%202001%20 %20 report%20brief.pdf.

Institute of Medicine. 2011. *The Future of Nursing: Leading Change, Advancing Health.* Washington, DC: The National Academies Press.

Jones, Jim. 1997. "Work for Elderly Earns Woman National Honor." *Fort Worth Star-Telegram,* April 19, 1997.

Judd, Deborah. 2014. In *A History of American Nursing: Trends and Eras.* 2nd ed. Edited by Deborah Judd and Kathleen Sitzman. Burlington, MA: Jones & Bartlett Learning.

Karger, Howard Jacob, and David Stoesz. 1990. *American Social Welfare Policy.* New York: Longman.

Keen-Payne, Rhonda. 1999. "We Must Have Nurses: Spanish Influenza in America." *Nursing History Review,* no. 7: 23-50.

"The Lady with the Lamp in Texas, May 5, 1967." 1967. *Harris Hospital News.* Fort Worth, TX.

Long, Kathleen Ann. 2004. "Preparing Nurses for the 21st Century: Re-envisioning Nursing Education and Practice." *Journal of Professional Nursing* 20, no. 2: 82–88.

Lynaugh, Joan E., and Barbara Bates. 1974. "Physical Diagnosis: A Skill for All Nurses?" *The American Journal of Nursing* 74, no. 1 (January): 58–59.

Mckinney, Harold. 1962. "Harris College of Nursing Desegregates as 6,200 Register in the Round." *The Daily Skiff,* 61, no. 2.

Miller, Patsy. 1978. "Right Prescription Found for Cultural Understanding." *Fort Worth Star-Telegram,* July 18, 1978, Living Section C: 1, 3.

Moore, L.S. and C.A. Irwin. 1990. "Quality control in Social Work: The Gatekeeping Role in Social Work Education." *Journal of Teaching in Social Work,* 4, 113–128.

Moore, L.S. and C.A. Irwin. 1991. "Gatekeeping: A Model for Screening Baccalaureate Students for Field Education." *Journal of Social Work Education,* 27, 8–17.

Moore, L.S., A.J. Detlaff, and T.J. Dietz. 2004. "Using the Myers-Briggs Type Indicator for Field Education Supervision." *Journal of Social Work Education,* 40, 337–349.

Moseley, George B. 2008. "The U.S. Health Care Non-system, 1908-2008." *AMA Journal of Ethics* 10, no. 5 (May): 324–31.

National Institute of Nursing Research. 2016. *The NINR Strategic Plan: Advancing Science, Improving Lives.* Bethesda, MD: 2, 4, 70, 72–5.

National League for Nursing. 2016. Research Priorities for 2016–2019. Retrieved from www.nln.org/research/research-priorities-in-nursing-education.

National League for Nursing. 2008. *National League for Nursing Research Grant Program Advances the Science of Nursing Education.*

Nursing Spectrum. 2005.

Popple, Phillip R., and Leslie Leighninger. 1990. *Social Work, Social Welfare, and American Society.* Boston: Allyn and Bacon.

Posluszny, Laura, and Diane A. Hawley. 2017. "Comparing Professional Values of Sophomore and Senior Baccalaureate Nursing Students." *Journal of Nursing Education* 56, no. 9 : 546–50. https://doi:org/10.3928/014834-20170817-06.

Quigley, Evelyn D. 2003. "Contributions of the Professional, Public, and Private Sectors in Promoting Patient Safety." *Online Journal of Issues in Nursing* 8, no. 3: 71–84.

Richards, M. Ann. 1977. "One Integrated Curriculum: An Empirical Evaluation." *Nursing Research* 26, no. 2 (March-April): 90–95.

Sabatino, Charles P. 2010. "The Evolution of Health Care Advance Planning Law and Policy." *The Milbank Quarterly* 88, no. 2 (June): 211–39.

Salinas, Meghan. 2017. "Susan Moore's 35 Years." *Harris Magazine of Harris College of Nursing & Health Sciences* 10:11.

Salmond, Susan W., and Mercedes Echevarria. 2017. "Healthcare Transformation and Changing Roles for Nursing." *Orthopedic Nursing* 36, no. 1 (January): 12–25.

Shaefor, Bradford W. 2014. "The Professionalization of Baccalaureate-Level Social Work." *Advances in Social Work* 15, no. 1: 196–206.

"Shaping the Future of Health Care." 2016. *Harris Magazine of the Harris College of Nursing & Health Sciences* 9.

Sherrod, Melissa. 2017. "The History of Cesarean Birth from 1900 to 2016." *Journal of Obstetric, Gynecologic & Neonatal Nursing* 46 : 628–36.

Sigma Theta Tau International Honor Society of Nursing. 2016. "STTI Organizational Fact Sheet." Sigma Theta Tau International Honor Society of Nursing. http://www.nursingsociety.org/connect-engage/about-stti/sigma-theta-tau-international-organizational-fact-sheet.

Sigma Theta Tau International Honor Society of Nursing. *Mission.* Retrieved from nursingsociety.org/connect-engage/about-stti/sigma, 2017.

Sigma Theta Tau International Honor Society of Nursing. *Mission.* Sigma Theta Tau International Honor Society of Nursing. nursingsociety.org/connect-engage/about-stti/sigma-theta-tau-international-organizational-fact-sheet, 2017.

Sigma Theta Tau International Honor Society of Nursing. 2016. *Sigma Theta Tau International, Inc. 1920–2007, Ruth Lilly Special Collections and Archives.* IUPUI University Library, Indiana University Purdue University, Indianapolis, IN. http://www.ulib.iupui.edu/collections/general/mss051.

Silvia, Mary Cipriano. 1974. "Science, Ethics, and Nursing." *The American Journal of Nursing* 74, no. 11 (November): 2004–7.

Smith, Andi. 2018. *TCU/DFW EBP Collaborative: EBP Fellowship Outcomes Summary Report.* (Fort Worth, TX: TCU, Harris College of Nursing & Health Sciences), 2008–18.

Stevens, Kathleen R. 2013. "The Impact of Evidence-Based Practice in Nursing and the Next Big Ideas." *Online Journal of Issues in Nursing* 18, no. 2: 1.

TCU 1993-1995 Undergraduate Catalog. 1993–1995. Fort Worth, TX: TCU, 239.

TCU 1995-1997 Undergraduate Catalog. 1995–1997. Fort Worth, TX: TCU, 252.

TCU 1998 Undergraduate Catalog. 1998. Fort Worth, TX: TCU, 260.

TCU 1999 Undergraduate Catalog. 1999. Fort Worth, TX: TCU, 270.

TCU Faculty and Staff Handbook. 1983. Fort Worth, TX: TCU.

TCU Nursing Faculty. 2018. *TCU Nursing: Vision, Mission and Core Values.* Texas Christian University, Harris College of Nursing & Health Sciences, Fort Worth, TX.

TCU (Texas Christian University). 2018. *Discover TCU Nursing.* Texas Christian University, Fort Worth, TX.

TCU (Texas Christian University). 1972. *THIS IS TCU: The Magazine of Texas Christian University.* Fort Worth, TX.

TCU (Texas Christian University). 1987. "Nursing College First to Add New Technology." *Horned Frog.* Texas Christian University. Fort Worth, TX.

TCU 360. 2013. "Colleagues Remember Professor for Devotion to Social Justice." January 2013. Retrieved from https://www.tcu360.com/story/16770colleagues-remember-professor-devotion-social-justice/.

Thompson, Patricia Eichelberger. 1978. "Stress in the Adoption Process: A Personal Account." *Social Work* 23, no. 3 (May): 248.

Trossman, Susan. "Handle with Care: The ANA Launches a Multifaceted Campaign to Prevent Workplace Injuries." *American Journal of Nursing* 104, no. 1: 73–75.

Van Meter, David. 2000. "Realizing the Possibilities." *TCU Magazine,* Winter 2000. Retrieved from https://magazine.tcu.edu/winter-2000/realizing the possibilities/ on Feb. 15, 2018. Fort Worth, TX, 2000.

Weeks, Susan Mace, June Marshall, and Paulette Burns. 2009. "Development of an Evidence-Based Practice and Research Collaborative Among Urban Hospitals." *Nursing Clinics of North America* 44 (March): 27–31.

Weeks, Susan. 2016. "From the Dean." *Harris Magazine: Magazine of Harris College of Nursing & Health Sciences,* 9: 2.

Weeks, Susan. 2015. "From the Dean." *Harris Magazine: Magazine of Harris College of Nursing & Health Sciences,* 8: 2.

World Health Organization. 2010. *WHO Definition of Interprofessional Education (IPE).* http://www.nationalacademies.org/hmd/~/media/Files/Activity%20Files/Global/InnovationHealthProfEducation/2012-AUG-29/0209-Spencer.pdf.

Zastrow, Charles. 2016. *Introduction to Social Work and Social Welfare: Empowering People.* 12th ed. Boston: Cengage Learning.

About the Authors

Mary Lou Bond is a graduate of Bethel Deaconess Hospital School of Nursing (diploma), Texas Christian University (bachelor of science nursing, master of religious education), University of Pittsburgh (master of nursing), the University of Texas at Austin (doctor of philosophy in nursing), and the School of Nurse Midwifery at El Centro Medico in Rio Piedras, Puerto Rico. She practiced nurse-midwifery in central Mexico before beginning her professional teaching career as a faculty member at Texas Christian University. As an educational administrator, she served as assistant dean and associate dean at the University of Texas at Arlington and as interim dean at the University of Arkansas for Medical Sciences. She was the founding associate dean of the PhD in Nursing Program at the University of Texas at Arlington (UTA).

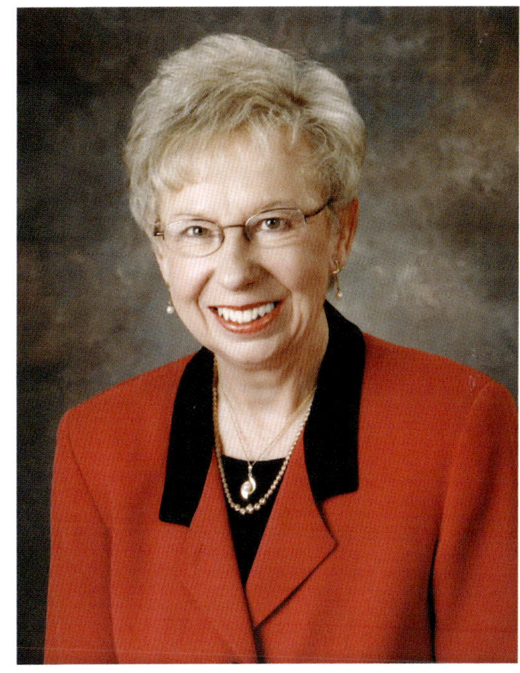

Dr. Mary Lou Bond.

Dr. Bond is professor emerita at the University of Texas at Arlington (UTA) College of Nursing and Health Innovation and currently adjunct faculty at TCU, Harris College of Nursing & Health Sciences. She has served as visiting director at Universidad Internacional in Cuernavaca, Morelos, Mexico, and as a visiting professor at Universidad Europea de Madrid. She was founder of the Challenge to Leadership Program, a forerunner of the UTA Hispanic Student Nurses' Association, and cofounder, in 1996, of UTA's Center for Hispanic Studies in Nursing and Health, which has the goal of fostering increased understanding between health providers and individuals of Hispanic origin. She has organized and led numerous educational programs to Mexico for health care students and professionals.

Bond has served on the Joint Commission on Accreditation of Hospitals and Organizations' Technical Advisory Panel on Culture, Language and Health; the Board of Trustees for the Commission of Graduates of Foreign Nursing Schools; and the

Board of Review for the National League for Nursing. She is an elected member of the American Academy of Nursing and the Academy of Nurse Educators of the National League for Nursing and Sigma Theta Tau International. She has been honored as a distinguished alumni of Bethel Deaconess Hospital, University of Pittsburgh, and the University of Texas at Austin and as an honorary alumni of the University of Arkansas for Medical Sciences.

Rhonda Keen-Payne obtained her bachelor of science in nursing from TCU; a master of nursing science with a specialty in maternal-fetal nursing from the University of Arkansas for Medical Sciences, Little Rock; and a PhD in Nursing from Texas Woman's University, Denton, TX. She also completed extensive course work in graduate studies in the Department of History at TCU between 1991 and 2007. Keen-Payne has practiced nursing in a variety of roles, including staff nurse, clinical nurse specialist, and Lamaze instructor at Harris Methodist Hospital, Fort Worth, Texas.

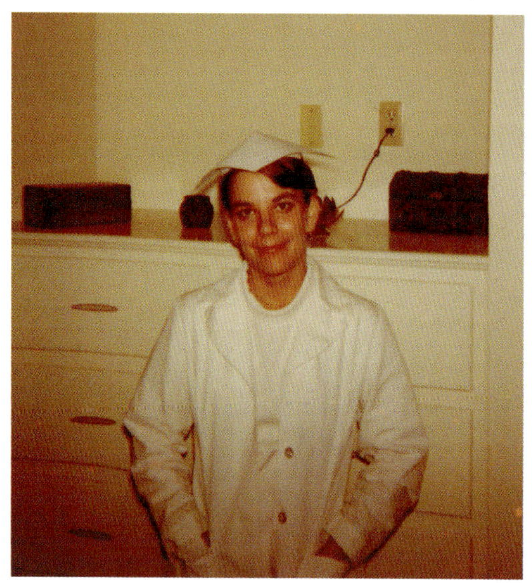

Rhonda Keen-Payne as a student, 1981.

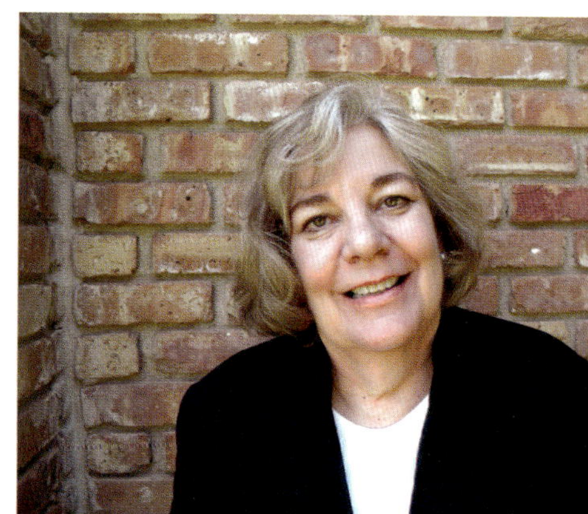

Dr. Rhonda Keen-Payne, Rankin Professor, 2015.

During her tenure at TCU (1982–present), she has served in multiple roles within the university and the college. At the university level, she has served on the faculty senate, as a member of multiple committees including the Women's Studies Minor Steering Committee, the Sexual Harassment Investigation Team, TCU's Commission on the Future, Faculty Equity Committee, and TCU Inclusiveness Committee. At the college level, she has served on numerous committees and served as interim associate dean (1994–95 and 1996–97), interim dean (1995–96), and dean (1999–2006).

Throughout the years, Dr. Keen-Payne has received many honors for her contributions to the nursing and education professions. She was named the Texas Woman's University Great 100 Alumni, is the recipient of the Ruth Eloise Sperry Teaching Award (1989, 1996), the Teaching Excellence Award from the Texas League for Nursing, the Burlington Northern Foundation Faculty Achievement Award, and the Mortar Board Preferred Professor. Keen-Payne currently holds the position of W. F. "Tex" and Pauline Curry Rankin Professor of Nursing (1998–present) at Harris College of Nursing & Health Sciences.

Contributing Authors

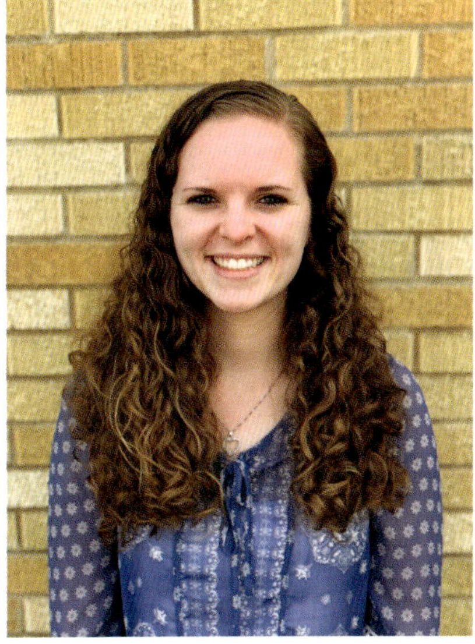

Katelyn Jones is a 2019 graduate of the TCU program and a member of the John V. Roach Honors College at Texas Christian University. She served as a peer educator and student worker for the Wellness Center on campus and is also involved in the TCU Rangers spirit organization. She has served as a teaching adviser for TCU's anatomy and physiology lab and as a team adviser for the nursing program as a part of the National Student Leadership Conference at Yale University. Jones assisted in writing this book as part of her honors thesis project.

Katelyn Jones,
Honors Student, BSN 2019.

Joel Mitchell was born in Alaska and grew up working as a deckhand on his father's commercial fishing boat, an activity that provided the means to attend Lewis and Clark College. In 1974, he completed a degree in psychology, but during his senior year, he discovered the field of kinesiology, an area of study that he pursued at the graduate level at the University of Maryland, College Park. After earning a master's degree with an emphasis in exercise physiology, Mitchell went on to earn his doctorate in human bioenergetics in the Human Performance Laboratory at Ball State University under the guidance of David Costill, a leader in the rapidly developing field of exercise science.

In 1988 Dr. Mitchell joined the faculty at TCU, where he spent thirty years teaching anatomical kinesiology and a variety of undergraduate and graduate courses in exercise physiology. He served as chair of the Department of Kinesiology for twenty-three years, overseeing the growth and evolution of the department that began prior to his tenure as chair. His research agenda included studies on fluid balance and thermoregulation during exercise as well as a secondary line of research examining the effect of exercise on the immune system in both athletic and general populations.

Following the 2018 spring semester, Mitchell and his wife Peggy, after almost forty years of marriage and adherence to the academic calendar, began enjoying the freedom of retirement. Travel, building a log cabin in Oregon, and spending more time with their children and grandchildren are just a few items that are on their agenda.

Linda Moore, professor emeritus in the TCU Department of Social Work, is the primary author of the chapter on social work. Moore served the department for over thirty years, helping to create a vibrant department with a strong history of university and community service. James Petrovich, associate professor and chair of the Department of Social Work, assisted with editing the chapter. Dr. Petrovich has been at TCU since 2010.

Kay Sanders retired after her sixteenth year as an anesthesia program director. She spent fifteen of those years at Texas Wesleyan University, where she started a distance education program, utilizing video teleconferencing and a human patient simulator lab, and brought on board more than sixty clinical sites. She was the founding director of the TCU School of Nurse Anesthesia. She received the American Nurse Anesthetists' Program Director of the Year Award in 2008. Dr. Sanders will be retiring June 1, 2020.

Dr. Sanders's professional roles include president of the Texas Association of Nurse Anesthetists; member of the American Nurse Anesthetists (AANA) education and finance committees and chair of the AANA nominating committee; member of the Texas Nurses Association Advanced Practice Committee; director of the Council on Accreditation of Nurse Anesthesia Educational Programs (COA) (2010–17) and served two years as COA president, two years as vice president, and one year as secretary-treasurer.

Sanders received a bachelor of science from Tulane University in 1965, a second bachelor of science from Texas Woman's University in 1980, a master of health science from Texas Wesleyan University in 1983, a certificate in nurse anesthesia from Texas Wesleyan University in 1984, and a doctor of nursing practice from Texas Christian University in 2009.

Christopher R. Watts, dean of the Harris College of Nursing & Health Sciences since June 1, 2019, previously served as professor and director of the Davies School of Communication Sciences and Disorders at TCU. His teaching, research, and clinical interests center on laryngeal function in voice and swallowing. Dr. Watts arrived at TCU in 2008 as department chair and served as assistant dean for Harris College from 2015 to 2018. Watts has published extensively in peer-reviewed scientific journals and is a regular speaker on laryngeal function at national and international scientific conferences. In 2012, he was the recipient of the Wassenich Award.

Index

A

B

C

F

G

H

I

J

K

L

M

N

O

P

Q

R

S

T

U